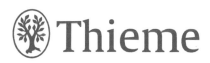

Medical Biochemistry Q&A

Joseph D. Fontes, PhD
Professor
Department of Biochemistry and Molecular Biology
Director of Foundational Sciences
Office of Medical Education
University of Kansas School of Medicine
Kansas City, Kansas

Darla L. McCarthy, PhD
Assistant Dean of Curriculum
Associate Teaching Professor–Biochemistry
Department of Basic Medical Sciences
University of Missouri-Kansas City School of Medicine
Kansas City, Missouri

239 illustrations

Thieme
New York • Stuttgart • Delhi • Rio de Janeiro

Acquisitions Editor: Delia DeTurris
Managing Editor: Apoorva Goel
Director, Editorial Services: Mary Jo Casey
Production Editor: Shivika
International Production Director: Andreas Schabert
Editorial Director: Sue Hodgson
International Marketing Director: Fiona Henderson
International Sales Director: Louisa Turrell
Senior Vice President and Chief Operating Officer:
    Sarah Vanderbilt
President: Brian D. Scanlan

Library of Congress Cataloging-in-Publication Data
Names: Fontes, Joseph D., author. | McCarthy, Darla L., author.
Title: Medical biochemistry Q&A / Joseph D. Fontes,
Darla L. McCarthy.
Other titles: Medical biochemistry Q & A
Description: New York : Thieme, [2019] | Includes bibliographical
references and index. |
Identifiers: LCCN 2018041620 (print) | LCCN 2018042494 (ebook) |
ISBN 9781626234642 | ISBN 9781626234635 (alk. paper) | ISBN
9781626234642 (eISBN)
Subjects: | MESH: Biochemical Phenomena |
Examination Questions
Classification: LCC QP518.5 (ebook) | LCC QP518.5 (print) | NLM
QU 18.2 | DDC 572.076—dc23
LC record available at https://lccn.loc.gov/2018041620

© 2019 Thieme Medical Publishers, Inc.
Thieme Publishers New York
333 Seventh Avenue, New York, NY 10001 USA
+1 800 782 3488, customerservice@thieme.com

Thieme Publishers Stuttgart
Rüdigerstrasse 14, 70469 Stuttgart, Germany
+49 [0]711 8931 421, customerservice@thieme.de

Thieme Publishers Delhi
A-12, Second Floor, Sector-2, Noida-201301
Uttar Pradesh, India
+91 120 45 566 00, customerservice@thieme.in

Thieme Publishers Rio de Janeiro, Thieme Publicações Ltda.
Edifício Rodolpho de Paoli, 25º andar
Av. Nilo Peçanha, 50 – Sala 2508
Rio de Janeiro 20020-906, Brasil
+55 21 3172 2297

Cover design: Thieme Publishing Group
Typesetting by Thomson Digital

Printed in USA by King Printing Company, Inc.   5 4 3 2 1

ISBN 978-1-62623-463-5

Also available as an e-book:
eISBN 978-1-62623-464-2

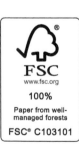

To the medical students who have taught me as much, if not more, than I have taught them.

— *Joseph D. Fontes*

To my husband, Jim, and to Natalie, John, and Hannah, for their endless and loving support.

— *Darla L. McCarthy*

Contents

Preface

For early-stage medical students, no assessment looms as large as early board examinations. Tools that make one competitive for these examinations must reflect the content and style of these examinations. This question bank is one such tool, and is suitable for use during either coursework or dedicated USMLE® Step 1 or COMLEX 1 board examination preparation.

The learning objectives at the beginning of each chapter are derived from objectives proposed by the Association of Biochemistry Educators—objectives that are adopted by numerous medical biochemistry instructors. The questions in this book have been written to test student mastery of the learning objectives. Many of the objectives are "high yielding" for board examinations, while others focus on foundational material that is crucial for understanding biochemistry, but is tested only during coursework.

Most of the high-yielding objectives and questions appear in *Metabolism* and *Molecular Biology*, although there is some high-yielding content in the *Foundational Principles and Protein Function* unit too. Students who are preparing for board examinations should readily be able to pick which chapters are relevant to use, and will find that a majority of questions in this book are useful for the initial stages of board preparation, while they are reviewing specific content areas before tackling questions that integrate multiple disciplines. Students in the first year of medical school, who are just beginning their journey toward mastery of medical biochemistry, will find that all of the questions in this book are helpful.

Joseph D. Fontes, PhD
Darla L. McCarthy, PhD

Acknowledgment

Lessons we have learned from our students, mentors, teachers, and colleagues have contributed greatly to the writing of this book. We would especially like to thank the following medical students who carefully reviewed the questions and provided helpful feedback: Ilham Boda, Paige Charboneau, Nikhil Dhall, Morgan Dresvyannikov, Elsa George, Chizitam Ibezim, Akash Jani, Athira Jayan, Robert Johnson, Diana Jung, Anusha Kodidhi, Brad Leupold, Rmaah Memon, Anthony Oyekan, Nikita Rafie, Adithi Reddy, Kavelin Rumalla, Mehr Zhara Shah, and Erica Swanson.

We would also like to thank our editorial team at Thieme. Delia DeTurris, Kenneth Schubach, and Apoorva Goel provided excellent support during the writing of this text.

How to Use This Series

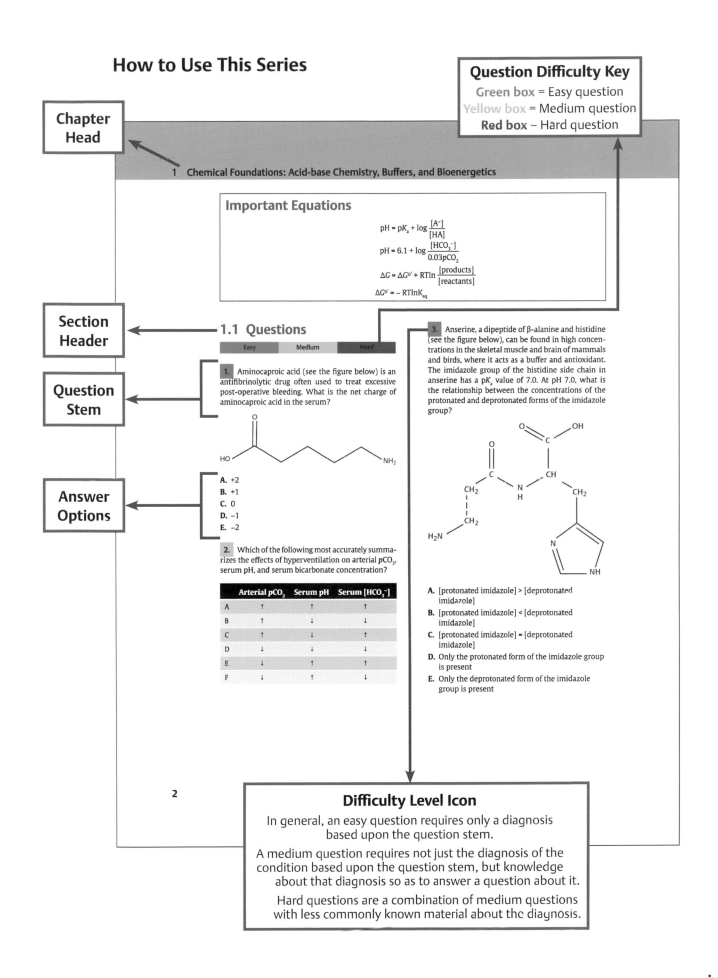

Chapter Head

Section Header

Question Stem

Answer Options

Question Difficulty Key

Green box = Easy question
Yellow box = Medium question
Red box – Hard question

1 Chemical Foundations: Acid-base Chemistry, Buffers, and Bioenergetics

Important Equations

$$pH = pK_a + \log \frac{[A^-]}{[HA]}$$

$$pH = 6.1 + \log \frac{[HCO_3^-]}{0.03 pCO_2}$$

$$\Delta G = \Delta G^{o'} + RT \ln \frac{[products]}{[reactants]}$$

$$\Delta G^{o'} = - RT \ln K_{eq}$$

1.1 Questions

Easy	Medium	Hard

1. Aminocaproic acid (see the figure below) is an antifibrinolytic drug often used to treat excessive post-operative bleeding. What is the net charge of aminocaproic acid in the serum?

A. +2
B. +1
C. 0
D. –1
E. –2

2. Which of the following most accurately summarizes the effects of hyperventilation on arterial pCO_2, serum pH, and serum bicarbonate concentration?

	Arterial pCO_2	Serum pH	Serum [HCO_3^-]
A	↑	↑	↑
B	↑	↓	↓
C	↑	↓	↑
D	↓	↓	↓
E	↓	↑	↑
F	↓	↑	↓

3. Anserine, a dipeptide of β-alanine and histidine (see the figure below), can be found in high concentrations in the skeletal muscle and brain of mammals and birds, where it acts as a buffer and antioxidant. The imidazole group of the histidine side chain in anserine has a pK_a value of 7.0. At pH 7.0, what is the relationship between the concentrations of the protonated and deprotonated forms of the imidazole group?

A. [protonated imidazole] > [deprotonated imidazole]
B. [protonated imidazole] < [deprotonated imidazole]
C. [protonated imidazole] = [deprotonated imidazole]
D. Only the protonated form of the imidazole group is present
E. Only the deprotonated form of the imidazole group is present

Difficulty Level Icon

In general, an easy question requires only a diagnosis based upon the question stem.

A medium question requires not just the diagnosis of the condition based upon the question stem, but knowledge about that diagnosis so as to answer a question about it.

Hard questions are a combination of medium questions with less commonly known material about the diagnosis.

Chapter Head

Question Difficulty Key
Green box = Easy question
Yellow box = Medium question
Red box = Hard question

Correct Answer

Correct Answer Explanation

Incorrect Answer Explanation

Indicates Question Difficulty

1.2 Answers and Explanations

| Easy | Medium | Hard |

1. Correct: C. 0 .

The net charge on aminocaproic at serum pH will be zero. Recall that when the solution pH is below the pK_a value of an ionizable group, the group will be predominantly protonated in solution. Conversely, when the solution pH is above the pK_a value of an ionizable group, the group will be predominantly deprotonated in solution. Normal serum pH is 7.4. The pK_a value of the carboxyl group on aminocaproic acid will be between 2 and 4 (typical values for carboxyl groups). This pK_a value is below the serum pH, so the group will exist predominantly in its deprotonated form, which for a carboxyl group is the negatively charged (–1) carboxylate ion. The pK_a value of the amino group on aminocaproic acid will be close to 9 (a typical value for an amino group). This pK_a value is higher than serum pH, so the group will exist predominantly in its protonated form, which for an amino group is the positively charged (+1) ammonium ion. Thus, at pH 7.4, the carboxyl group of aminocaproic acid will be negatively charged, and the amino group will be positively charged. This results in a net charge of zero.

2. Correct: F ↓ ↑ ↓ .

During hyperventilation, serum pCO_2 decreases, serum pH increases, and serum bicarbonate concentration decreases. Hyperventilation causes a decrease in serum pCO_2, as the lungs exhale more CO_2 than in normal ventilation. According to Le Chatelier's principle, the decreased serum CO_2 level will drive the bicarbonate buffering system equilibrium (see the figure below) toward the left in an attempt to replace the lost CO_2 and re-establish equilibrium.

$$CO_2 + H_2O \rightleftharpoons H_2CO_3 \rightleftharpoons H^+ + HCO_3^-$$

As the equilibrium shifts to the left, the concentration of H^+ will drop, resulting in an increase in pH. (Recall that pH –log[H^+]; an increase in [H^+] results in a decrease in pH, and a decrease in [H^+] results in an increase in pH.) The leftward shift in equilibrium will also consume bicarbonate ions (HCO_3^-), thus decreasing serum [HCO_3^-]. Furthermore, renal compensation will result in greater loss of bicarbonate ions from the serum, as the kidneys decrease the amount of bicarbonate resorption in an attempt to drive the equilibrium back to the right. (The kidneys will also decrease elimination of H^+ but not enough so as to bring serum pH back down to normal.)

Choices A, B, and C are all incorrect, as they all indicate an increase in serum pCO_2, which would occur with *hypo*ventilation when the lungs exhale less CO_2 than in normal ventilation.

Choice D is incorrect because it indicates a drop in pH; the decrease in pCO_2 during hyperventilation causes a decrease in serum H^+ and an increase in pH.

Choice E is incorrect. Although this choice correctly indicates a decrease in pCO_2 and an increase in pH, it incorrectly indicates an increase in bicarbonate.

3. Correct: C. [protonated imidazole] = [deprotonated imidazole].

There will be equal concentrations of the protonated and deprotonated forms of the imidazole group at pH 7.0. The answer to this question is obtained from the Henderson–Hasselbalch equation:

$$pH = pK_a + \log \frac{[A^-]}{[HA]},$$

where the term [HA] refers to the molar concentration of a weak acid (protonated imidazole, in this case), and [A^-] refers to the molar concentration of its corresponding conjugate base (deprotonated imidazole, in this case). According to this equation, when the pH of a solution is equal to the pK_a of an ionizable group, as is the case described in this question, the term log([A^-]/[HA]) must be equal to zero. Recall that log(1) = 0; therefore, when the pH of the solution is equal to the pK_a of an ionizable group, there will be a 1:1 ratio of the protonated (HA) and deprotonated (A^-) forms of the ionizable group.

Choice A is incorrect; for the concentration of protonated imidazole to be greater than the concentration of deprotonated imidazole, the solution pH would have to be less than the imidazole pK_a.

Choice B is incorrect; for the concentration of protonated imidazole to be less than the concentration of deprotonated imidazole, the solution pH would have to be greater than the imidazole pK_a.

Choices D and E are incorrect, as the solution pH would need to be more than 3 units away for one of the two forms of the ionizable group to be essentially undetectable; i.e., pH < 4 for <0.1% of the deprotonated form to be present, and pH > 10 for <0.1% of the protonated form to be present.

4. Correct: E. 100:1.

The ratio of ionized to un-ionized naproxen is will be approximately 100:1 at serum pH. This problem is solved using the Henderson–Hasselbalch equation,

$$pH = pK_a + \log \frac{[A^-]}{[HA]},$$

which allows us to determine the proportion of protonated and deprotonated forms of a molecule at any pH when we know the pK_a value of the molecule's ionizable group. In this case, the pH of our solution is 7.4, normal serum pH. However, because we are only doing an estimation for this problem, we can use a pH value of 7.2 in order to make our calculation easier. The pK_a of the carboxyl group on naproxen is

Chapter 1

Chemical Foundations: Acid–Base Chemistry, Buffers, and Bioenergetics

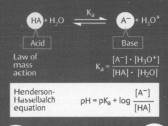

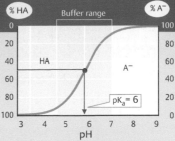

LEARNING OBJECTIVES

▶ Define and explain pH and pK_a.

▶ Apply the Henderson–Hasselbalch equation to solve pH problems.

▶ Determine the charge on a peptide or small molecule at a given pH.

▶ Explain the bicarbonate buffer system, and how it is influenced by respiratory and metabolic changes.

▶ Differentiate between various physiological causes of acid-base disturbance, recognizing how disturbances will influence arterial pH, carbon dioxide partial pressure (pCO_2), and bicarbonate concentrations.

▶ Explain and calculate Gibbs free energy, standard Gibbs free energy, and the equilibrium constant as they apply to biochemical reactions.

▶ Calculate free energy and equilibrium in coupled reactions.

▶ Apply Le Chatelier's principle to explain how the equilibria of biochemical reactions can be manipulated.

Important Equations

$$pH = pK_a + \log \frac{[A^-]}{[HA]}$$

$$pH = 6.1 + \log \frac{[HCO_3^-]}{0.03pCO_2}$$

$$\Delta G = \Delta G^{o'} + RT\ln \frac{[products]}{[reactants]}$$

$$\Delta G^{o'} = -RT\ln K_{eq}$$

1.1 Questions

Easy	Medium	Hard

1. Aminocaproic acid (see the figure below) is an antifibrinolytic drug often used to treat excessive post-operative bleeding. What is the net charge of aminocaproic acid in the serum?

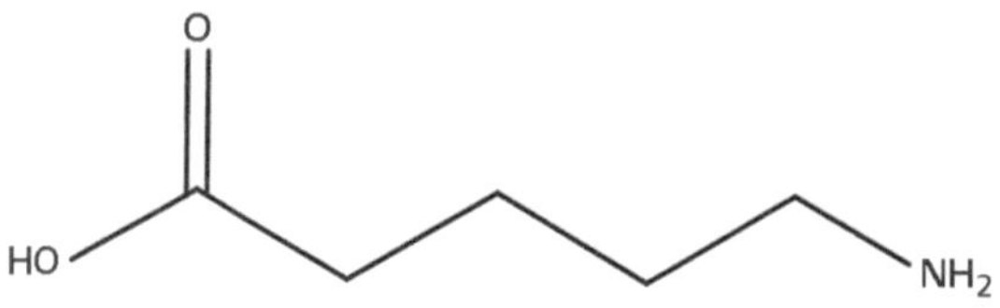

A. +2

B. +1

C. 0

D. −1

E. −2

2. Which of the following most accurately summarizes the effects of hyperventilation on arterial pCO_2, serum pH, and serum bicarbonate concentration?

	Arterial pCO_2	Serum pH	Serum $[HCO_3^-]$
A	↑	↑	↑
B	↑	↓	↓
C	↑	↓	↑
D	↓	↓	↓
E	↓	↑	↑
F	↓	↑	↓

3. Anserine, a dipeptide of β-alanine and histidine (see the figure below), can be found in high concentrations in the skeletal muscle and brain of mammals and birds, where it acts as a buffer and antioxidant. The imidazole group of the histidine side chain in anserine has a pK_a value of 7.0. At pH 7.0, what is the relationship between the concentrations of the protonated and deprotonated forms of the imidazole group?

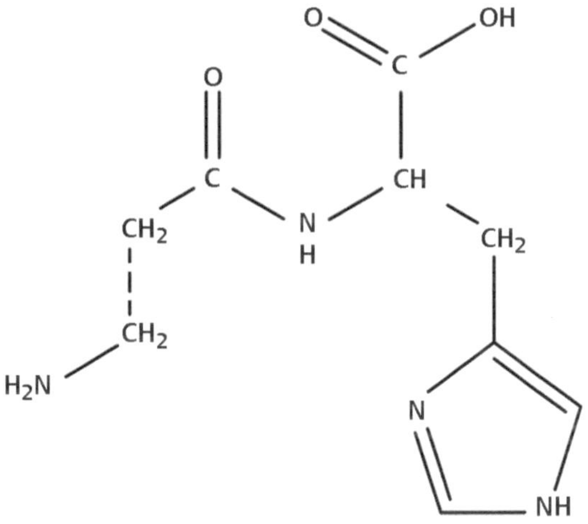

A. [protonated imidazole] > [deprotonated imidazole]

B. [protonated imidazole] < [deprotonated imidazole]

C. [protonated imidazole] = [deprotonated imidazole]

D. Only the protonated form of the imidazole group is present

E. Only the deprotonated form of the imidazole group is present

4. The structure of naproxen, a nonsteroidal anti-inflammatory drug, is shown in the figure below. Naproxen has a pK_a value of 5.2, and its solubility is very sensitive to pH. What would be the approximate ratio of the ionized to unionized forms of the drug at serum pH?

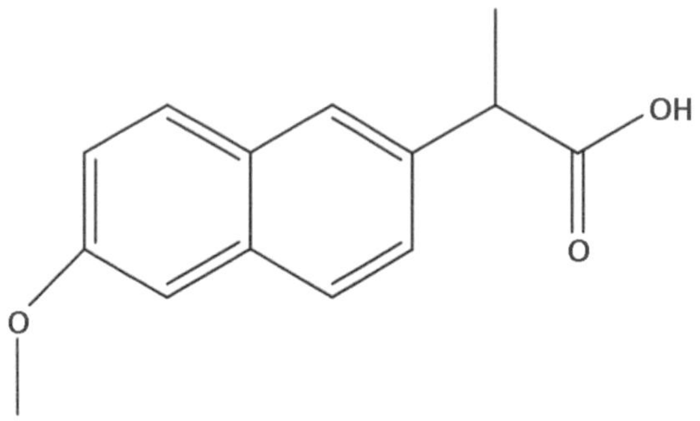

A. 1:100

B. 1:10

C. 1:1

D. 10:1

E. 100:1

5. While doing some yardwork at home, a teenage boy fell into some underbrush. Recognizing that there were poison ivy vines in the brush, the boy rushed indoors, removed his clothing, and washed thoroughly. The chemical irritant in poison ivy is urushiol, a mixture of catechols substituted with long-chain alkyl groups, like the one shown in the figure below. Which of the following household products should the boy use when washing his skin?

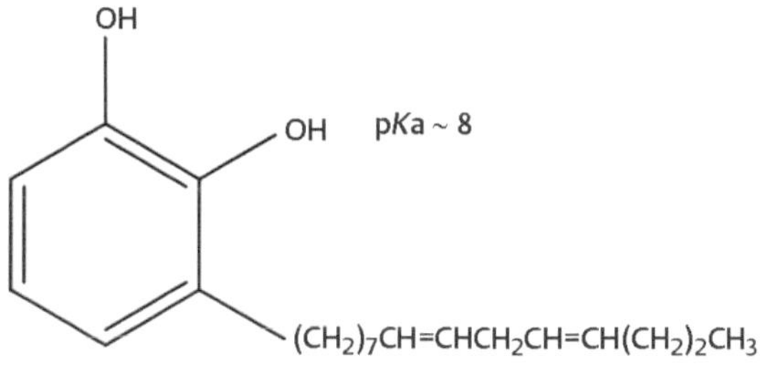

A. Vinegar

B. Ammonia

C. Soapy water

D. Water

E. Sugar water

6. A 20-year-old female visits an urgent care clinic complaining of recent weight loss, fatigue, thirst, and increased urinary frequency. Physical examination reveals shallow, rapid breathing and a faint ketotic odor. The physician assistant on duty suspects new-onset type I diabetes and orders a basic metabolic panel, arterial blood gases (ABGs), and urinalysis. Which of the following blood values is most compatible with this patient's probable illness?

	pH	Bicarbonate (mEq/L)	Arterial pCO_2 (mm Hg)
A	7.27	13	30
B	7.27	27	60
C	7.40	24	40
D	7.52	24	30
E	7.52	35	45

7. A 20-year-old female is brought to an emergency department by her roommate, who found her lying semi-conscious on the floor with an empty bottle of aspirin by her side. The patient indicated that she had consumed the aspirin in a suicide attempt. At the hospital, the patient reports severe abdominal pain and nausea and appears to be confused and lethargic. Physical examination reveals hyperventilation, which is characteristic of the initial stages of salicylate poisoning. The physician on duty orders administration of activated charcoal, as well as a basic metabolic panel and measurements of serum salicylate levels and ABGs. Which of the following blood values is most compatible with the respiratory alteration this patient is exhibiting?

	pH	Bicarbonate (mEq/L)	Arterial pCO_2 (mm Hg)
A	7.27	13	30
B	7.27	27	60
C	7.40	24	40
D	7.52	24	30
E	7.52	35	45

8. A 23-year-old man who had recently immigrated from Syria presented at the emergency room with severe hypertension, hypokalemia, and quadriparesis. He had no prior medical history, but mentioned that he had been fasting during the last 3 weeks in observation of Ramadan. He indicated that during that time, he was drinking about 1 L of erk soos daily. Erk soos is a drink made of licorice plant extract, which contains a compound that mimics mineralocorticoids. Excessive intake can cause renal wasting of potassium and protons, resulting in metabolic alkalosis. Which of the following blood values is most compatible with licorice toxicity?

	pH	Bicarbonate (mEq/L)	Arterial pCO_2 (mm Hg)
A	7.25	13	30
B	7.25	23	55
C	7.40	24	40
D	7.55	25	30
E	7.55	44	52

9. A 23-year-old man was brought to the emergency room after he was found unconscious in his home following a possible methadone overdose. In addition to his lack of consciousness, the patient also had pinpoint pupils. His respiratory rate was 9 breaths per minute (normal: 12–18), and his percutaneous oxygen saturation was 75% (normal: >95%). The attending resident ordered an ABG measurement, which indicated a partial oxygen pressure of 56 mm Hg. Which of the following values would also most likely appear on the ABG?

	pH	Bicarbonate (mEq/L)	Arterial pCO_2 (mm Hg)
A	7.25	13	30
B	7.25	23	55
C	7.40	24	40
D	7.55	25	30
E	7.55	44	52

10. Following a major earthquake in a rural area of Peru, a 15-year-old boy who suffered chest trauma was treated at a field hospital. He was placed on a mechanical ventilator, and his ABGs were regularly monitored to ensure that adequate ventilation was occurring. Unfortunately, the thermal printer on the hospital's semi-automatic chemistry analyzer was in need of repair, and often one or more of the reported measurements was unreadable. The results for the most recent ABG reading indicated a serum pH of 7.49, and a bicarbonate concentration of 22 mEq/L, but the arterial pCO_2 was unreadable. Based on the reported pH and bicarbonate values, what is this patient's pCO_2?

A. 43 mm Hg

B. 40 mm Hg

C. 37 mm Hg

D. 34 mm Hg

E. 30 mm Hg

11. A 35-year-old female who lost consciousness due to a severe case of diabetic ketoacidosis has been admitted to an intensive care unit (ICU). While reviewing the patient's charts, the attending physician noticed a significant discrepancy between the laboratory's reported serum bicarbonate values. The patient's basic metabolic panel, where the venous bicarbonate concentration is measured directly, was 17 mEq/L, but the ABG measure, where the arterial bicarbonate concentration is calculated from the measured arterial serum pH and pCO_2 values, was 22 mEq/L. Normally, the two bicarbonate values differ by 2 mEq/L or less. Before asking for re-analysis of the blood samples, the physician decided to determine if the discrepancy was due to an error in calculation. Assuming that the reported values for arterial pH (7.24) and pCO_2 (36 mm Hg) are correct, what is this patient's arterial bicarbonate concentration?

A. 22 mEq/L

B. 19 mEq/L

C. 17 mEq/L

D. 15 mEq/L

E. 12 mEq/L

12. An 84-year-old woman of Japanese origin was recently prescribed a diuretic to treat her worsening essential hypertension. In addition to the prescribed diuretic, the woman began consuming traditional Japanese herbal medications that contain extracts of licorice root, which is known to contain a chemical with significant mineralocorticoid activity. A few weeks later, she developed severe hypokalemia and metabolic alkalosis, with a serum pH of 7.58. In an attempt to compensate for metabolic alkalosis, the woman's respiratory pattern changed. Which of the following statements most accurately explains how her altered respiration influences the serum bicarbonate buffering system?

A. It increases the dissociation of $H_2CO_3 \rightarrow H^+ + HCO_3^-$

B. It increases the dissociation of $H_2CO_3 \rightarrow H_2O + CO_2$

C. It increases association of $H^+ + HCO_3^- \rightarrow H_2CO_3$

D. It increases the pK_a of carbonic acid

E. It increases expression of carbonic anhydrase in erythrocytes

13. A 45-year-old female presented at her primary care physician's office with a complaint of abdominal cramping and intermittent abdominal and flank pain which, after appropriate examination and testing, was attributed to a renal uric acid stone. The structure and pK_a value of uric acid are shown below. The patient was prescribed pain medication, as well as an antispasmodic to facilitate stone passage. After the stone passed, she was instructed to make dietary changes and take an oral supplement with the goal of altering her urine pH in order to prevent formation of additional uric acid stones. Which of the conditions listed below most accurately describes a situation in which urinary uric acid solubility increases from about 50 to 90%, as would be a desirable outcome for this patient?

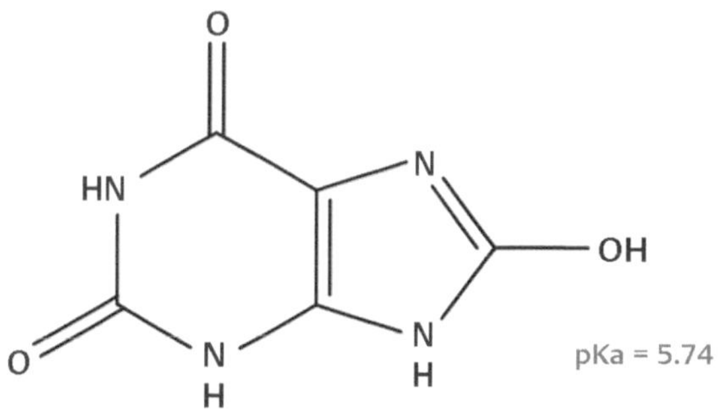

pKa = 5.74

	Urinary pH prior to treatment	Urinary pH after treatment
A	4.7	5.7
B	5.7	6.7
C	6.7	5.7
D	5.7	4.7
E	4.7	6.7
F	6.7	4.7

14. The preferred method for confirming placement of nasogastric feeding tubes in the stomach, as opposed to the lung or esophagus, is to obtain a chest X-ray. However, in some cases, placement is confirmed by aspirating fluid from the placed tube and by checking the aspirate pH. Which of the following proton concentrations would most likely be found in aspirate obtained from a patient whose nasogastric tube has been correctly placed?

A. 3.2×10^{-5} M

B. 1.5×10^{2} M

C. 1.0×10^{-7} M

D. 5.0×10^{-3} M

E. 9.3×10^{1} M

15. A 65-year-old female with a history of hypertension, type II diabetes, and one myocardial infarction develops congestive heart failure. She is prescribed oral ethacrynic acid (see the figure below), a loop diuretic, in order to reduce significant edema in her lower legs and feet. As this drug moves through the digestive tract, from which organ will it most rapidly diffuse across epithelial cell membranes?

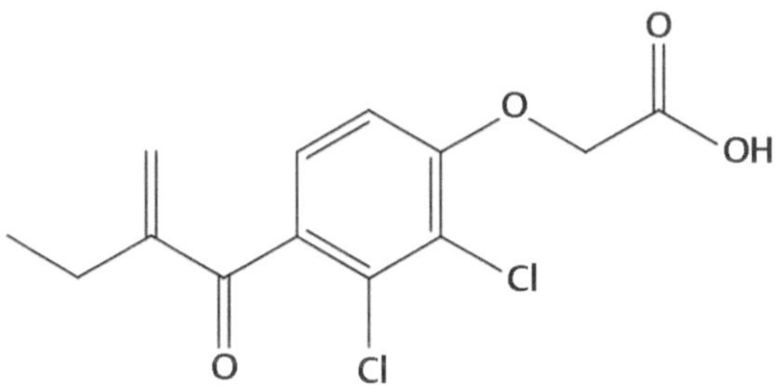

A. The stomach, because the lower pH increases the hydrophobicity of ethacrynic acid

B. The stomach, because the lower pH decreases the hydrophobicity of ethacrynic acid

C. The duodenum, because the higher pH increases the hydrophobicity of ethacrynic acid

D. The duodenum, because the higher pH decreases the hydrophobicity of ethacrynic acid

16. A 6-month-old infant with developmental delays and hypotonia presented at the emergency department in respiratory distress. Laboratory results at this hospital visit were indicative of lactic acidosis, and eventually a diagnosis of pyruvate dehydrogenase deficiency was made. If the patient's serum pH during her episode of lactic acidosis was 7.10, what was the approximate ratio of lactate:lactic acid in her serum at that time? The pK_a value for lactic acid is 3.9.

A. 1.8:1

B. 1:1.8

C. 3.2:1

D. 1:3.2

E. 160:1

F. 1:160

G. 1600:1

H. 1:1600

Consider the following narrative and figure for questions 17 to 19.

The figure below represents a simplified version of calcium cycling in myocytes. Recall that during myocyte contraction, calcium ions are released from the sarcoplasmic reticulum (SR) into the myoplasm, where they bind to troponin, thus initiating the processes involved in contraction. Calcium also activates enzymes involved in glycogenolysis and the citric acid cycle. As illustrated in the figure, myoplasmic and SR calcium concentrations are determined by the SR calcium ATPase (SRCA), which pumps calcium ions into the SR, and the ryanodine receptor (RyR), which upon activation by neural stimulus of myocytes allows calcium ions to flow into the myoplasm. There are other pumps and channels involved in this system, but for the following questions, assume that the SRCA pump and RyR are the only important factors.

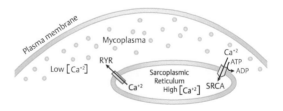

17. Movement of calcium ions from a low concentration in the myoplasm to a high concentration in the SR lumen is driven by adenosine triphosphate (ATP) hydrolysis. In resting myocytes, the ΔG for ATP hydrolysis is approximately –65 kJ/mol. The $\Delta G^{o'}$ for ATP hydrolysis, however, is –30.5 kJ/mol. Which of the following can we most reasonably assume, based on the observed difference between ΔG and $\Delta G^{o'}$?

A. The ATP concentration is higher in myocytes than in other cell types

B. In the myoplasm, the concentration of ATP is higher than the product of the adenosine diphosphate (ADP) and phosphate ion concentrations

C. In the myoplasm, ATP is in equilibrium with ADP and phosphate ions

D. In the myoplasm, the concentration of ATP is lower than the product of the ADP and phosphate ion concentrations

E. ATP synthase works at a faster rate in myocytes than in other cell types

18. The energy required to support the calcium ion gradient across the SR membrane is defined as

$$\Delta G = -2RT \ln([Ca^{2+}]_{cyt}/[Ca^{2+}]_{SR}),$$

where $[Ca^{2+}]_{SR}$ is the SR $[Ca^{2+}]$ and $[Ca^{2+}]_{cyt}$ is the cytosolic $[Ca^{2+}]$. (Recall that R, the gas constant, is 0.008314 kJ/mol-K, and that physiological temperature is 310 K.) A typical concentration of calcium ions in the SR is about 1 mM. Assuming that the only protein involved in establishing the calcium ion concentrations in the SR, and the myoplasm is the SRCA pump, that the RyR is closed, and that energy transfer is 100% efficient, what is the lowest possible myoplasmic calcium ion concentration that could be obtained if ΔG for ATP hydrolysis is –65 kJ/mol?

A. 1 mM

B. 80 μM

C. 55 μM

D. 350 nM

E. 3.3 nM

19. Some individuals inherit mutations in RyR that trigger it to release calcium ions into the myoplasm in response to certain anesthetics, such as halothane. These individuals are at risk of developing malignant hyperthermia when exposed to triggering anesthetic agents. The symptoms of malignant hyperthermia include a rapid rise in body temperature. Why does increased myoplasmic $[Ca^{+2}]$ cause excess heat generation in these individuals?

A. It increases ΔG for the reaction catalyzed by the SRCA pump, thus necessitating additional heat-generating ATP synthesis and hydrolysis

B. It increases ΔG for the reaction catalyzed by the SRCA pump, thus increasing the amount of heat generated as the pump works

C. It increases ΔG for metabolic reactions, thus increasing the amount of heat released in the process of generating ATP

D. It decreases ΔG for metabolic reactions, thus increasing the amount of heat released in the process of generating ATP

E. It increases the rates of metabolic processes, thus increasing the amount of heat released in the process of generating ATP

Refer to the following table while answering questions 20 to 23.

Reaction	$\Delta G^{o'}$
Glutamate + NAD$^+$ + H$_2$O → α-ketoglutarate + NADH + H$^+$ + NH$_4^+$	+80.5 kJ/mol
Glutamine + H$_2$O → glutamate + NH$_4^+$	–14.2 kJ/mol
ATP + H$_2$O → ADP + Pi	–30.5 kJ/mol
Glutamate + ATP → γ-glutamyl phosphate + ADP	+17.5 kJ/mol

Abbreviations: ADP, adenosine diphosphate; ATP, adenosine triphosphate NAD$^+$, nicotinamide adenine dinucleotide oxidized; NADH, nicotinamide adenine dinucleotide hydrogen.

20. Ammonia is a potent neurotoxin. One possible explanation for its severe toxicity is that high concentrations of ammonia drive the reaction catalyzed by glutamate dehydrogenase (see the figure below) to the left, thus consuming large quantities of neuronal α-ketoglutarate and depleting the mitochondrial pool of citric acid cycle intermediates. This results in cellular energy depletion. In an experiment in which hyperammonemia was induced in rats, the following metabolite concentrations were measured in neuronal mitochondria. What is the ΔG for the deamination of glutamate by glutamate dehydrogenase in these neurons? (Recall that the gas constant R = 0.008314kJ/mol-K, and that physiological temperature is 310 K.)

Ammonium ion	1.5×10^{-3} M
Glutamate	7.5×10^{-3} M
α-ketoglutarate	3.0×10^{-5} M
NAD$^+$	3.0×10^{-4} M
NADH	5.0×10^{-5} M

Abbreviations: NAD$^+$, nicotinamide adenine dinucleotide oxidized; NADH, nicotinamide adenine dinucleotide hydrogen.

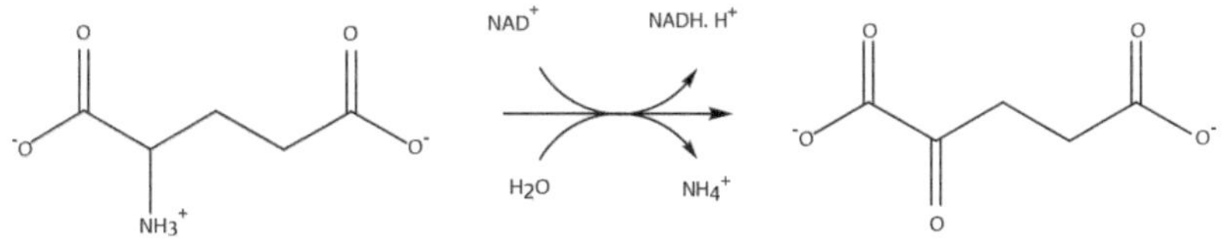

NAD$^+$ NADH. H$^+$

H$_2$O   NH$_4^+$

NH$_3^+$

A. +116 kJ/mol
B. +80.5 kJ/mol
C. +45 kJ/mol
D. –45 kJ/mol
E. –80.5 kJ/mol
F. –116 kJ/mol

21. Do the experimental results described in the previous question support the hypothesis that the neurotoxicity of ammonia is due to depletion of the neuronal mitochondrial pool of α-ketoglutarate?

A. No, the measured concentration of α-ketoglutarate is too high

B. No, the glutamate dehydrogenase reaction is not being driven toward glutamate deamination

C. Yes, the glutamate concentration is high

D. Yes, the glutamate dehydrogenase reaction is being driven toward glutamate synthesis

22. A second important reaction that is stimulated under conditions of hyperammonemia is the one catalyzed by glutamine synthetase (see the figure below). This reaction may contribute to the neural toxicity of ammonia because it results in the consumption of large quantities of glutamate, a neurotransmitter, and the production of large quantities of glutamine. High intracellular glutamine concentrations result in osmolar imbalance and subsequent swelling and death of cells. What is the equilibrium constant of the reaction catalyzed by glutamine synthetase? (Recall that the gas constant R = 0.008314 kJ/mol-K, and that physiological temperature is 310 K.)

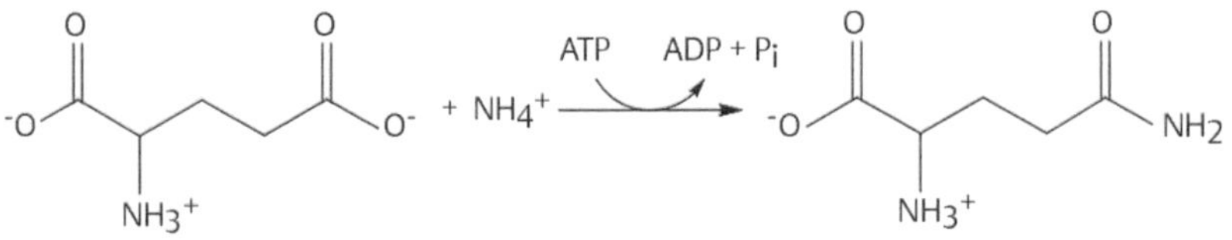

A. 1.4×10^5

B. 5.6×10^2

C. 2.5×10^2

D. 1.8×10^{-3}

E. 4.0×10^{-3}

F. 7.2×10^{-6}

23. The reaction catalyzed by glutamine synthetase is a two-step reaction involving the formation of a γ-glutamyl phosphate intermediate:

Step 1: glutamate + ATP → γ-glutamyl phosphate + ADP

Step 2: γ-glutamyl phosphate + NH_4^+ → glutamine + Pi

What is the $\Delta G^{\circ'}$ for Step 2 in this reaction sequence?

A. +33.8 kJ/mol

B. +17.5 kJ/mol

C. +14.2 kJ/mol

D. +1.2 kJ/mol

E. -16.3 kJ/mol

24. Congenital glutamine synthetase deficiency results in hyperammonemia and elevated glutamine levels in body fluids. Its phenotype is characterized by severe neonatal encephalopathy and brain malformations. In an individual with only 10% of normal glutamine synthetase activity, the equilibrium constant for the glutamine synthetase reaction would change in which of the following ways?

A. It would decrease by 90%

B. It would decrease by 10%

C. It would remain the same

D. It would increase by 10%

E. It would increase by 90%

1.2 Answers and Explanations

Easy	Medium	Hard

1.   Correct: C. 0.

The net charge on aminocaproic at serum pH will be zero. Recall that when the solution pH is below the pK_a value of an ionizable group, the group will be predominantly protonated in solution. Conversely, when the solution pH is above the pK_a value of an ionizable group, the group will be predominantly deprotonated in solution. Normal serum pH is 7.4. The pK_a value of the carboxyl group on aminocaproic acid will be between 2 and 4 (typical values for carboxyl groups). This pK_a value is below the serum pH, so the group will exist predominantly in its deprotonated form, which for a carboxyl group is the negatively charged (–1) carboxylate ion. The pK_a value of the amino group on aminocaproic acid will be close to 9 (a typical value for an amino group). This pK_a value is higher than serum pH, so the group will exist predominantly in its protonated form, which for an amino group is the positively charged (+1) ammonium ion. Thus, at pH 7.4, the carboxyl group of aminocaproic acid will be negatively charged, and the amino group will be positively charged. This results in a net charge of zero.

2.   Correct: F. Arterial pCO_2 ↓; Serum pH ↑; Serum [HCO_3^-] ↓

During hyperventilation, serum pCO_2 decreases, serum pH increases, and serum bicarbonate concentration decreases. Hyperventilation causes a decrease in serum pCO_2, as the lungs exhale more CO_2 than in normal ventilation. According to Le Chatelier's principle, the decreased serum CO_2 level will drive the bicarbonate buffering system equilibrium (see the figure below) toward the left in an attempt to replace the lost CO_2 and re-establish equilibrium.

$$CO_2 + H_2O \rightleftharpoons H_2CO_3 \rightleftharpoons H^+ + HCO_3^-$$

As the equilibrium shifts to the left, the concentration of H⁺ will drop, resulting in an increase in pH. (Recall that pH –log[H⁺]; an increase in [H⁺] results in a decrease in pH, and a decrease in [H⁺] results in an increase in pH.) The leftward shift in equilibrium will also consume bicarbonate ions (HCO_3^-), thus decreasing serum [HCO_3^-]. Furthermore, renal compensation will result in greater loss of bicarbonate ions from the serum, as the kidneys decrease the amount of bicarbonate resorption in an attempt to drive the equilibrium back to the right. (The kidneys will also decrease elimination of H⁺ but not enough so as to bring serum pH back down to normal.)

Choices A, B, and C are all incorrect, as they all indicate an increase in serum pCO_2, which would occur with *hypo*ventilation–when the lungs exhale less CO_2 than in normal ventilation.

Choice D is incorrect because it indicates a drop in pH; the decrease in pCO_2 during hyperventilation causes a decrease in serum H⁺ and an increase in pH.

Choice E is incorrect. Although this choice correctly indicates a decrease in pCO_2 and an increase in pH, it incorrectly indicates an increase in bicarbonate.

3.   Correct: C. [protonated imidazole] = [deprotonated imidazole].

There will be equal concentrations of the protonated and deprotonated forms of the imidazole group at pH 7.0. The answer to this question is obtained from the Henderson–Hasselbalch equation:

$$pH = pK_a + \log \frac{[A^-]}{[HA]},$$

where the term [HA] refers to the molar concentration of a weak acid (protonated imidazole, in this case), and [A⁻] refers to the molar concentration of its corresponding conjugate base (deprotonated imidazole, in this case). According to this equation, when the pH of a solution is equal to the pK_a of an ionizable group, as is the case described in this question, the term log([A⁻]/[HA]) must be equal to zero. Recall that log(1) = 0; therefore, when the pH of the solution is equal to the pK_a of an ionizable group, there will be a 1:1 ratio of the protonated (HA) and deprotonated (A⁻) forms of the ionizable group.

Choice A is incorrect; for the concentration of protonated imidazole to be greater than the concentration of deprotonated imidazole, the solution pH would have to be less than the imidazole pK_a.

Choice B is incorrect; for the concentration of protonated imidazole to be less than the concentration of deprotonated imidazole, the solution pH would have to be greater than the imidazole pK_a.

Choices D and E are incorrect, as the solution pH would need to be more than 3 units away for one of the two forms of the ionizable group to be essentially undetectable; i.e., pH < 4 for <0.1% of the deprotonated form to be present, and pH > 10 for <0.1% of the protonated form to be present.

4.   Correct: E. 100:1.

The ratio of ionized to un-ionized naproxen is will be approximately 100:1 at serum pH. This problem is solved using the Henderson–Hasselbalch equation,

$$pH = pK_a + \log \frac{[A^-]}{[HA]},$$

which allows us to determine the proportion of protonated and deprotonated forms of a molecule at any pH when we know the pK_a value of the molecule's ionizable group. In this case, the pH of our solution is 7.4, normal serum pH. However, because we are only doing an estimation for this problem, we can use a pH value of 7.2 in order to make our calculation easier. The pK_a of the carboxyl group on naproxen is

5.2. Substituting in 7.2 for pH, and 5.2 for pK_a, the Henderson–Hasselbalch equation becomes

$$7.2 = 5.2 + \log \frac{[A^-]}{[HA]},$$

$$2 = \log \frac{[A^-]}{[HA]},$$

$$10^2 = \frac{[A^-]}{[HA]},$$

So, the ratio of A^-: HA is 100:1. In the case of naproxen, the conjugate base (A^-) is the deprotonated or ionized form of the molecule, and the acid (HA) is the unionized form (i.e., the structure shown in the figure with Question 4), so the ratio of ionized to unionized naproxen is 100:1.

---

5. Correct: C. Soapy water.

The boy would be best served by washing with soapy water. The goal here is to facilitate the removal of urushiol from the skin. The long hydrocarbon chain on urushiol makes it very hydrophobic or "greasy." Soap, which is amphipathic, is able to interact with the hydrophobic urushiol and facilitates the suspension of urushiol. Furthermore, soapy water is basic, with a normal pH of about 9 to 10. The pK_a value of the central hydroxyl group on urushiol is close to 8. Because the pH of soapy water is higher than the pK_a value of this hydroxyl group, the group will be deprotonated and thus, negatively charged. This will additionally increase the solubility of urushiol.

A is incorrect. Vinegar is 5 to 20% acetic acid and will have a pH value close to 3. Because this pH is below the pK_a of the ionizable hydroxyl group on urushiol, the group will remain protonated, thus decreasing the solubility of urushiol and decreasing the effectiveness of the wash solution to remove the hydrophobic molecule.

B is incorrect. The pH of household ammonia is well above the pK_a value of the ionizable hydroxyl group on urushiol, so the group would be deprotonated and thus, slightly more soluble in solution than the protonated form. However, the increase in solubility gained by deprotonating the hydroxyl group will not be significant enough to facilitate removal of urushiol from the skin; the hydrophobic carbon chain provides too much non-polar surface area to be suspended in water.

D is incorrect. Plain water will not dissolve the hydrophobic urushiol.

E is incorrect. Adding sugar to water will have no effect on the ability of water to dissolve urushiol.

---

6. Correct: A. pH = 7.27; Bicarbonate = 13; Arterial pCO_2 = 30.

Diabetic ketoacidosis is a metabolic acidosis; it will cause a decrease in serum pH below the normal value of 7.4, with a decrease in serum bicarbonate below the normal value of 24 mEq/L. The figure in the next column shows a mathematical simplification of the Henderson–Hasselbalch for the serum bicarbonate buffering system that is helpful to use while thinking about metabolic and respiratory disturbances in serum acid–base balance.

In the case described here, we know that the serum pH will be lower than 7.4, because we're told that the patient has a metabolic acidosis. As we see in the simplified expression of the Henderson–Hasselbalch equation, there are two ways to decrease serum pH; either the serum bicarbonate level decreases, or the CO_2 level increases. (Normal serum bicarbonate concentration is 24 mEq/L, and a normal serum pCO_2 is 40 mm Hg.) *A decrease in bicarbonate occurs under conditions of metabolic acidosis, and an increase in CO_2 pressure occurs under conditions of respiratory acidosis.* This patient's serum pCO_2 is lower than normal because she is hyperventilating to "blow off" acid (H_2CO_3) from her serum.

B is incorrect. This combination of bicarbonate concentration (close to normal) and CO_2 pressure (higher than normal) is consistent with a respiratory acidosis.

C is incorrect. This combination of parameters represents normal conditions.

D is incorrect. This combination of parameters represents a respiratory alkalosis.

E is incorrect. This combination of parameters represents a metabolic alkalosis.

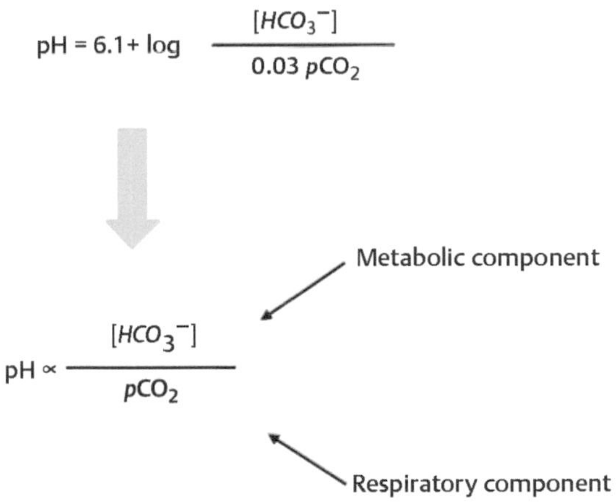

$$pH = 6.1 + \log \frac{[HCO_3^-]}{0.03\, pCO_2}$$

$$pH \propto \frac{[HCO_3^-]}{pCO_2}$$

Metabolic component

Respiratory component

---

7. Correct: D. pH = 7.52; Bicarbonate = 24; Arterial pCO_2 = 30.

Hyperventilation, induced by salicylate activation of the respiratory center in this case, causes respiratory alkalosis; it will cause an increase in serum pH above the normal value of 7.4, with a decrease in serum CO_2 pressure below the normal value of 40 mm Hg. The figure shown in Answer 6 shows a mathematical simplification of the Henderson–Hasselbalch equation that is helpful to use while thinking about metabolic and respiratory disturbances in serum acid–base balance. The direction of the primary cause of acid–base imbalance (i.e., either an increase or decrease in bicarbonate, or an increase or decrease in CO_2) will dictate the direction of the change in pH. In the case

11

described here, we know that the driving force for the acid–base disturbance is hyperventilation. Therefore, we know that the major determinant of the serum pH change will be a decrease in serum pCO_2 as the patient "blows off" more CO_2. As we see in the simplified version of the Henderson–Hasselbalch equation, a decrease in CO_2 level will result in an increase in pH. In cases of hyperventilation, serum bicarbonate levels are either normal, as is the case here, or decreased if there has been adequate time for the kidneys to reduce the level of bicarbonate resorption (i.e., if renal compensation has commenced).

A is incorrect. This combination of parameters represents a metabolic acidosis.

B is incorrect. This combination of parameters represents a respiratory acidosis.

C is incorrect. This combination of parameters represents normal conditions.

E is incorrect. This combination of parameters represents a metabolic alkalosis.

8.   Correct: E. pH = 7.55; Bicarbonate = 44; Arterial pCO_2 = 52

Metabolic alkalosis will cause an increase in serum pH above the normal value of 7.4, with an increase in serum bicarbonate above the normal value of 24 mEq/L. Figure in Answer 6 shows a mathematical simplification of the Henderson–Hasselbalch equation for the serum bicarbonate buffering system that is helpful to use while thinking about metabolic and respiratory disturbances in serum acid–base balance. In the case described here, we know that the serum pH will be higher than 7.4, because we are told that the patient has a metabolic alkalosis. As we see in the simplified expression the Henderson–Hasselbalch equation, there are two ways to increase serum pH; either the serum bicarbonate level increases, or the CO_2 level decreases. (Normal serum bicarbonate concentration is 24 mEq/L, and a normal serum pCO_2 is 40 mm Hg.) *An increase in bicarbonate occurs under conditions of metabolic alkalosis, and a decrease in CO_2 pressure occurs under conditions of respiratory alkalosis.*

A is incorrect. This combination of parameters represents a metabolic acidosis.

B is incorrect. This combination of parameters represents a respiratory acidosis.

C is incorrect. This combination of parameters represents normal conditions.

D is incorrect. This combination of parameters represents a respiratory alkalosis. (Although the bicarbonate level here is slightly higher than normal, it is within the normal reference range and is much less deviant than is the CO_2 pressure.)

9.   Correct: B. pH = 7.25; Bicarbonate = 23; Arterial pCO_2 = 55.

Respiratory depression resulting in hypoventilation will cause respiratory acidosis: a decrease in serum

pH (below the normal value of 7.4), with an increase in arterial pCO_2 above the normal value of 40 mm Hg. Figure in Answer 6 shows a mathematical simplification of the Henderson–Hasselbalch equation that is helpful to use while thinking about metabolic and respiratory disturbances in serum acid–base balance. The direction of the primary cause of acid–base imbalance (i.e., either an increase or decrease in bicarbonate, or an increase or decrease in CO_2) will dictate the direction of the change in pH. In the case described here, we know that the driving force for the acid–base disturbance is hypoventilation. Therefore, we know that the major determinant of the serum pH change will be an increase in serum pCO_2. As we see in the simplified version of the Henderson–Hasselbalch equation, an increase in CO_2 level will result in a decrease in pH.

A is incorrect. This combination of parameters represents a metabolic acidosis.

C is incorrect. This combination of parameters represents normal conditions.

D is incorrect. This combination of parameters represents a respiratory alkalosis.

E is incorrect. This combination of parameters represents a metabolic alkalosis.

10.   Correct: E. 30 mm Hg.

The patient's pCO_2 can be determined from the pH and bicarbonate concentration using the Henderson–Hasselbalch equation for the blood bicarbonate buffering system, where the units on $[HCO_3^-]$ are either mEq/L or mmol/L, and the units on pCO_2 are mm Hg:

$$pH = 6.1 + \log \frac{[HCO_3^-]}{0.03pCO_2}.$$

Using the pH value of 7.49 and a bicarbonate concentration of 22 mEq/L, one can solve the equation for pCO_2.

$$7.49 = 6.1 + \log \frac{[22mEq/L]}{0.03pCO_2}$$

$$1.39 = \log \frac{22}{0.03pCO_2}$$

$$24.5 = \frac{22}{0.03pCO_2}$$

$$0.74 \, pCO_2 = 22$$

$$pCO_2 = 30 \text{ mm Hg}$$

11.   Correct: D. 15 mEq/L.

The patient's arterial bicarbonate concentration can be determined from the pH and arterial pCO_2 using the Henderson–Hasselbalch equation for the blood bicarbonate buffering system, where the units on $[HCO_3^-]$ are either mEq/L or mmol/L, and the units on pCO_2 are mm Hg:

$$pH = 6.1 + \log \frac{[HCO_3^-]}{0.03pCO_2}$$

Using the pH value of 7.24 and a pCO_2 of 36 mm Hg, one can solve the equation for $[HCO_3^-]$:

$$7.24 = 6.1 + \log \frac{[HCO_3^-]}{0.03 \, (36 \text{ mm Hg})}$$

$$1.14 = \log \frac{[HCO_3^-]}{1.08}$$

$$13.8 = \log \frac{[HCO_3^-]}{1.08}$$

$[HCO_3^-] = 14.9$ mEq/L

12. Correct: A. It increases the dissociation of $H_2CO_3 \rightarrow H^+ + HCO_3^-$.

Her respiratory compensation will increase the dissociation of $H_2CO_3 \rightarrow H^+ + HCO_3^-$. In response to metabolic alkalosis, the respiratory system will compensate by hypoventilating. Hypoventilation causes less CO_2 gas to be blown out of the lungs, thus resulting in more retention of CO_2 and an increase in carbonic acid concentration (see figure in Answer 2, the equilibrium shifts to the right when pCO_2 increases). This increased carbonic acid concentration results in increased dissociation of carbonic acid to produce bicarbonate ions and protons. Serum pH is determined by the proton concentration (recall that pH = $-\log[H^+]$), so the increased proton concentration will help to decrease the serum pH.

B is incorrect. Retention of CO_2 gas during hypoventilation would increase the *association* of $H_2O + CO_2 \rightarrow H_2CO_3$; the reverse of what is stated here.

C is incorrect. Retention of CO_2 gas during hypoventilation would increase the *dissociation* of $H_2CO_3 \rightarrow H^+ + HCO_3^-$; the reverse of what is stated here.

D is incorrect. The pK_a of a weak acid is not affected by changes in the concentrations of reactants or products of the equilibrium reaction involving the weak acid. The pK_a can only be changed by altering the chemical structure of the acid in question or by changing the temperature.

E is incorrect. Mature erythrocytes lack nuclei, and, therefore, are unable to alter the level of carbonic anhydrase by regulating its expression.

13. Correct: B. Urinary pH prior to treatment = 5.7; Urinary pH after treatment = 6.7.

The more water-soluble form of uric acid is the deprotonated form, which carries a negative charge. When urine pH is equal to 5.7, the pK_a of the ionizable hydroxyl group on uric acid, the ratio of protonated:deprotonated species will be 1:1. Fifty percent of the molecules will be in the more soluble, deprotonated form. As urinary pH increases, more of the uric acid adopts the deprotonated, soluble form. When the pH is 1 unit higher than the pK_a, i.e., when the pH is 6.7, approximately 90% of the molecules will be deprotonated. (This can be shown using the Henderson–Hasselbalch equation, pH = pK_a + $\log([A^-]/[HA])$; if you use a pH value of 6.7 and a pK_a of 5.7, the equation shows that the ratio $[A^-]/[HA]$ is 10:1, or 91% A^-.)

A is incorrect. In this scenario, the solubility increases from about 10% to 50%.

C is incorrect. In this scenario, the solubility decreases from about 90 to 50%.

D is incorrect. In this scenario, the solubility decreases from 50 to about 10%.

E is incorrect. In this scenario, the solubility increases from about 10 to about 90%.

F is incorrect. In this scenario, the solubility decreases from about 90 to about 10%.

14. Correct: D. 5.0×10^{-3} M.

If the nasogastric tube is placed correctly, the aspirate proton concentration will be closest to 5.0×10^{-3} M. If the nasogastric tube is placed in the stomach, the aspirate should have a pH between 1 and 3. This correlates to a proton ion concentration between 1.0×10^{-1} M and 1.0×10^{-3} M. (Recall that pH = $-\log[H^+]$, where the $[H^+]$ units are M.) 5.0×10^{-3} M is in that range.

A is incorrect; this proton concentration corresponds to pH 4.5, which is too high.

B is incorrect; this proton concentration corresponds to pH –2.1, which is too low.

C is incorrect; this proton concentration corresponds to pH 7.0, which is too high.

E is incorrect; this proton concentration corresponds to pH –2.0, which is too low.

15. Correct: A. The stomach, because the lower pH increases the hydrophobicity of ethacrynic acid.

Ethacrynic acid will more rapidly diffuse across epithelial cell membranes in the stomach, because the lower pH increases the hydrophobicity of ethacrynic acid. Hydrophobic, uncharged molecules diffuse across nonpolar cell membranes more readily than do charged molecules. Ethacrynic acid contains a carboxyl functional group, which has a pK_a of 2.5. (Recall that most carboxylic acids have a pK_a value in the range of 2–4.) Thus, at a pH value of 2.5, 50% of the ethacrynic acid will be protonated and uncharged, as shown in figure in Answer 15, and the remaining 50% will be deprotonated and negatively charged. At pH values below 2.5, more than 50% of the ethacrynic acid will be protonated and uncharged; at pH values above 2.5, more than 50% of the ethacrynic acid will be deprotonated and charged. Thus, in the stomach, where pH ranges generally between 1 and 3, a larger percentage of the ethacrynic acid molecules will be uncharged and able to diffuse across epithelial membranes than in the duodenum, where the pH is higher.

B is incorrect. At lower pH values, more ethacrynic acid will be protonated, and thus have increased, not decreased, hydrophobic character.

C is incorrect. Duodenal pH, which generally ranges between 5.5 and 6.1, is significantly higher than the pK_a value of the carboxyl group on ethacrynic acid. In the duodenum, then, most of the ethacrynic acid will be deprotonated and negatively charged, thus decreasing its hydrophobicity and therefore its ability to diffuse across nonpolar epithelial membranes.

D is incorrect. Duodenal pH, which generally ranges between 5.5 and 6.1, is significantly higher than the pK_a value of the carboxyl group on ethacrynic acid. Thus, in the duodenum, most of the ethacrynic acid will be deprotonated and negatively charged, thus decreasing its hydrophobicity and therefore its ability to diffuse across non-polar epithelial membranes.

16. Correct: G. 1600:1.

This question can be answered using the Henderson-Hasselbalch equation:

$$pH = pK_a + \log \frac{[A^-]}{[HA]}.$$

(A good mnemonic device for remembering how to arrange the variables in this equation is to link pK_a, where the subscript a stands for *acid* dissociation constant, and [acid] as being on the same side of the equation. Furthermore, just as the a in pK_a is a subscript, the [acid] is below the [conjugate base] in the ratio.) In this case, the conjugate base (A^-) is lactate ion, and the weak acid (HA) is lactic acid. Using a pH value of 7.1, and a pK_a value of 3.9, we can solve for the ratio [conjugate base]/[acid].

$$7.1 = 3.9 + \log \frac{[A^-]}{[HA]}$$

$$3.2 = \log \frac{[A^-]}{[HA]}$$

$$1584 = \log \frac{[A^-]}{[HA]}$$

17. Correct: B. In the myoplasm, the concentration of ATP is higher than the product of the adenosine diphosphate (ADP) and phosphate ion concentrations.

We can assume that in the myoplasm, the concentration of ATP is higher than the product of the ADP and phosphate ion concentrations. $\Delta G^{o'}$ is the Gibbs free energy change of a reaction under standard conditions: pH 7.0, 1 M concentrations of reactants and products, and 298 K. Under these standard conditions, the free energy change for the reaction

$$ATP + H_2O \rightarrow ADP + phosphate$$

is –30.5 kJ/mol. The reaction is favorable and releases 30.5 kJ of energy/mol of ATP hydrolyzed. The following equation allows us to calculate ΔG, the Gibbs free energy change under nonstandard conditions (i.e., when we are not starting with 1 M concentrations of reactants and products, and the temperature is not 298 K).

$$\Delta G = \Delta G^{o'} + RT\ln \frac{[ADP][phosphate]}{[ATP]}$$

Plugging in the given values for ΔG and $\Delta G'$, we see that

$$-65 \text{ kJ/mol} = -30.5 \text{ kJ/mol} + RT\ln \frac{[ADP][phosphate]}{[ATP]}$$

$$-95.5 \text{ kJ/mol} = RT\ln \frac{[ADP][phosphate]}{[ATP]}$$

Thus, the ratio of [ADP] (phosphate]/[ATP] must be <1. For that to be the case, the concentration of ATP must be higher than the product of the ADP and phosphate ion concentrations.

A is incorrect. The numerical values of reaction Gibbs free energy changes (ΔG values) do not reveal anything about absolute reactant or product concentrations.

C is incorrect. If ATP were in equilibrium with ADP and phosphate ions, the value of ΔG would be zero.

D is incorrect. If the concentration of ATP were lower than the product of the ADP and phosphate ion concentrations, the ΔG for ATP hydrolysis in these cells would be greater, not less, than –30.5 kJ/mol.

E. Thermodynamic values, such as Gibbs free energy changes, do not provide information regarding reaction rates.

18. Correct: E. 3.3 nM.

The lowest possible myoplasmic calcium ion concentration that could be obtained is 3.3 nM. In this system, the energy that is released during ATP hydrolysis is coupled, via the SRCA pump, to the movement of calcium ions across the SR against their concentration gradient. Thus, the energy available for moving the calcium ions is –65 kJ/mol, the ΔG for ATP hydrolysis. To determine the lowest possible calcium ion concentration that can be achieved in the myoplasm, use the equation

$$\Delta G = -2RT \ln ([Ca^{2+}]_{cyt}/[Ca^{2+}]_{SR})$$

Substitute in the following values and then solve for $[Ca^{2+}]_{cyt}$.

$$-65 \text{ kJ/mol} = -2(0.008314 \text{ kJ/mol-K})(310 \text{ K})\ln([Ca^{2+}]_{cyt}/[1 \text{ mM}])$$

$$-65 \text{ kJ/mol} = -5.15 \ln([Ca^{2+}]_{cyt}/[1 \text{ mM}])$$

$$12.6 = \ln([Ca^{2+}]_{cyt}/[1 \text{ mM}])$$

$$3.33 \times 10^{-6} = [Ca^{2+}]_{cyt}/[1 \text{ mM}])$$

$$3.33 \times 10^{-6} \text{mM} = [Ca^{2+}]_{cyt}$$

$$3.33 \text{ nM} = [Ca^{2+}]_{cyt}$$

19. Correct: E. It increases the rates of metabolic processes, thus increasing the amount of heat released in the process of generating ATP.

Increased cytosolic calcium concentration increases the rates of metabolic processes, thus increasing the amount of heat released in the process of generating ATP. The excess cytosolic calcium ions activate enzymes in glycogenolysis and the citric acid cycle, as stated in the introductory vignette. The increased flux of metabolites through these pathways and oxidative phosphorylation will generate additional heat, as most biochemical reactions are only about 40 to 50% thermodynamically efficient; a significant amount of the available chemical energy from these metabolic reactions is released as heat. The heat generated is a result primarily of increased flux of metabolites through the pathways and not due to alterations in thermodynamic parameters such as changes in ΔG.

A and B are incorrect. The increased cytosolic $[Ca^{2+}]$ will decrease the ΔG for the SRCA pump.

C and D are incorrect. The increased cytosolic $[Ca^{2+}]$ will activate metabolic pathways, such as glycogenolysis and the citric acid cycle. This is a kinetic phenomenon, not a thermodynamic one. Thus, the ΔG values for these reactions will not change, except to the extent that the concentrations of relevant reactants and products might slightly change.

20. Correct: C. +45 kJ/mol.

Using the observed concentrations of reactants and products, along with the $\Delta G^{o'}$ provided in the table, we can calculate the ΔG for the reaction:

$$\Delta G = \Delta G^{o'} + RT\ln \frac{[\alpha \text{ ketoglutarate}][NADH][\text{ammonium ion}]}{[\text{glutamate}][NAD^+]}$$

$\Delta G = 80.5\,kJ/mol + (0.008314\,kJ/mol)(310K)\ln$

$$\frac{[3.0 \times 10^{-5}\,M][5.0 \times 10^{-5}\,M][1.5 \times 10^{-3}\,M]}{[7.5 \times 10^{-3}\,M][3 \times 10^{-4}\,M]}$$

$$\Delta G = +45\,kJ/mol$$

Note that in the convention used by biochemists, when H_2O, H^+, and/or Mg^{2+} are reactants or products, their concentrations are not included in these calculations, but rather are incorporated into the constant $\Delta G^{o'}$.

21. Correct: D. Yes. The glutamate dehydrogenase reaction is being driven toward glutamate synthesis.

Yes, the experimental results indicate that the glutamate dehydrogenase is being driven toward glutamate synthesis, thus depleting the mitochondrial pool of α-ketoglutarate. The ΔG (+45 kJ/mol) calculated based on the observed neuronal mitochondrial concentrations of the various metabolites indicates that the reaction in which glutamate is oxidized to α-ketoglutarate and ammonium ion is released is energetically unfavorable in these mitochondria. The reverse reaction, in which ammonium ion combines with α-ketoglutarate to form glutamate must have a $\Delta G = -45$ kJ/mol and is energetically favorable. Thus, when metabolite concentrations are as described by these experimental results, the glutamate dehydrogenase reaction will be driven in the direction of α-ketoglutarate consumption.

A and C are incorrect. It is not possible to determine the direction of a chemical reaction based only on the concentration of a single reactant or product. The reaction direction is determined by calculating ΔG, which depends on $\Delta G^{o'}$ and the concentrations of reactants and products.

B is incorrect. Calculation of the reaction ΔG under the measured mitochondrial metabolite concentrations indicates that the reaction is unfavorable in the direction of glutamate deamination.

22. Correct: B. 5.6 × 10².

The equilibrium constant, K_{eq}, can be calculated using the formula $\Delta G^{o'} = -RT\ln K_{eq}$. $\Delta G^{o'}$ for the glutamine synthase reaction is determined by combining the $\Delta G^{o'}$ values for the following reactions that are shown in the table

$$\text{glutamate} + NH_4^+ \rightarrow \text{glutamine} + H_2O$$

$\Delta G^{o'} = +14.2$ kJ/mol (reverse the sign on $\Delta G^{o'}$ since the reaction direction is opposite that shown in the table)

$$ATP + H_2O \rightarrow ADP + Pi$$

$$\Delta G^{o'} = -30.5 \text{ kJ/mol}$$

Reaction sum: glutamate + ATP + NH_4 → glutamine + ADP + Pi

$\Delta G^{o'}$ sum: 14.2 kJ/mol – 30.5 kJ/mol = –16.3 kJ/mol

Now, we can calculate K_{eq}:

$$\Delta G^{o'} = -RT\ln K_{eq}$$

$$-16.3 \text{ kJ/mol} = -(0.008314 \text{ kJ/mol-K})(310 \text{ K})\ln K_{eq}$$

$$6.32 = \ln K_{eq}$$

$$K_{eq} = 560$$

23. Correct: A. +33.8 kJ/mol.

Combining these two reaction steps yields the net reaction catalyzed by glutamine synthase. Because thermodynamic parameters of a reaction depend only on the free energy of the reactants and products, and not on the identities of the reaction intermediates, we know that the sum of the Gibbs free energy values for these two reaction steps will be equal to the Gibbs free energy of the glutamine synthetase reaction that can be calculated from the second two reactions shown in the table:

$$\text{glutamate} + NH_4^+ \rightarrow \text{glutamine} + H_2O$$

$\Delta G^{o'}$ = +14.2 kJ/mol (reverse the sign on $\Delta G^{o'}$ since the reaction direction is opposite that shown in the table)

$$ATP + H_2O \rightarrow ADP + Pi$$

$$\Delta G^{o'} = -30.5 \text{ kJ/mol}$$

Reaction sum: glutamate + ATP + NH_4 → glutamine + ADP + Pi

$\Delta G^{o'}$ sum: 14.2 kJ/mol – 30.5 kJ/mol = -16.3 kJ/mol.

Thus, the sum of the Gibb's free energy two steps for the glutamate synthetase reaction must equal –16.3 kJ/mol.

Step 1: glutamate + ATP → γ-glutamyl phosphate + ADP
$\Delta G^{o'}$ = +17.5 kJ/mol.

Step 2: γ-glutamyl phosphate + NH_4^+ → glutamine + Pi
$\Delta G^{o'}$ = X.

Sum: glutamate + ATP + NH_4^+ → glutamine + ADP + Pi
$\Delta G^{o'}$ = –16.3 kJ/mol.

Solving for X, we find that $\Delta G^{o'}$ for Step 2 is +33.8 kJ/mol.

---

24.   Correct: C. It would remain the same.

The equilibrium constant will remain the same. The thermodynamic properties (Gibbs free energy, equilibrium constant, etc.) of a reaction are not influenced by the presence of a catalyst. Enzymes and other catalysts only change the kinetic properties of the reaction. Thus, a deficiency in glutamine synthetase will have no effect on the equilibrium constant of the reaction catalyzed by glutamine synthetase. The deficiency will only slow down the rate at which equilibrium is reached.

A, B, D, and E are incorrect. Changes in the amount of active catalyst will alter the rate at which equilibrium is reached, but will not affect the equilibrium constant.

Chapter 2

Chemistry of Carbohydrates, Lipids, Proteins, and Nucleotides

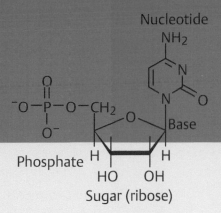

LEARNING OBJECTIVES

▶ List the 20 amino acids, knowing the appropriate three-letter codes, and classify them according to the chemical properties of their side chains.

▶ List the essential and conditionally essential amino acids.

▶ Calculate the isoelectric point (pI) of a small peptide and know the significance of the pI value.

▶ Define, discuss, and identify the following: peptide bond, peptide backbone, N-terminus, C-terminus, and disulfide bridge, as well as common post-translational modifications.

▶ Analyze experimental data obtained by protein chromatography (size exclusion, ion exchange, and affinity), dialysis, sodium dodecyl sulfate-polyacrylamide gel electrophoresis (SDS-PAGE), two-dimensional (2D) electrophoresis, isoelectric focusing, Western blots, enzyme-linked immunosorbent assay (ELISA), and mass spectrometry.

▶ Describe the structures and dietary sources of the major mono-, di-, and polysaccharides: glucose, galactose, fructose, lactose, sucrose, starch, glycogen, and cellulose.

▶ Describe the structures and functions of the major lipids: saturated and unsaturated fatty acids, triglycerides, glycerophospholipids, sphingolipids, and sterols.

▶ Name the major purine and pyrimidine bases, and use the correct terminology while discussing structural features that distinguish different classes of nucleotide metabolites.

2.1 Questions

| Easy | Medium | Hard |

1. A 63-year-old male is placed on total parenteral nutrition (TPN) after he experiences complications following a small bowel resection. Which of the following amino acids has a polar and uncharged side chain *and* must be included in the TPN solution?

A. Serine

B. Lysine

C. Tryptophan

D. Threonine

E. Glutamine

2. A 15-year-old girl was admitted to a hospital for treatment of pneumonia. During the hospitalization, her urine was found to be positive for reducing sugars, although the girl had no history or symptoms of diabetes. Further testing resulted in a diagnosis of essential benign fructosuria. What is the primary dietary source of the sugar in this patient's urine?

A. Milk

B. Potatoes

C. Fruit juice

D. Whole wheat bread

E. Chicken

3. A medical researcher who is studying the effects of glutathione (GSH) on aging needs to do an experimental procedure during which the net charge on GSH should be zero. What should be the pH of the solution she uses for the procedure? Refer to the image below for the structure and pK_a values of GSH.

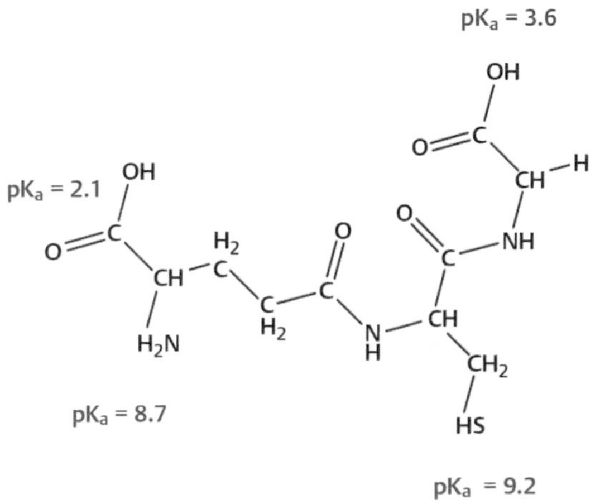

pK_a = 3.6

pK_a = 2.1

pK_a = 8.7

pK_a = 9.2

A. 2.1

B. 2.9

C. 3.6

D. 5.9

E. 6.2

4. Gamma-glutamyl transpeptidase (GGT) catalyzes the cleavage of the peptide bond between cysteine and γ-glutamate in GSH and is expressed at high levels in the liver. Measurement of serum GGT levels is frequently used in the diagnosis and monitoring of certain diseases of the liver. Which of the following shows the product(s) of the GGT-catalyzed reaction with GSH? Refer to the figure in Question 3 for the structure of GSH.

A.

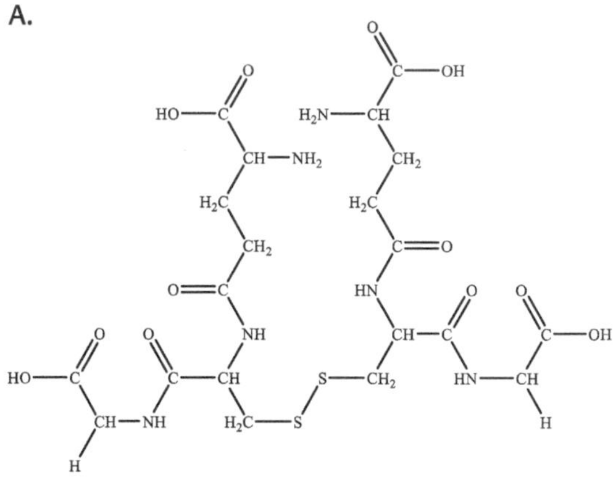

B.

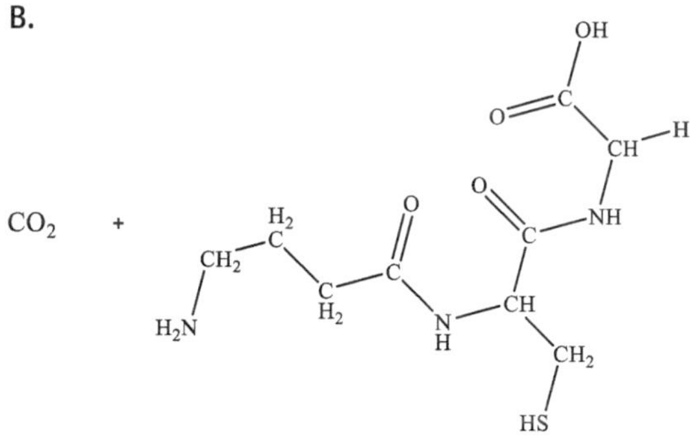

C.

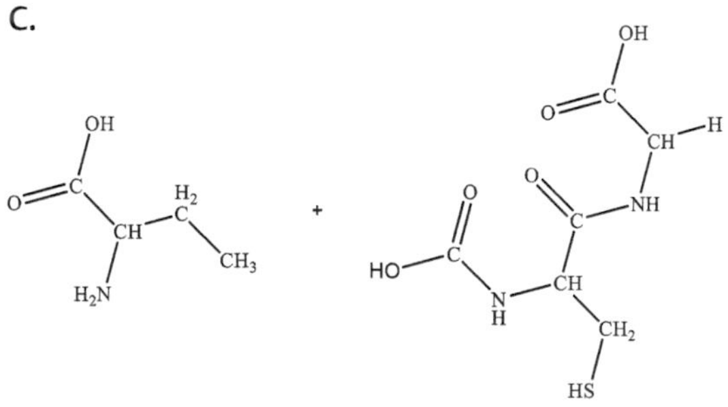

D.

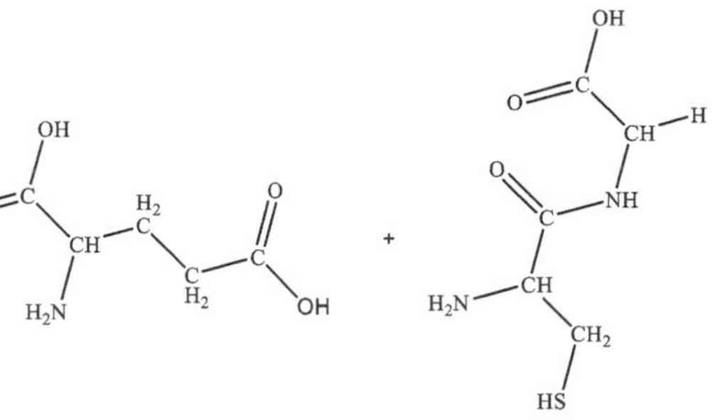

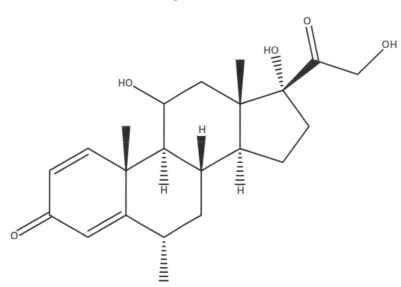

E.

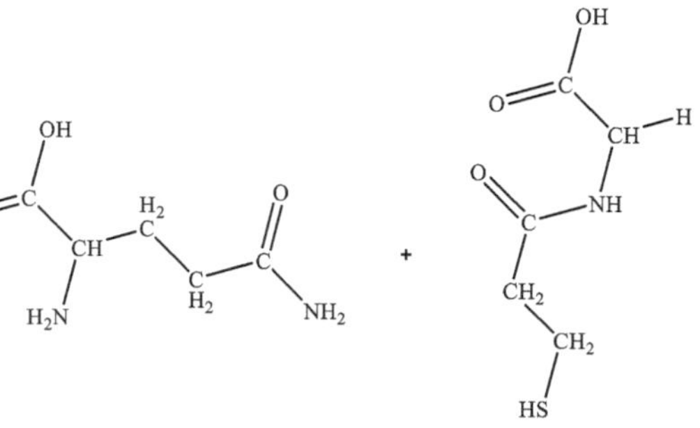

5. The ratio of glutathione:glutathione disulfide (GSH:GSSG) in young adults (average age = 33) is approximately 48:1, while the GSH:GSSG ratio in older adults (average age = 77) is approximately 35:1.[1] What does this indicate about the intercellular environment in the erythrocytes of older adults compared to younger adults?

A. It is more oxidizing

B. It is more reducing

C. It is more acidic

D. It is more basic

E. It has a higher adenosine triphosphate:adenosine diphosphate (ATP:ADP) ratio

F. It has a lower ATP:ADP ratio

6. A 40-year-old woman who was diagnosed with multiple sclerosis 15 years ago visits her primary care provider for evaluation of a recent flare-up of her symptoms, including fatigue, blurred vision, and difficulty walking. The physician prescribed a 5-day course of intravenous SoluMedrol. The structure of the active component in SoluMedrol is shown in the figure below.

The mechanism by which SoluMedrol enters the cells in which it acts is most likely which one of the following?

A. Simple diffusion

B. Facilitated diffusion

C. Primary active transport

D. Secondary active transport

E. Endocytosis

[1] Kosenko EA, Tikhonova LA, Li Y, et al. Antioxidant status and energy state of erythrocytes in Alzheimer dementia—potential probing for markers. Syst Biol Free Radic Antioxid. 2012:2289–2304. doi:10.1007/978-3-642-30018-9_202.

7. A 2-year-old boy is brought to the pediatrician by his mother, who has noticed that the boy generally seems pale and lethargic. Physical examination and laboratory testing eventually result in the diagnosis of a rare hemoglobinopathy. Which of the following mutations would you expect to cause the most drastic alteration in the functional performance of hemoglobin, or any other protein, assuming the replacement is not necessarily at a substrate binding site or active site?

A. Replacement of valine with leucine

B. Replacement of aspartic acid with glutamate

C. Replacement of lysine with arginine

D. Replacement of serine with threonine

E. Replacement of glutamate with lysine

8. A 27-year-old woman was referred to a neurologist after complaining of extreme fatigue, visual disturbances, and unexplained pain. After a careful examination, the neurologist ordered a magnetic resonance imaging (MRI) of the patient's head and neck, as well as a lumbar puncture and analysis of cerebrospinal fluid (CSF). The CSF was analyzed for evidence of myelin basic protein (MBP), which is often elevated in the CSF of individuals who have multiple sclerosis. MBP is unusual in that it has a very high pI value. Which of the following amino acids are likely to be highly represented in the primary sequence of MBP?

A. Aspartate and glutamate

B. Serine, threonine, and tyrosine

C. Tryptophan, valine, leucine, and isoleucine

D. Arginine and lysine

E. Cysteine and methionine

9. Recently, some scientists reported the discovery of a new drug that may be useful in the treatment of gout.[2] The structure of the drug, referred to as Compound 48, is shown in the figure below. Compound 48 is a derivative of which of the following classes of biomolecules?

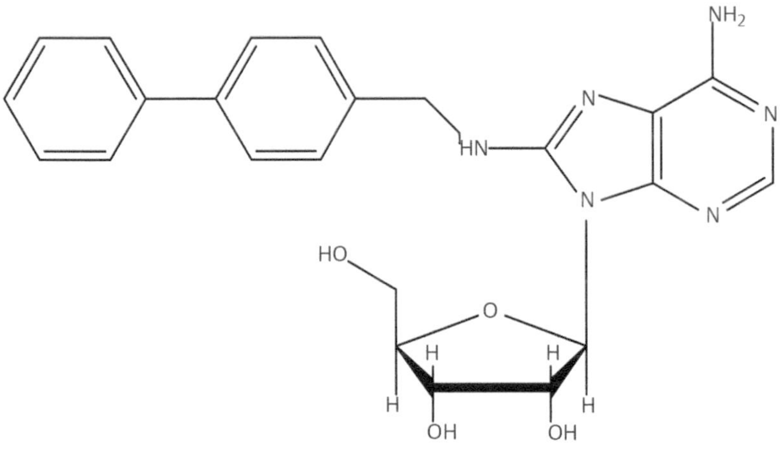

A. Pyrimidine nucleotide

B. Pyrimidine nucleoside

C. Pyrimidine base

D. Purine nucleotide

E. Purine nucleoside

F. Purine base

[2]Tatani K, Masahiro H, Yoshinori N, Masayuki I, Satoshi S. Identification of 8-aminoadenosine derivatives as a new class of human concentrative nucleoside transporter 2 inhibitors. ACS Med Chem Lett. 2015:244–248. Web.

10. Researchers recently reported two novel cases of a rare autosomal recessive disorder in steroid hormone synthesis.[3] The patients they described had a mutation in the *CYP11A1* gene, which encodes the enzyme that catalyzes the first step in the synthesis of all steroid hormones. The novel mutation resulted in a partial loss-of-function due to a conformational change and involved a mutation that replaced a positively charged amino acid with a large nonpolar one. Which of the following mutations did they most likely observe?

A. Valine replaced with amino acid

B. Aspartate replaced with isoleucine

C. Lysine replaced with glutamate

D. Arginine replaced with tryptophan

E. Glutamine replaced with valine

11. Myelin Basic Protein (MBP) is often elevated in the cerebral spinal fluid (CSF) of individuals who have multiple sclerosis. Based on its primary sequence, the calculated pI of the most predominant isoform of MBP is 11.7. MBP undergoes extensive post-translational modifications, which include phosphorylations, methylation of arginine residues, deamidation of glutamine residues, and N-terminal acetylation. What will be the effect of these post-translational modifications on the pI of MBP?

A. Increased pI

B. Decreased pI

C. No change in pI

12. Cancerous cells generally have a high demand for the amino acid glutamine, and thus often up-regulate expression of proteins that mediate glutamine transport. In the rat C6 glioma cell line, for example, the alanine/serine/cysteine transporter 2 (ASCT2) glutamine transporter is up-regulated. In an effort to develop an inhibitor of glutamine transport by ASCT2 that could potentially function as an anti-tumor drug, some researchers recently studied the biochemical properties of the transporter.[4] As part of their studies, they examined the ability of different amino acids to compete with glutamine for transport into C6 glioma cells. Some of their results are shown in the figure below. Which of the following is the most reasonable interpretation of these results?

A. ASCT2 has a higher binding affinity for glutamic acid than for glutamate

B. ASCT2 has a protonizable amino acid residue that plays a key role in binding to transport inhibitors

C. ASCT2 has a higher binding affinity for amino acids with short side chains

D. ASCT2 has a higher binding affinity for amino acids that contain sulfhydryl groups

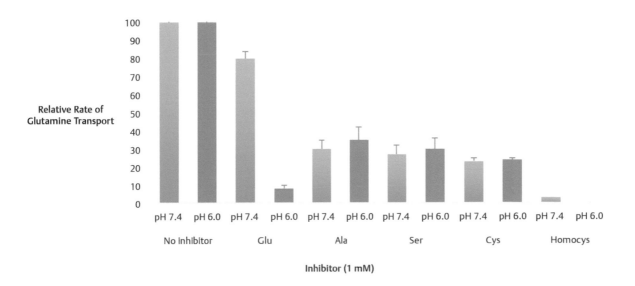

[3]Parajes S, Kamrath C, Rose IT, et al. A novel entity of clinically isolated adrenal insufficiency caused by a partially inactivating mutation of the gene encoding for P450 side chain cleavage enzyme (CYP11A1) J Clin Endocrinol Metab. 2011;96(11). doi:10.1210/jc.2011-1277.

[4]Esslinger CS, Cybulski KA, Rhoderick JF. Nγ-Aryl glutamine analogues as probes of the ASCT2 neutral amino acid transporter binding site. Bioorg Med Chem. 2005;13(4):1111–1118. doi:10.1016/j.bmc.2004.11.028.

Consider the following vignette for questions 13 to 15.

A 16-year-old female presented at the emergency department with nausea, vomiting, and excruciating right flank pain that radiated to her upper lumbar region. She reported that she had two urinary tract infections in the past 4 months, with the most recent one diagnosed 4 days ago. Urinalysis revealed microscopic hematuria, and microscopic cystine crystals were noted. Imaging studies and family history substantiated a diagnosis of cystinuria, an autosomal recessive disorder in cystine and basic amino acid renal reabsorption. Extracorporeal shock wave lithotripsy was used to dissolve a 1.2 cm stone that had lodged in her upper right ureter. The patient was instructed to maintain adequate hydration and eat a low-protein, low-sodium diet in order to decrease her urinary cystine concentration. She was also prescribed potassium citrate to alkalinize her urine. The four pK_a values of the ionizable groups on cystine are 9.2, 8.3, 2.1, and 1.8.

13. What is the net charge on the cystine in this patient's urine if her urinary pH is 6.0?

A. +2

B. +1

C. 0

D. −1

E. −2

14. The patient was prescribed potassium citrate in order to alkalinize her urine, with the goal of increasing the solubility of cystine and preventing formation of new crystals. At what urinary pH will approximately 10% of the urinary cystine carry a net negative (−1) charge?

A. 7.0

B. 7.3

C. 8.2

D. 8.3

E. 9.2

15. During a follow-up visit 2 weeks later, the patient's urinary levels of cystine were still significantly elevated, and microscopic cystine crystals were again observed. Her physician prescribed α-mercaptopropionylglycine. What is the *most likely* mechanism by which α-mercaptopropionylglycine helps to decrease cystine crystallization in this patient's urine?

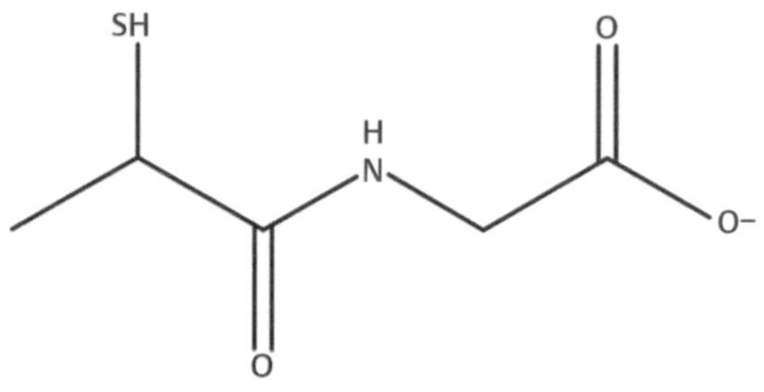

A. It produces a soluble disulfide complex

B. It decreases urinary pH

C. It inhibits the amino acid transporter that is mutated in most individuals with cystinuria

D. It increases urinary pH

16. A 3-month-old girl with a history of hemolytic anemia from birth was recently diagnosed with pyruvate kinase deficiency. Genetic testing indicates that she has a mutation in which the arginine residue at position 532 in the pyruvate kinase amino acid sequence is changed to a tryptophan. This particular mutation results in the loss of activation of pyruvate kinase by fructose-1,6-bisphosphate (FBP), an allosteric activator. What is the most likely role of arginine 532 in binding to FBP?

A. It forms an ionic interaction with a positively charged group on FBP

B. It forms a hydrophobic interaction with a nonpolar region on FBP

C. It forms a hydrophobic interaction with a hydroxyl group on FBP

D. It forms a disulfide bond with FBP

E. It forms an ionic interaction with a negatively charged group on FBP

17. During his annual physical examination, a 30-year-old man complains to his physician that he has been experiencing extreme fatigue over the last few months. During the last week, he has also noticed a numb sensation in his left hand and has on occasion had to balance himself by leaning on a chair or desk after rising from a seated position. The primary care physician refers the patient to a neurologist. After a thorough examination, the neurologist orders an MRI of the head and neck, as well as lumbar puncture and CSF analysis. The CSF analysis included isoelectric focusing of proteins, followed by immunoblotting to detect immunoglobulin G (IgG). During this process, the proteins will be separated according to which of the following properties?

A. A pH at which they have no ionized groups

B. A pH at which they have no positively charged groups

C. A pH at which they have no negatively charged groups

D. A pH at which they have equal numbers of positively and negatively charged groups

E. A pH at which they have an increased affinity for substrate

18. Three isoforms of cardiac troponin (cTn), cardiac troponin I (cTnI), cardiac troponin T (cTnT), and cardiac troponin C (cTnC), are released into serum within a few hours of a myocardial infarction. cTnI and cTnC are frequently used as biomarkers for the diagnosis of myocardial infarction. The figure below shows the results of a sodium dodecyl sulfate polyacrylamide gel electrophoresis (SDS-PAGE) experiment in which all three of the cTn isoforms were analyzed. From these results, what can we conclude regarding cTnC?

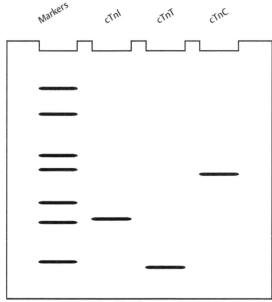

Source: Shi Q, Ling M, Zhang X, et al. Degradation of Cardiac Troponin I in Serum Complicates Comparisons of Cardiac Troponin I Assays. Clinical Chemistry. 1999.

A. cTnC is a heterodimer

B. cTnC contains more basic, positively charged, amino acids than either cTnI or cTnT

C. cTnC has a lower molecular weight than either cTnI or cTnT

D. cTnC is more highly glycosylated than either cTnI or cTnT

E. cTnC is composed primarily of alpha helices

19. Anandamide is an endogenous ligand for endocannabinoid receptors, which function primarily in the nervous system. Like other endocannabinoids, anandamide functions to elicit a natural analgesic effect. The substrate and products of the two-step pathway for synthesis of anandamide are shown in the figure below. To which class of biomolecules does the substrate for anandamide synthesis belong, and what is the identity of the portion of the molecule colored pink?

	Biomolecule class	Pink structure
A	Sphingolipid	Palmitic acid
B	Sphingolipid	Stearic acid
C	Glycerophospholipid	Palmitic acid
D	Glycerophospholipid	Stearic acid
E	Triglyceride	Palmitic acid
F	Triglyceride	Stearic acid

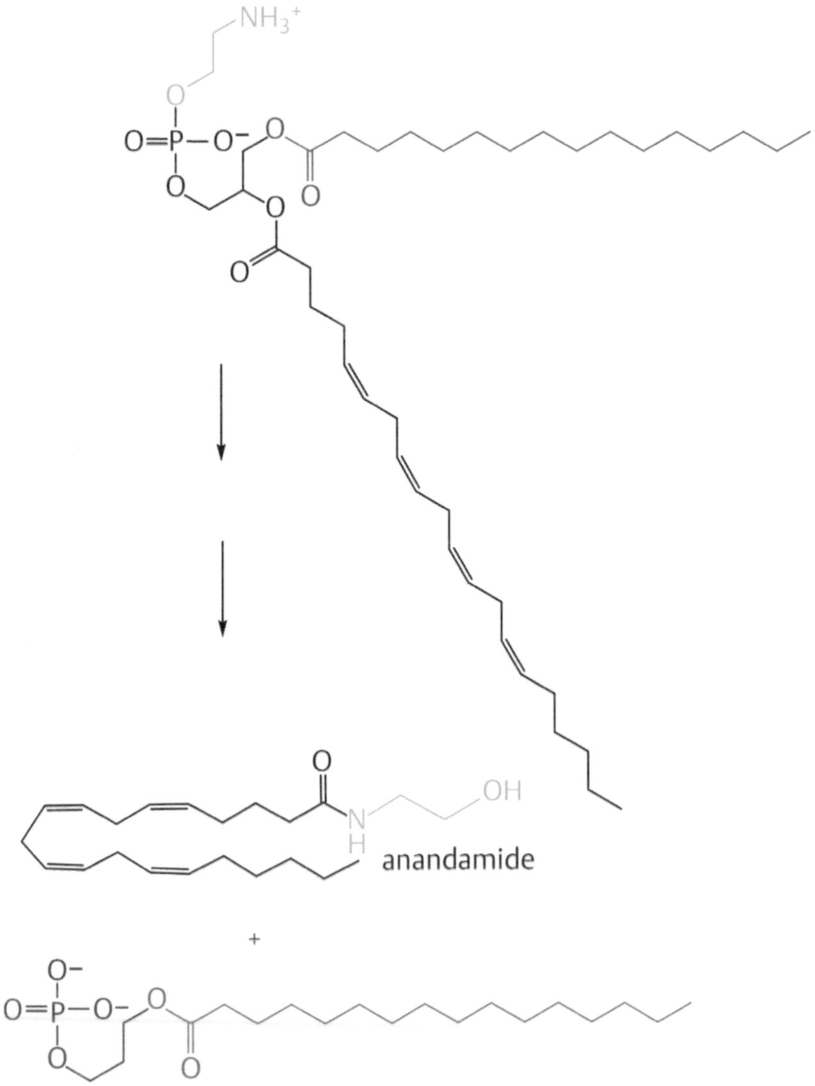

20. A young man gets lost while hiking in the Appalachian Mountains. After 3 days without food, he begins to eat tree leaves, which contain between 20 and 30% carbohydrate by mass. This diet provides only 4 calories of dietary energy per cup of shredded leaves; much less than the 30 to 40 calories expected based on carbohydrate content. Why is this man unable to obtain significant calories by eating the leaves?

A. Plant leaves do not contain glucose

B. This man is probably lactose intolerant

C. The glucose in the leaves is largely incorporated into homopolysaccharide chains with α-1,6 linkages

D. The glucose in the leaves is largely incorporated into homopolysaccharide chains with β-1,4 linkages

E. The carbohydrates in the leaves are mostly glycosaminoglycans

anandamide

21. A woman with severe hypochondriasis is certain that she has undiagnosed phenylketonuria. She self-prescribes a nearly protein-free diet and begins taking a dietary supplement containing all of the essential amino acids, but phenylalanine. If she continues with this diet, she will develop a deficiency in which of the following amino acids?

A. Alanine

B. Tyrosine

C. Histidine

D. Serine

E. Tryptophan

22. The newborn screening results for a 2-day-old infant indicate that the child has classical galactosemia; consumption of dietary galactose could result in severe liver damage and death. Which of the following should be eliminated from this child's diet?

A. Table sugar

B. Gluten

C. Eggs

D. Dairy products

E. Gelatin

23. A 23-year-old homeless woman presents at an emergency department complaining of severe flu-like symptoms for at least 3 weeks. History reveals that she has lost a significant amount of weight (she estimates that she has dropped at least 3 pant sizes) in the last 2 months, and that she occasionally works as a prostitute. Subsequent testing reveals a sexually transmitted disease, and she is placed on a multi-drug regimen that includes a 2'-deoxythymidine analog. Which of the following structures most likely represents the drug?

A. Structure A

B. Structure B

C. Structure C

D. Structure D

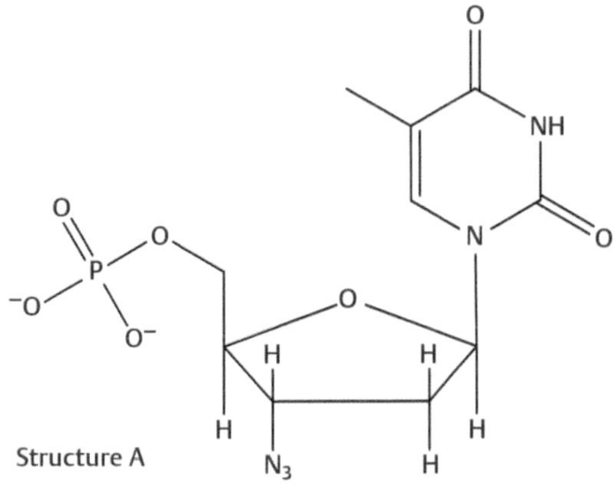

Structure A

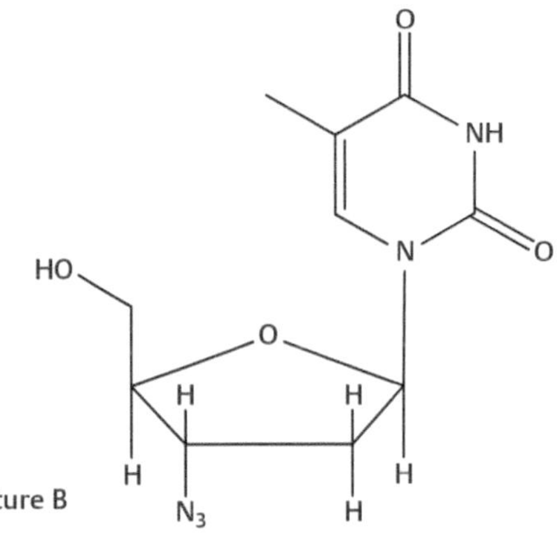

Structure B

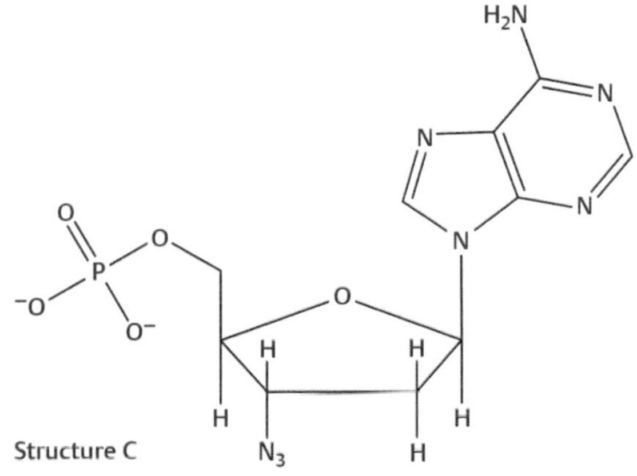

Structure C

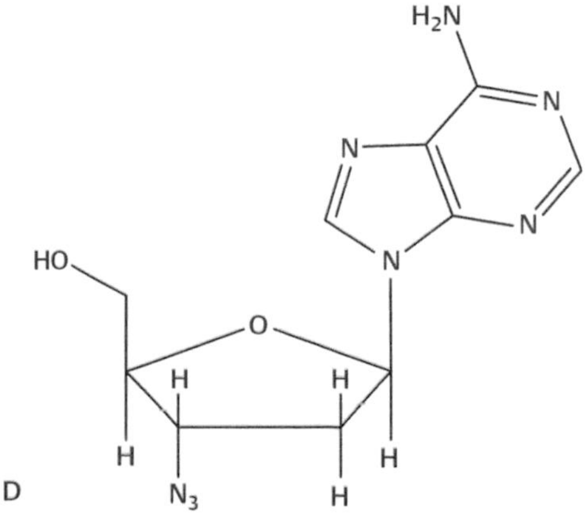

Structure D

25

2.2 Answers and Explanations

| Easy | Medium | Hard |

1. Correct: D. Threonine

Threonine has a polar, uncharged side chain, and is one of the nine essential amino acids. TPN solution must contain all of the essential amino acids, which cannot be made by the human body so must be provided in the diet. The essential amino acids are as follows: phenylalanine, valine, threonine, tyrosine, isoleucine, methionine, histidine, leucine, and lysine. (Private Tim Hill—PVT TIM HiLL—is a mnemonic for remembering these.) Cysteine, tyrosine, and arginine are conditionally essential amino acids; cysteine is made from methionine and tyrosine from phenylalanine, so a diet deficient in the essential amino acids methionine or phenylalanine will eventually result in insufficient levels of cysteine and tyrosine. Arginine is made in the urea cycle and is considered conditionally essential because the body sometimes cannot keep up with the demand for arginine simply by making its own. Of the amino acids listed here, only threonine meets the criteria of being essential *and* having a polar uncharged side chain.

A is incorrect. Although it is polar and uncharged, serine is not one of the nine essential amino acids.

B is incorrect. Although lysine is an essential amino acid, its side chain is charged.

C is incorrect. Although tryptophan is an essential amino acid, its side chain is nonpolar.

Choice E is incorrect. Although it is polar and uncharged, glutamine is not one of the nine essential amino acids.

2. Correct: C. Fruit juice

Fruit juice is a source of fructose. In fructosuria, fructose is eliminated in the urine. Fructose is a component of sucrose (also known as table sugar; a disaccharide composed of glucose and fructose), which is found in fruit and sweetened foods. Sucrose is digested to glucose and fructose by intestinal sucrase. Fructose may also be found as a free sugar in honey and in foods containing high fructose corn syrup. Fructose is intestinally absorbed and primarily metabolized in the liver via a pathway that is initiated by phosphorylation of fructose using the enzyme fructokinase. Fructokinase activity is impaired in benign essential fructosuria, resulting in accumulation of fructose in the serum, and eventual elimination in the urine.

A is incorrect. The sugar contained in milk is lactose, a disaccharide composed of glucose and galactose.

B is incorrect. Potatoes are rich in starch, a polymer of glucose that is digested to glucose monomers in the intestine.

D is incorrect. Whole wheat bread is rich in starch, a polymer of glucose that is digested to glucose monomers in the intestine.

E is incorrect. Meat contains very little carbohydrate, which will be in the form of glycogen, not sucrose.

3. Correct: B. 2.9

The solution pH should be 2.9. The solution pH at which a peptide will carry a net charge of zero is known as the pI value of the peptide. To determine the pI value, you first need to determine the various ionization states of the peptide. For GSH, the first four ionizations states, as they would appear in solution from low to high pH, are shown in the figure on the next page. The pI is calculated as the average of the two pK_a values for the equilibria on either side of the species with a net charge of zero. In this case, the two pK_a values that should be used are 2.1 (deprotonation of the γ-glutamate carboxyl group) and 3.6 (deprotonation of the terminal carboxyl group). $(2.1 + 3.6)/2 = 2.9$.

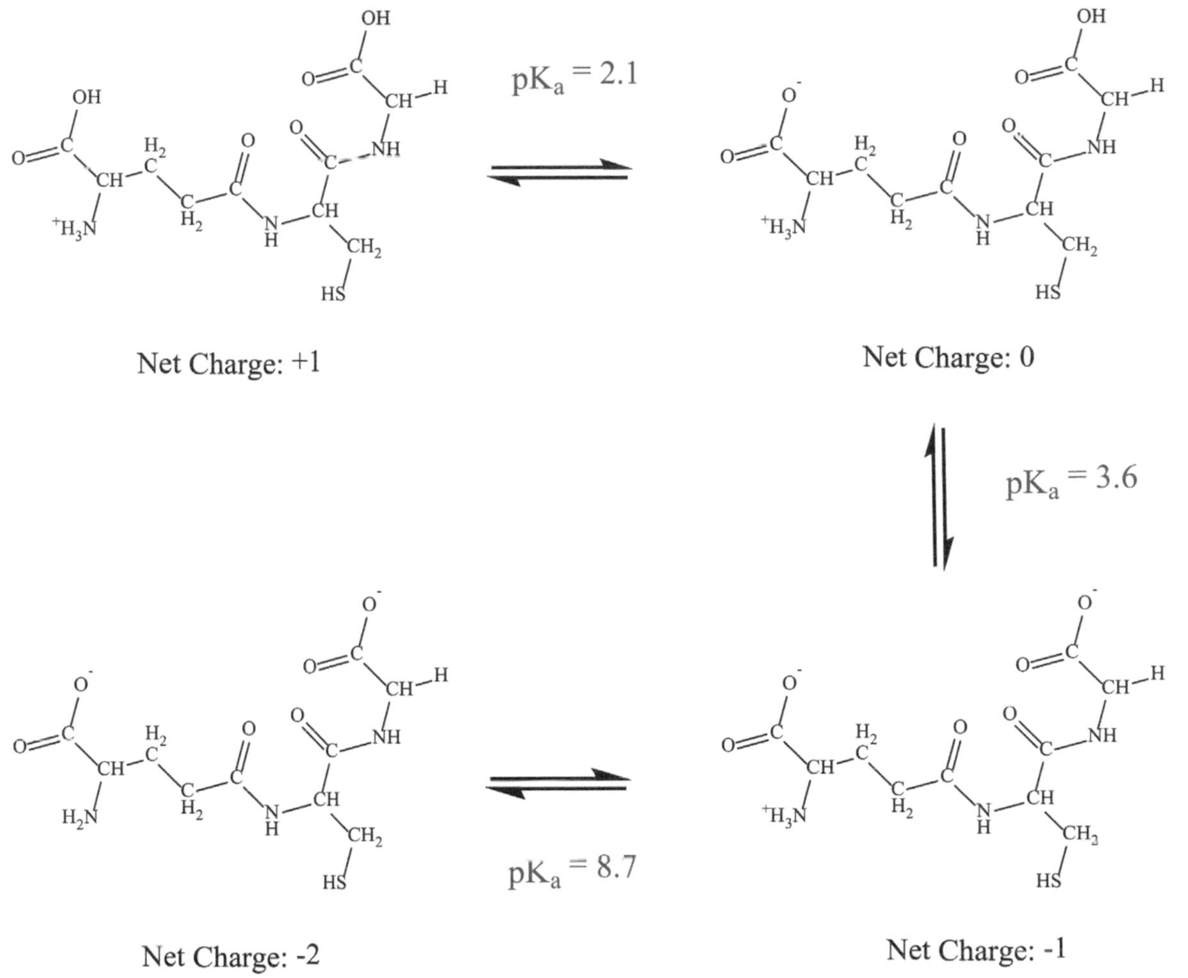

$pK_a = 2.1$

Net Charge: +1

Net Charge: 0

$pK_a = 3.6$

$pK_a = 8.7$

Net Charge: -2

Net Charge: -1

4. Correct: D.

GGT cleaves peptide bonds, which link carboxyl and amino groups of amino acids to each other. During peptide synthesis, when amino acid carboxyl and amino groups condense, they form an amide functional group, also known as a peptide bond. The two peptide bonds in GSH are shown in red in the figure given below.

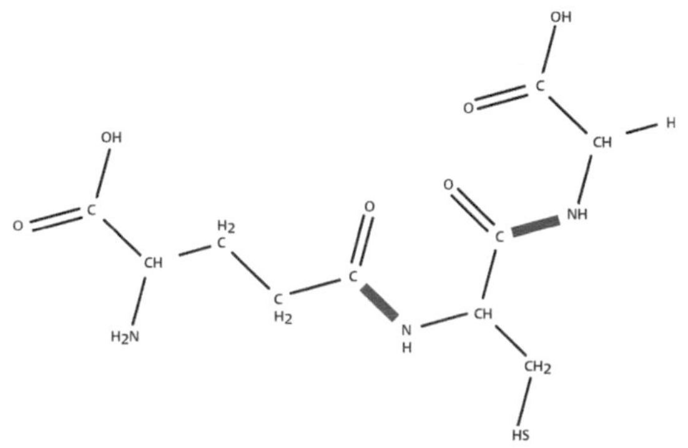

Hydrolysis of the peptide bond produces a free amino group on one product and a free carboxyl group on the other. The molecules shown in choice D are produced by hydrolysis of the γ-glutamyl peptide bond in GSH. The products are glutamate and cysteinylglycine.

A is incorrect. The structure shown is GSH disulfide, the product of oxidation of GSH.

B is incorrect. This would be the product of a decarboxylation reaction.

C is incorrect. These products result from cleavage of an unreactive C–C bond, which generally does not occur in biological systems, and is not catalyzed by proteases like GGT.

E is incorrect. These products result from cleavage of an unreactive C–N bond, which generally does not occur in biological systems, and is not catalyzed by proteases like GGT.

5. Correct: A. It is more oxidizing.

The intercellular environment in older adults is more oxidizing than that of younger adults. The formation of a disulfide bond between two free thiol groups, as occurs when GSH is converted to GSSG, is an oxidation reaction, as illustrated in (i) below.

(i) GSH + GSH $\xrightleftharpoons[[R]]{[O]}$ GSSG

During the course of this reaction the sulfur atoms lose electrons, which are used to reduce co-reactants (indicated by [O], for oxidant, in the reaction above) in the process. An important example is the reaction catalyzed by GSH peroxidase, shown in (ii), where electrons are removed from GSH and are used to reduce peroxide.

(ii) $2\,GSH + H_2O_2 \rightleftharpoons GSSG + 2\,H_2O$

GSH plays an important role in protecting cells from oxidative stress, by inactivating hydrogen peroxide and other potent oxidants. The decreased GSH:GSSG ratio in the erythrocytes of older adults indicates that the cytosol contains relatively large amounts of oxidants that shift the equilibria of these redox reactions toward generation of GSSG.

B is incorrect. The conversion of GSSG to GSH is a reduction reaction; the reverse of the reaction shown in (ii).

C is incorrect. The ratio of GSH to GSSG is primarily dependent on the redox status of the cell, and not on pH.

D is incorrect. The ratio of GSH to GSSG is primarily dependent on the redox status of the cell, and not on pH.

E and F are incorrect. The ATP:ADP ratio does not directly influence the GSH:GSSG ratio. However, a low ATP:ADP ratio may have an adverse effect on the cell's ability to generate nicotinamide adenine dinucleotide phosphate (NADPH) via the pentose phosphate pathway, as more glucose will be required for energy generation. If his happens, the GSH:GSSG ratio will drop, as GSH reductase requires NADPH to reduce GSSG. However, the net effect of this will be that the cytosol will become a more oxidizing environment. Thus choice A is a better answer than choice F.

6. Correct: A. Simple diffusion.

SoluMedrol enters cells by simple diffusion. The structure shown is that of a typical steroid. SoluMedrol is the brand name of methylprednisolone, a corticosteroid. Steroids are lipophilic; as with other lipophilic or small uncharged substances, the primary mechanism by which they enter the cell is by simple diffusion. As illustrated in the image below, lipophilic and small, polar uncharged molecules diffuse through the plasma membrane in the same direction as their concentration gradient. Once inside the cell, steroids bind nuclear receptors which regulate gene expression.

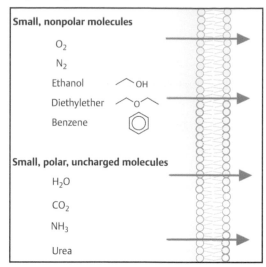

Source: Panini S. Medical Biochemistry - An Illustrated Review. 1st Edition. Thieme; 2013.

B is incorrect. Facilitated diffusion, which is illustrated in the image below, involves the use of protein carriers that facilitate the movement of polar and charged molecules across the membrane. The molecules move in the same direction as their concentration gradients, so the process does not require an input of energy. Lipophilic molecules, such as steroids, move freely across the lipid bilayer, and thus do not require facilitation of diffusion.

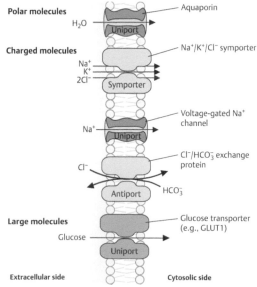

Source: Panini S. Medical Biochemistry - An Illustrated Review. 1st Edition. Thieme; 2013.

C and D are both incorrect. Active transport, as illustrated in the two figures on the next page, is used to move molecules across the plasma membrane in the direction that opposes their concentration gradient. This is not necessary for steroids, which have significantly lower intracellular concentrations than extracellular concentrations. Primary active transport uses energy generated from the direct hydrolysis of ATP by the transport protein, while secondary active transport uses energy generated by coupling transport with the movement of different molecule down its concentration gradient.

Primary active transport (movement from low to high concentration; energy-dependent)

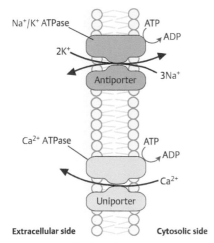

Source: Panini S. Medical Biochemistry - An Illustrated Review. 1st Edition. Thieme; 2013.

Secondary active transport (movement from low to high concentration AND high to low concentration; energy-dependent)

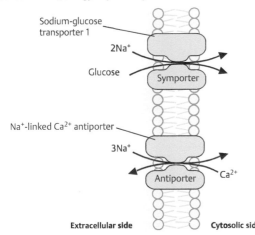

Source: Panini S. Medical Biochemistry - An Illustrated Review. 1st Edition. Thieme; 2013.

E is incorrect. Endocytosis is triggered by the binding of a receptor to its ligand. As stated earlier, steroids, in general, do not bind to plasma membrane receptors. Rather, they diffuse across the lipid membrane.

7. Correct: E. Replacement of glutamate with lysine.

Replacement of glutamate, which carries a negative charge on its side chain at physiological pH, with lysine, which carries a positive charge on its side chain at physiological pH, may disrupt the formation of ionic bonds that frequently stabilize the tertiary and quaternary structures of proteins.

A is incorrect. Valine and leucine both have hydrophobic side chains; this is a conservative mutation. Although leucine is slightly larger in size than valine is, its substitution for valine in most proteins is not detrimental to stability or function.

B is incorrect. Glutamic acid and aspartic acid both have carboxyl side chains that will be negatively charged at physiological pH. The only difference between these amino acids is that glutamate contains an additional methylene group. This conservative mutation will rarely affect the stability or function of a protein, except in some circumstances where the mutation occurs in the active site or substrate binding site.

C is incorrect. Lysine and arginine are similar in that they both carry a positive charge at physiological pH. This conservative mutation will rarely affect the stability or function of a protein, except in some circumstances where the mutation occurs in the active site or substrate binding site.

D is incorrect. Serine and threonine are both polar, uncharged, amino acids that contain a hydroxyl group. Although threonine carries an additional methyl group, generally, substitution of a serine with threonine will not significantly affect protein structure, function, or stability.

8. Correct: D. Arginine and lysine.

MBP contains many arginine and lysine residues. The pI value is the pH at which a molecule carries no net electrical charge. The charge on a peptide changes as the pH of the solution in which it is suspended changes. At very low pH values, peptide ionizable functional groups are protonated and either have no charge (carboxyl groups, found at the C-terminus and on aspartate and glutamate residue side chains) or a positive charge (amino, guanidino, or imidazolium groups, found at the N-terminus and on lysine, arginine, and histidine residue side chains). As the pH increases above the pK_a values of the carboxyl groups, they become deprotonated to form negatively charged carboxylate ions, and the net charge on the peptide becomes less positive. As the pH continues to increase above the pK_a values of the imidazolium, amino, and guanidine groups, protons on the positively charged functional groups begin to dissociate, and the net charge becomes more negative. Polypeptide chains that have a greater number of positively charged functional groups, such as arginine and lysine, will necessarily require higher solution pH values in order to become neutral or negatively charged.

A is incorrect. Aspartate and glutamate have low pK_a values. A polypeptide chain that is very rich in these amino acids and poor in basic amino acids, such as arginine and lysine, will become electrically neutral at a relatively low pH.

B is incorrect. Serine, threonine, and tyrosine are polar, uncharged amino acids. The pK_a values of their side chains are so high that their ionization state of their side chains does not factor into the peptide pI value.

C is incorrect. Tryptophan, valine, leucine, and isoleucine are nonpolar amino acids with unionizable side chains. They do not contribute to the peptide pI value.

E is incorrect. Methionine has a nonpolar, unionizable side chain and will not contribute to the peptide pI value. The pK_a value for the cysteine side chain is generally around 8. When the solution pH is above the cysteine pK_a value, the side chain becomes negatively charged. Thus, a peptide very rich in cysteine residues will not necessarily have a very high pI value.

9. Correct: E. Purine nucleoside.

Compound 48 is a derivative of adenosine; a purine nucleoside. Comparison of Compound 48 with the structures shown in (i) below shows that the absence of a phosphate group on the 5'-ribose hydroxyl group makes Compound 48 a nucleoside. Comparison with the structures shown in (ii) below reveals that the nucleotide base, adenine, is a purine. Recall that purines have the larger structure (two rings), but the shorter name. Pyrimidines have the smaller structure (one ring), but the longer name.

A is incorrect. Pyrimidines have only one ring in the nucleotide base structure.

B is incorrect. Pyrimidines have only one ring in the nucleotide base structure.

C is incorrect. Pyrimidines have only one ring in the nucleotide base structure.

D is incorrect. Nucleotides have phosphate attached to the 5'-hydroxyl group on the ribose ring.

F is incorrect. Once a ribose ring is attached to the nucleotide base; the structure is referred to as either a nucleoside (no phosphate added) or a nucleotide.

10. Correct: D. Arginine replaced with tryptophan.

An arginine to tryptophan mutation involves replacing a positively charged side chain with a large nonpolar side chain. Only three amino acids may carry a positive charge on the side chain: arginine, histidine, and lysine. Thus, only choices C and D identify an appropriate amino acid for the wild-type enzyme. The mutation involved the replacement of a positively charged amino acid with a large nonpolar amino acid. The large nonpolar amino acids are isoleucine, leucine, methionine, phenylalanine, tryptophan, and valine. Choice D, then, indicates a change from a positively charged amino acid residue to a large nonpolar one.

A is incorrect. Valine is a large nonpolar amino acid.

B is incorrect. Aspartate is a negatively charged amino acid.

C is incorrect. Although lysine is a positively charged amino acid, and glutamate is negatively charged, not large and nonpolar.

E is incorrect. Glutamine is a polar uncharged amino acid.

11. Correct: B. Decreased pI.

These post-translational modifications will decrease the pI value. The pI value is the pH at which a molecule carries no net electrical charge. Polypeptide chains that have a large number of positively charged functional groups, such as arginine and lysine, will necessarily require higher solution pH values in order to become neutral or negatively charged (at

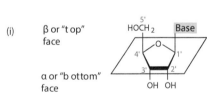

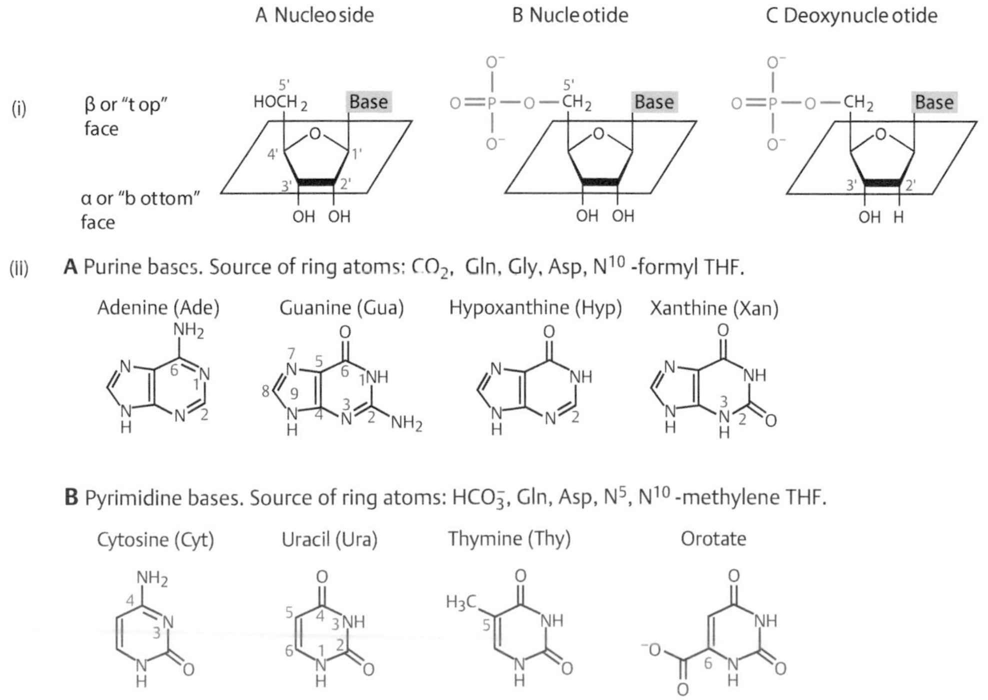

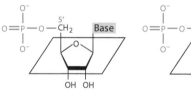

(i)   β or "top" face

α or "bottom" face

A Nucleoside   B Nucleotide   C Deoxynucleotide

(ii)   **A** Purine bases. Source of ring atoms: CO_2, Gln, Gly, Asp, N^{10}-formyl THF.

Adenine (Ade)   Guanine (Gua)   Hypoxanthine (Hyp)   Xanthine (Xan)

B Pyrimidine bases. Source of ring atoms: HCO_3^-, Gln, Asp, N^5, N^{10}-methylene THF.

Cytosine (Cyt)   Uracil (Ura)   Thymine (Thy)   Orotate

Source: Panini S. Medical Biochemistry - An Illustrated Review. 1st Edition. Thieme; 2013.

high solution pH, the positively charged amino acid residues are deprotonated and become neutral). These peptides, like MBP, have high pI values. Post-translational modifications, such as methylation of arginine residues and acetylation of N-terminal amino groups, decrease the amount of positive charge on the peptide chain. In addition, phosphorylation of side chains and deamidation of glutamine residues will increase the amount of negative charge on the peptide chain. The net effect is that the peptide chain will carry a neutral charge at lower pH values; thus, the pI will decrease.

12. Correct: A. ASCT2 has a higher binding affinity for glutamic acid than for glutamate.

The data suggest that ASCT2 has a higher binding affinity for glutamic acid than for glutamate. Glutamate is a very poor inhibitor of transport by ASCT2 at pH 7.4, with about 80% of the control level of glutamine transport occurring when 1 mM glutamate is present. However, when the pH is dropped to 6.0, much greater inhibition is observed (<10% of the control level of glutamine transport is observed). At this lower pH, more of the carboxyl side chain of glutamate, which has a pK_a value of 4.1, will be protonated than at pH 7.4. This suggests that the protonated form of glutamate, i.e., glutamic acid, is a better inhibitor of glutamine transport, and thus that ASCT2 has a higher binding affinity for glutamic acid than for glutamate.

B is incorrect. While the data shown for inhibition of glutamine transport by glutamate do indicate pH dependence, inhibition of transport by the other amino acids is not pH dependent. Furthermore, transport of glutamine is not pH dependent. Thus, it is unlikely that the pH dependence of inhibition by glutamate is due to changes in the protonation state of an ionizable amino acid residue on ASCT2. Rather, the pH dependence is more likely to reflect the protonation state of glutamate.

C is incorrect. The ASCT2 transporter has a higher affinity for amino acids with *longer* side chains, as shown by the difference in inhibition between cysteine and homocysteine. The side chain of homocysteine contains one more methylene group than does cysteine, and the data indicate that homocysteine is a significantly better inhibitor of glutamine transport than is cysteine.

D is incorrect. The ASCT2 transporter binding affinity for inhibitor is not affected by the presence of a sulfhydryl group. The data show that cysteine and serine are equally potent inhibitors; these amino acids are identical except that cysteine contains a sulfhydryl group while serine contains a hydroxyl group.

13. Correct: C. 0

At pH 6.0, the net charge on cysteine is zero. The structure of cystine is shown in the figure below. The two carboxyl groups have pK_a values of 1.8 and 2.1. The patient's urinary pH is 6.0, which is well above these pK_a values; the carboxyl groups will be fully deprotonated, each providing a –1 charge. The two amino groups have pK_a values of 8.3 and 9.2. The patient's urinary pH is well below these pK_a values; they will be fully protonated, each providing a +1 charge. So, the ionization state will be as shown in the figure below, with a net charge of zero. Cystine is least soluble in urine when its net charge is zero. The treating physician will attempt to alkalinize this patient's urine in order to increase cystine solubility.

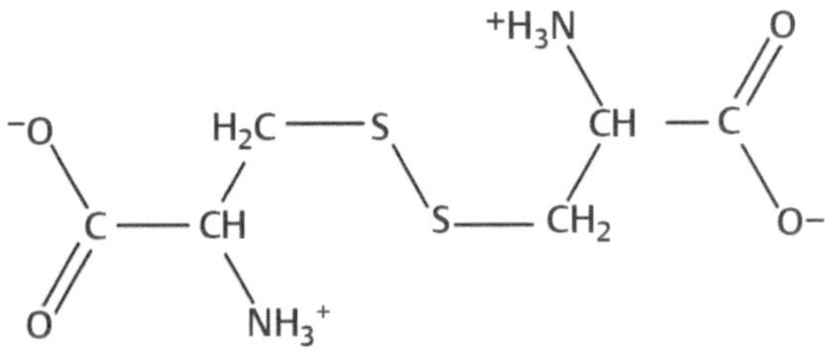

14. Correct: B. 7.3.

Approximately 10% of the cysteine will carry a net negative (–1) charge at pH 7.3. This question can be solved using the Henderson–Hasselbalch equation: pH: $pK_a + \log([A^-]/[HA])$. We established in the previous question that at pH 6.0, cystine has a net zero charge. As the urine pH is raised by treatment with potassium citrate, the cystine amino group with the lowest pK_a value, 8.3, will begin to be deprotonated. These deprotonated cystine molecules will carry a net –1 charge (i.e., both carboxyl groups will be deprotonated and will each have a –1 charge; the amino group with the highest pK_a will be protonated and have a +1 charge, and the amino group with pK_a 8.3 will be deprotonated and have no charge). In this this (de)ionization event, the acid (HA) is the protonated amino group, and the conjugate base (A−) is the deprotonated amino group. We are trying to determine the pH at which approximately 10% of the cystine molecules carry a –1 charge; i.e., the pH at which the ratio of [A−]/[HA] is 1:10. Using the Henderson–Hasselbalch equation, we see that

$$pH: pK_a + \log([A^-]/[HA])$$

$$pH: 8.3 + \log(1/10)$$

$$pH: 7.3.$$

This problem can also be quickly solved using the rule-of-thumb that 90% of an ionizable species will be protonated when the pH of the solution is 1 pH unit lower than the pK_a of the ionizable group.

15. Correct: A. It produces a soluble disulfide complex.

α-Mercaptopropionylglycine forms soluble disulfide bonds. Cystine, like all disulfides, readily undergoes disulfide exchange reactions with other thiols. As shown in the figure below, cystine will react with α-mercaptopropionylglycine to form free cysteine and cysteine-mercaptopropionylglycine disulfide. Cysteine-mercaptopropionylglycine disulfide has a net –1 charge at pH values lower than 8 and is thus much more soluble in the urine than is cystine.

B is incorrect. α-Mercaptopropionylglycine will not alter urinary pH.

C is incorrect. Inhibition of the amino acid transporter in question will only further inhibit renal reabsorption of cystine and may increase urinary cystine concentrations, thus aggravating the condition.

D is incorrect. α-Mercaptopropionylglycine will not alter urinary pH.

α - mercaptopropionylglycine

cystine

cysteine

cysteine-mercaptopropionylglycine disulfide

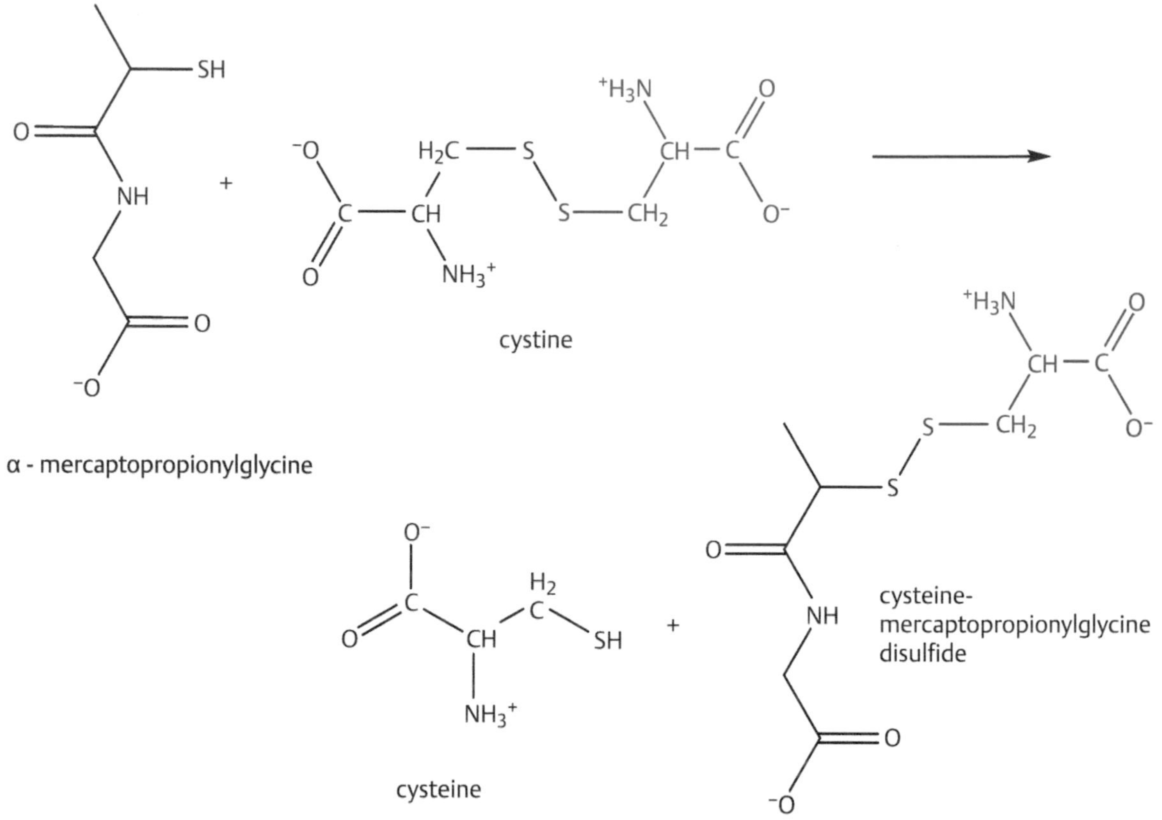

16.   Correct: E. It forms an ionic interaction with a negatively charged group on FBP.

Arginine has a positively charged side chain that can form an ionic interaction with a negatively charged phosphate group on FBP.

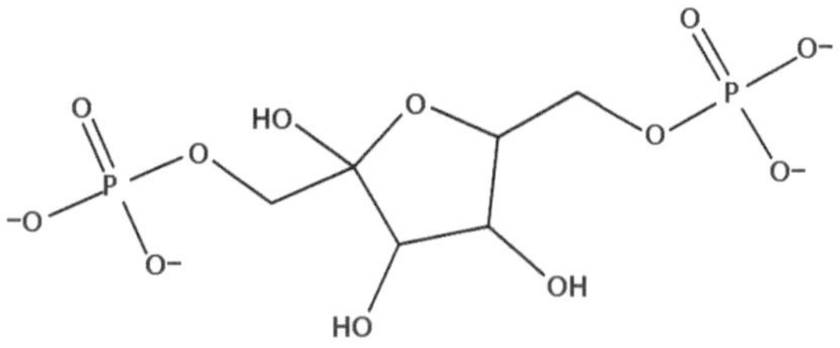

A is incorrect. FBP does not contain any positively charged functional groups. Furthermore, arginine carries a positive charge that would repel a positive charge on FBP, if it had one.

B is incorrect. Arginine has a positively charged side chain and would not form hydrophobic interactions. Furthermore, FBP is a phosphorylated carbohydrate that does not have significant nonpolar character.

C is incorrect. Hydroxyl groups do not form non polar interactions.

D is incorrect. Neither arginine nor FBP contains sulfhydryl groups that could form disulfide bonds.

17.   Correct: D. A pH at which they have equal numbers of positively and negatively charged groups.

During isoelectric focusing, proteins are separated according to the pH at which they have an equal number of positively and negatively charged groups. A mixture of proteins is electrophoresed through a solution or gel that has a stable pH gradient in which the pH smoothly increases from the cathode to the anode. If the protein mixture is placed at the cathode, the pH will be low and most of the peptide chains will carry a net positive charge. When electrophoresis begins, the positively charged proteins migrate toward the anode. However, as the proteins migrate, the pH increases, and some of the ionizable groups are deprotonated. At the area of the solution or gel where the pH is equal to the peptide pI, the net charge on the peptide will be zero, and it will no longer migrate. Thus, the procedure separates proteins based on differences in pI value; the pH at which a protein has equal numbers of positively and negatively charged functional groups, resulting in a net neutral electrical charge.

A is incorrect. Isoelectric focusing separates proteins according to the pH at which they have no net electrical charge (i.e., the pI value). This means that they have equal numbers of positively and negatively charged groups, not that there are no ionized groups.

B is incorrect. Isoelectric focusing separates proteins according to the pH at which they have no net electrical charge (i.e., the pI value). This means that they have equal numbers of positively and negatively charged groups, not that there are positively charged groups.

C is incorrect. Isoelectric focusing separates proteins according to the pH at which they have no net electrical charge (i.e., the pI value). This means that they have equal numbers of positively and negatively charged groups, not that there are no negatively charged groups.

D is incorrect. Isoelectric focusing does not involve separation according to substrate affinity.

18.   Correct: C. cTnC has a lower molecular weight than either cTnI or cTnT.

cTnC has a lower molecular weight than either cTnI or cTnT. SDS-PAGE separates proteins according to molecular weight, with longer peptide chains moving more slowly, and thus migrating a shorter distance, through the gel. Thus, because it migrated a longer distance down the gel, we can conclude that cTnC is a smaller peptide and has a lower molecular weight.

A is incorrect. If cTnC were a heterodimer, we would expect to see two bands in lane 3, assuming that the two peptide chains composing the dimer were of significantly different molecular weights.

B is incorrect. SDS-PAGE separates proteins only based on size and not differences in charge.

D is incorrect. SDS-PAGE separates proteins only based on size and not differences in charge. A high degree of glycosylation would increase both the degree of negative charge on cTnC and its molecular weight. Neither of these can be supported by the evidence provided in this gel.

E is incorrect. Proteins are denatured during SDS-PAGE, so the composition of their secondary structure will have no effect on migration.

19.   Correct: C Glycerophospholipid Palmitic acid.

The substrate is phosphatidylethanolamine, a glycerophospholipid, and the pink structure is palmitic acid. As illustrated in the figure below, panel 3, glycerophospholipids, also known as phosphoglycolipids, are composed of a glycerol backbone with ester linkages to two fatty acid chains and a phosphate, to which is attached a head group. The fatty acid shown in pink in the figure given in the question is saturated, meaning it has no double bonds, and is composed of 16 carbons. Thus, it can be identified as palmitic acid.

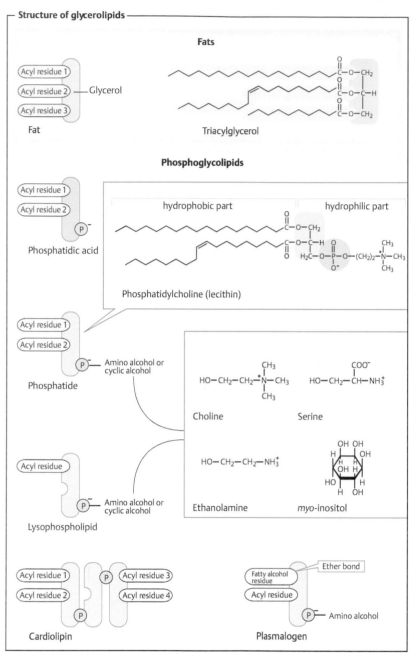

Structure of glycerolipids

Fats

Fat

Triacylglycerol

Phosphoglycolipids

Phosphatidic acid

hydrophobic part   hydrophilic part

Phosphatidylcholine (lecithin)

Phosphatide

Amino alcohol or cyclic alcohol

Choline

Serine

Ethanolamine

myo-inositol

Lysophospholipid

Amino alcohol or cyclic alcohol

Cardiolipin

Plasmalogen

Ether bond

Fatty alcohol residue

Acyl residue

Amino alcohol

Source: Koolman J, Röhm K. Color Atlas of Biochemistry. 3rd Edition. Thieme; 2012.

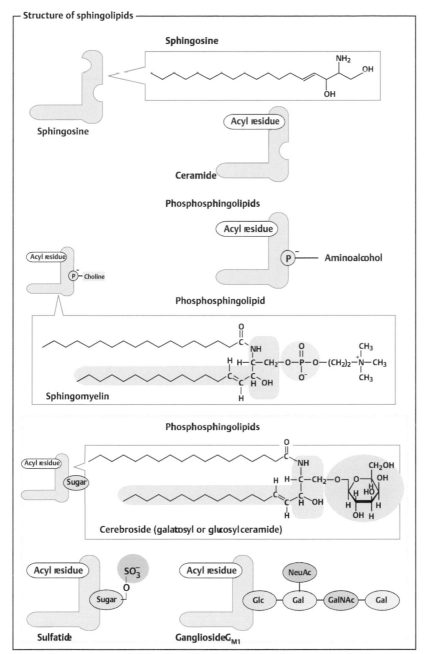

Source: Koolman J, Röhm K. Color Atlas of Biochemistry. 3rd Edition. Thieme; 2012.

A and B are incorrect. Sphingolipids are composed of a sphingosine backbone, connected via an amide bond to one fatty acid chain, and to a phosphate to which is also attached a head group. See the figure below for a review of sphingolipid structure.

D is incorrect. The fatty acid chain in question contains 16 carbons and is thus palmitic acid. Stearic acid contains 18 carbons.

E and F are incorrect. Triglycerides are composed of a glycerol backbone with three fatty acids attached via ester linkages, as reviewed in panel 1 in the figure shown with option C.

20. Correct: D. The glucose in the leaves is largely incorporated into homopolysaccharide chains with β-1,4 linkages.

Cellulose, a polymer of glucose molecules connected by β-1,4 linkages, is the primary carbohydrate found in plant leaves. As illustrated in the figure below, cellulose is a homopolymer of glucose residues linked by β-1,4 glycosidic bonds. Humans, like most animals (other than termites), do not express digestive cellulase, an enzyme that hydrolyzes β-1,4 glycosidic bonds. Plant leaves do contain a small amount of starch, which is composed of amylopectin, a homopolymer of glucose residues linked by α-1,4 glycosidic bonds and containing α-1,6 branching glycosidic bonds, and amylose, a homopolymer of glucose residues linked by α-1,4 glycosidic bonds with no branch points. The small amount of starch in the leaves is the primary source of calories this man obtains.

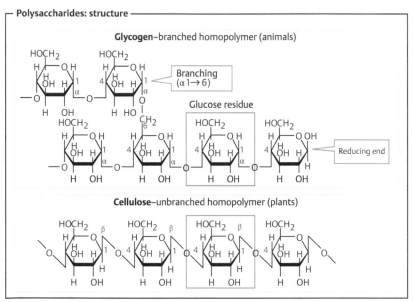

Polysaccharides: structure

Glycogen–branched homopolymer (animals)

Branching (α1→6)

Glucose residue

Reducing end

Cellulose–unbranched homopolymer (plants)

Important polysaccharides

Poly-saccharide	Mono-saccharide 1	Mono-saccharide 2	Linkage	Branching	Occurrence	Function
Bacteria						
Murein	D-GlcNAc	D-MurNAc	β 1→ 4	—	Cell wall	SC
Dextran	D-Glc	—	α 1→ 6	α1→ 3	Slime	WB
Plants						
Agarose	D-Gal	L-aGal	β 1→ 4	α1→ 3	Red algae (agar)	WB
Carrageenan	D-Gal	—	β 1→ 3	α1→ 4	Red algae	WB
Cellulose	D-Glc	—	β 1→ 4	—	Cell wall	SC
Xyloglucan	D-Glc	D-Xyl (D-Gal, L-Fuc)	β 1→ 4	β 1→ 6 (β 1→ 2)	Cell wall (Hemicellulose)	SC
Arabinan	L-Ara	—	α 1→ 5	α1→ 3	Cell wall (pectin)	SC
Amylose	D-Glc	—	α 1→ 4	—	Amyloplasts	RC
Amylopectin	D-Glc	—	α 1→ 4	α1→ 6	Amyloplasts	RC
Inulin	D-Fru	—	β 2→ 1	—	Storage cells	RC
Animals						
Chitin	D-GlcNAc	—	β 1→ 4	—	Insects, crabs	SC
Glycogen	D-Glc	—	α 1→ 4	α1→ 6	Liver, muscle	RC
Hyaluronic acid	D-GlcUA	D-GlcNAc	β 1→ 4 β 1→ 3	—	Connective tissue	SC,WB

SC= structural carbohydrate, RC= reserve carbohydrate,
WB = water-binding carbohydrate; N-acetylmuramic acid, 3,6-anhydrogalactose

Source: Koolman J, Röhm K. Color Atlas of Biochemistry. 3rd Edition. Thieme; 2012.

A is incorrect. Most of the carbohydrate in the leaves is indeed glucose; it is simply tied up in cellulose rather than in starch.

B is incorrect. Plant leaves do not contain lactose, which is also known as milk sugar.

C is incorrect. Glucose polymers containing α-1,6 linkages, such as starch and glycogen, are readily digested by humans and thus provide the expected 4 calories/g of dietary energy.

E is incorrect. Cellulose is the primary carbohydrate found in leaves.

21. Correct: B. Tyrosine.

Although tyrosine is not essential, it is synthesized from phenylalanine and is thus considered a conditionally essential amino acid; a deficiency in phenylalanine will result in a deficiency in tyrosine. Recall that the essential amino acids are as follows: phenylalanine, valine, threonine, tyrosine, isoleucine, methionine, histidine, leucine, and lysine. Cysteine, tyrosine, and arginine are conditionally essential amino acids. (A helpful mnemonic for remembering these is: PVT TIM HiLL has a CAT that says ARGH. Phenylalanine, Valine, Threonine, Tryptophan, Isoleucine, Methionine, Histidine, Leucine, Lysine, Cysteine, Arginine (ARGH), and Tyrosine.)

A is incorrect. Alanine is nonessential, and its synthesis in the human body is not conditional on the availability of an essential amino acid.

C is incorrect. Although histidine is one of the essential amino acids, it will be present in the dietary supplement.

D is incorrect. Serine is nonessential, and its synthesis in the human body is not conditional on the availability of an essential amino acid.

E is incorrect. Although tryptophan is essential, it will be present in the dietary supplement.

22. Correct: D. Dairy products.

Dairy products contain lactose, a disaccharide of glucose and galactose, and should be eliminated from this child's diet. During digestion, lactose is hydrolyzed, releasing glucose and galactose. The figure given in the next column provides a review of the most common dietary disaccharides.

Maltose (D-Glucose + D-Glucose)

(α–1, 4 linkage)

Lactose (D-Galactose + D-Glucose)

(β–1, 4 linkage)

Sucrose (D-Glucose + D-Fructose)

α–1, β–2 linkage

Source: Panini S. Medical Biochemistry - An Illustrated Review. 1st Edition. Thieme; 2013.

A is incorrect. Table sugar is composed of sucrose, a disaccharide of glucose and fructose; it does not contain galactose.

B is incorrect. Gluten is a protein found in certain grains. Its consumption is not concomitant with consumption of galactose, which is a carbohydrate found primarily in milk products.

C is incorrect. Eggs do not contain lactose or milk sugar; the primary dietary source of galactose.

E is incorrect. Gelatin is the hydrolysis product of collagen, a protein. Its consumption is not concomitant with consumption of galactose, which is a carbohydrate found primarily in milk products.

23. Correct: D. Structure D.

This structure represents azidothymidine (AZT), a deoxythymidine analog. The features of this molecule that indicate that it is a deoxythymidine analog are that it contains a pyrimidine base (thymine is a pyrimidine base), it does not contain a hydroxyl group at the 2' position, and there are no phosphates attached at the 5'-carbon. Helpful mnemonic devices to remember which bases are purines and which are pyrimidines are PURe As Gold (PURines are Adenine and Guanine) and CUT the PY(pie) (Cytosine, Uracil, and Thymine are Pyrimidines). Recall that thymidine is the correct name for the thymine-containing nucleoside, while the nucleotide name would be thymidine 5'-monophosphate, diphosphate, or triphosphate.

A is incorrect. This molecule is a pyrimidine nucleotide analog.

B is incorrect. This molecule is a purine nucleotide analog.

C is incorrect. This molecule is a purine nucleoside analog.

Chapter 3

Biochemical Reactions and Catalysis

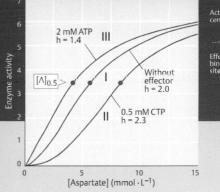

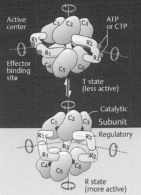

LEARNING OBJECTIVES

► Describe the basic type of reaction catalyzed by each of the six classes of enzymes, and recognize common names (dehydrogenase, peptidase, etc.) associated with important subclasses within each class.

► Define and describe the following: zymogen, proenzyme, coenzyme, cofactor, prosthetic group, apoenzyme, holoenzyme, and isozyme.

► Use the Michaelis–Menten equation to calculate reaction velocity and the constants V_{max} and K_m; understand the significance of V_{max} and K_m in metabolic systems.

► Analyze Michaelis–Menten and Lineweaver–Burk plots to estimate V_{max} and K_m and to distinguish between competitive, uncompetitive, mixed, and noncompetitive reversible inhibition.

► Compare and contrast different types of enzyme inhibitors.

► Explain positive and negative allostery, and be able to recognize it on substrate versus velocity curves.

► Recognize the roles of common coenzymes in enzyme-catalyzed reactions.

Michaelis-Menten Equation

$$v_o = \frac{V_{max}\,[S]}{K_m + [S]}$$

3.1 Questions

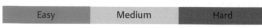

1. A 56-year-old man with severe hypertension is prescribed captopril, an angiotensin converting enzyme (ACE) inhibitor. In laboratory experiments, captopril has been shown to bind tightly to the active site of ACE, thus preventing binding of its normal substrates, angiotensin I and bradykinin. In the graph below, which of the curves most likely represent kinetic data obtained while monitoring the activity of ACE in the presence of an inhibitory amount of captopril and varying concentrations of angiotensin I? Note that one of the curves represents data obtained in the absence of captopril.

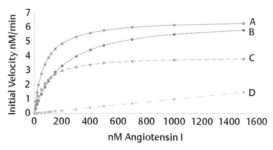

A. Curve A

B. Curve B

C. Curve C

D. Curve D

2. Indolethylamine-*N*-methyltransferase (INMT) catalyzes the transfer a methyl group from *S*-adenosylmethinone to amino groups on indole-containing molecules and plays a key role in the generation of a minor metabolite of tryptophan that has psychoactive effects. Increased INMT activity may play a role in the development of schizophrenia, thus efforts have been made to generate inhibitors of INMT activity. Recently, a group of researchers obtained the kinetic data shown in the graph below when they measured the velocity of the INMT-catalyzed reaction at various substrate concentrations in the presence and absence of propyl dimethyl aminotryptamine (PDAT), a reversible inhibitor of INMT. How does PDAT most likely interact with INMT?

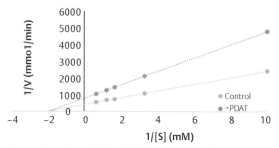

Source: Chu, Uyen B., Sevahn K. Vorperian, et al. Noncompetitive Inhibition of Indolethylamine-N-methyltransferase by N , N-Dimethyltryptamine and N , N-Dimethylaminopropyltryptamine. Biochemistry. 2014.

A. PDAT binds only to the substrate binding site of free INMT

B. PDAT binds to INMT only after substrate is bound in the active site

C. PDAT binds with equal affinity to both free and substrate-bound enzyme

D. PDAT binds only to free INMT, at a site other than the substrate binding site

3. *Porphyromonas gingivalis* is one of the pathogens associated with the development of adult periodontitis. This bacterium expresses several cysteine proteases called gingipains that play a major role in the destruction of periodontal tissue and deregulation of the inflammatory response. In order to understand the function of gingipain HRgpA, which cleaves between arginine (R) and serine (S) residues in its substrates, researchers performed kinetic studies with several different substrates.[1] Which amino acid, when placed at the fifth position of these hexapeptide substrates, reduces the affinity of HRgpA for the substrate?

Substrate	K_m (µM)	V_{max} (nM/sec)
GPRSFL	20.5	0.256
GPRSLL	26.2	0.281
GPRSNL	15.6	0.081
GPRSTL	39.1	0.317
GPRSIL	77.9	0.236

A. Phenylalanine (F)

B. Leucine (L)

C. Asparagine (N)

D. Threonine (T)

E. Isoleucine (I)

4. A 4-year-old boy who is undergoing treatment for T-cell acute lymphoblastomic leukemia becomes severely hyperuricemic as a result of rapid lysis of cancer cells. In order to prevent the development of renal uric acid crystals and subsequent renal complications, the boy is injected with rasburicase, a preparation of recombinant urate oxidase. If the boy is administered a dose of rasburicase that results in a maximal reaction velocity of 10 nmol/min, and the K_m for rasburicase under the conditions present in the boy's serum is 130 µmol/L, what will be the initial rate at which rasburicase degrades uric acid if the boy's serum uric acid concentration is 700 µmol/L?

A. 700 µmol/min

B. 10 vmol/min

C. 5 vmol/min

D. 8.4 vmol/min

E. 4.6 µmol/min

5. Researchers recently reported two novel cases of a rare autosomal recessive disorder in steroid hormone synthesis. The patients they described had a mutation in the *CYP11A1* gene, which encodes the enzyme that catalyzes the first step in the synthesis of all steroid hormones; conversion of cholesterol to pregnenolone. In order to better understand the disease-causing mutation, the investigators carried out kinetic studies of the wild-type and mutant enzymes. They obtained the results shown in the graph below. What is the effect of the mutation on the maximal rate and substrate affinity of CYP11A1?

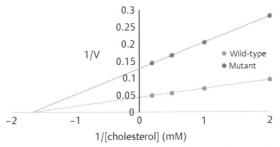

Source: Parajes S, Kamrath C, Rose IT, et al. A Novel Entity of Clinically Isolated Adrenal Insufficiency Caused by a Partially Inactivating Mutation of the Gene Encoding for P450 Side Chain Cleavage Enzyme (CYP11A1). The Journal of Clinical Endocrinology & Metabolism. 2011.

	Maximal rate	Substrate affinity
A.	Increase	Increase
B.	Increase	Decrease
C.	Decrease	Increase
D.	Decrease	Decrease
E.	No change	Decrease
F.	No change	Increase
G.	Decrease	No change
H.	Increase	No change

[1] (Reproduced from Ally N, Whisstock JC, Sieprawska-Lupa M, et al. Characterization of the specificity of arginine-specific gingipains from Porphyromonas gingivalis reveals active site differences between different forms of the enzymes. Biochem 2003;42(40):11693–11700.)

6. A researcher who was investigating hepatic tumorigenesis in mice discovered that an enzyme that catalyzes the reaction, shown in the figure below, is expressed at higher levels in hepatic tumor cells than in healthy hepatocytes. To which class does this enzyme belong?

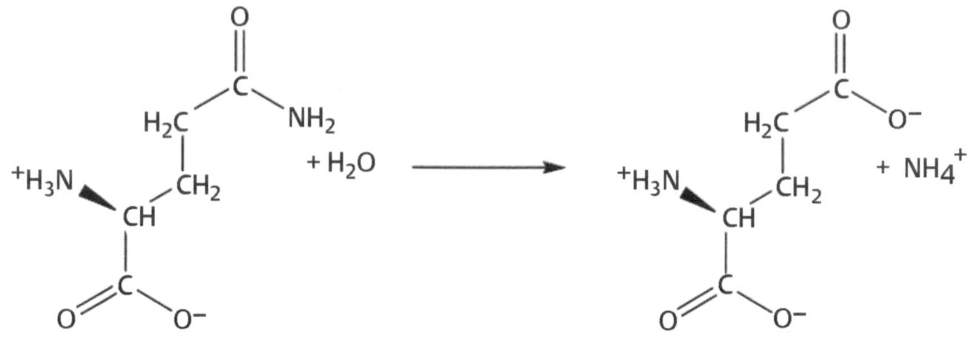

A. Oxidoreductase
B. Transferase
C. Hydrolase
D. Isomerase
E. Lyase
F. Ligase

7. Histidinemia, a usually asymptomatic autosomal recessive disorder with an incidence rate as high as 1 in 10,000 newborns, is caused by a deficiency in the enzyme that catalyzes the first step in the degradation of histidine, as shown in the figure below. To which class does this enzyme belong?

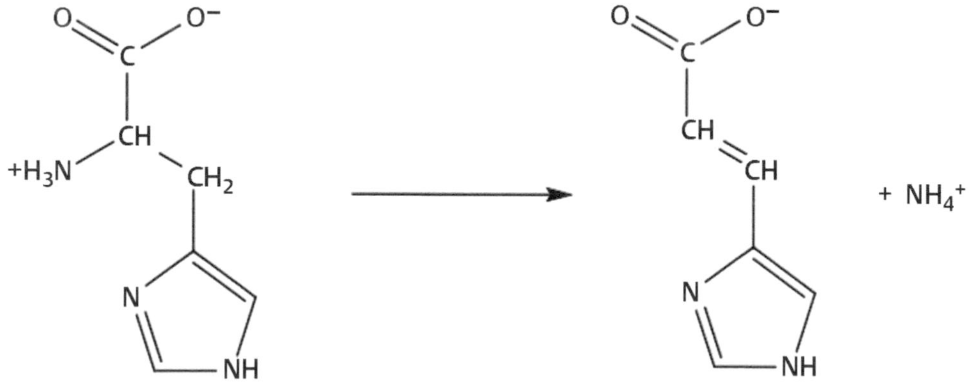

A. Oxidoreductase
B. Transferase
C. Hydrolase
D. Isomerase
E. Lyase
F. Ligase

8. Cancerous cells generally have a high demand for the amino acid glutamine, and thus often upregulate expression of proteins that mediate glutamine transport. In the rat C6 glioma cell line, for example, the ASCT2 glutamine transporter is upregulated. In an effort to develop a potential anticancer drug, some researchers recently synthesized and characterized an inhibitor of glutamine transport by ASCT2, γ- L-glutamyl-p-nitroanilide (GPN). Results of kinetic data from an experiment in which the researchers measured the rate of transport of glutamine into C6 glioma cells at varying concentrations of glutamine in the presence and absence of GPN are shown in the graph below. What type of inhibitor is GPN?

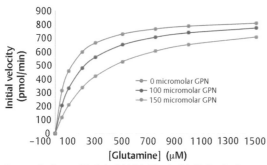

Source: Esslinger CS, Cybulski KA, Rhoderick JF. Nγ-Aryl glutamine analogues as probes of the ASCT2 neutral amino acid transporter binding site. Bioorganic & Medicinal Chemistry. 2005.

A. Irreversible

B. Competitive

C. Uncompetitive

D. Noncompetitive

Consider to the following narrative for questions 9 and 10.

A 3-month-old girl with a history of hemolytic anemia from birth was recently diagnosed with pyruvate kinase deficiency. Genetic testing indicates that she has a mutation in which the arginine residue at position 532 in the pyruvate kinase amino acid sequence is changed to a tryptophan.

9. To which class of enzymes does pyruvate kinase belong?

A. Hydrolase

B. Ligase

C. Lyase

D. Oxidoreductase

E. Transferase

10. Kinetic data obtained with normal (wild-type, WT) and mutant (R532W) pyruvate kinase in the presence and absence of fructose 1,6-bisphosphate (FBP), excess ADP, and varying concentrations of phosphoenolpyruvate are shown in the graph below. What do these data indicate regarding the role of FBP and the effect of the R532W mutation?

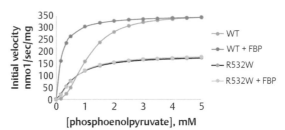

Source: Valentini G, Chiarelli LR, Fortin R, et al. Structure and Function of Human Erythrocyte Pyruvate Kinase. Molecular Basis of Nonspherocytic Hemolytic Anemia. Journal of Biological Chemistry. 2002.

	Role of FBP	Effect of R532W
A.	Allosteric activator	Decreased phosphoenol-pyruvate binding affinity
B.	Allosteric activator	Loss of FBP responsiveness
C.	Allosteric inhibitor	Decreased phosphoenol-pyruvate binding affinity
D.	Allosteric inhibitor	Loss of FBP responsiveness
E.	Cosubstrate	Decreased phosphoenol-pyruvate binding affinity
F.	Cosubstrate	Loss of FBP binding affinity

11. An 11-year-old boy is admitted to the emergency department due to severe mid-abdominal pain that radiates to his mid-back. The pain has persisted for about 7 hours. The boy's parents report that he has had similar episodes, which were less severe and lasted only a few hours, at least 4 times in the last year. The last episode was 1 week ago. Laboratory results indicate that his serum lipase and amylase levels are elevated. An abdominal CT scan is shown in the figure below. Based on these findings and the patient's family history, his physician orders genetic testing which indicates a mutation in *PRSS1*, one of three genes encoding trypsinogen isoforms. Which of the following is the most likely consequence of this patient's *PRSS1* mutation, leading to the symptoms and findings described here?

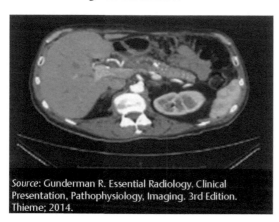

Source: Gunderman R. Essential Radiology. Clinical Presentation, Pathophysiology, Imaging. 3rd Edition. Thieme; 2014.

A. Increased trypsin activity in the small intestine

B. Decreased pancreatic lipase secretion

C. Increased pancreatic zymogen activation

D. Increased trypsinogen K_m

E. Decreased trypsinogen V_{max}

12. The analgesic drug codeine has no physiological effect until it is converted to morphine in the liver by Cytochrome P450 2D6 (CYP2D6). Approximately 7% of the Caucasian population, referred to as "poor metabolizers" express an isozyme of CYP2D6 that is much less active than the isozyme expressed by 80% of the Caucasian population, referred to as "extensive metabolizers." Kinetic parameters for the two isozymes are shown below.

Isozyme	V_{max} (nmol/h/mg protein)	K_m (mM)
A	0.4	0.026
B	6.4	8.5

Assuming that both poor and extensive metabolizers express similar concentrations of CYP2D6, and that hepatic codeine concentrations are in the low µM range, which of the following sets of conditions best describe poor metabolizers?

	Isozyme expressed	Effectiveness of codeine for pain relief
A.	A	weak
B.	B	weak
C.	A	strong
D.	B	strong

13. Myoplasmic Ca^{+2} concentrations are regulated in large part by the sarcoplasmic reticulum calcium ATPase (SRCA), which pumps Ca^{+2} into the sarcoplasmic reticulum (SR), and by the ryanodine receptor (SR), which releases Ca^{+2} from the SR into the myoplasm upon stimulation (see the figure below). Central core disease is a rare congenital muscle disorder involving mutations in the ryanodine receptor (RyR). Individuals harboring these mutations have "leaky" RyR, resulting in slightly higher-than-normal resting-state myoplasmic Ca^{+2} concentrations. Biochemical studies with myocytes obtained from patients with central core disease show that in order to compensate for leaky RyR, expression of the SRCA pump is increased. Kinetic experiments in which the SRCA pump activity in intact SR isolated from diseased subjects would be expected to show which of the following effects on the SRCA pump kinetic parameters compared to those observed in intact SR isolated from control subjects?

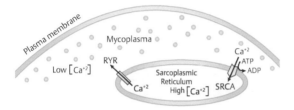

	V_{max}	K_m
A.	Decreased	Decreased
B.	No change	Increased
C.	Increased	Decreased
D.	No change	No change
E.	Increased	No change
F.	Increased	Increased

14. Glutamate dehydrogenase (GDH) plays essential roles in nitrogen metabolism and in the regulation of pancreatic insulin secretion. Mutations in the enzyme are associated with hyperinsulinemia and hyperammonemia. Regulation of GDH is quite complex and involves several modulators including GTP, ADP, Zn^{+2}, palmitoyl CoA, and leucine. At pH 7.2 in the absence of any regulators, the maximal velocity of GDH is 20 nmol/min/mg protein. At a glutamate concentration of 3 mM, the initial velocity of the GDH-catalyzed reaction is 10 mmol/min/mg protein. In the presence of leucine, the maximal velocity is still 20 nmol/min/mg protein, but when the glutamate concentration is 3 mM, the initial velocity is 15 mmol/min/mg protein. Which of the following most correctly describes the role of leucine in the GDH-catalyzed reaction?

A. It is an allosteric inhibitor of GDH

B. It is a pure noncompetitive (mixed) inhibitor of GDH

C. It is a competitive inhibitor of GDH

D. It is an allosteric activator of GDH

E. It is a competitive activator of GDH

15 The human genome contains two genes for pyruvate kinase (PK), the last enzyme in the glycolytic pathway. The *PK-LR* gene is expressed primarily in hepatocytes and erythrocytes. The *PK-M* gene is expressed in most other tissues, generating the enzyme pyruvate kinase M1 (PK M1). Cancer cells generally express the *PK-M* gene, but generate pyruvate kinase M2 (PK M2), rather than PK M1, by alternative splicing. PK M2 has decreased catalytic activity relative to PK M1, and also moonlights as a transcription factor that stimulates cell growth. Which of the following most accurately describes the relationship between PK M1 and PK M2?

A. PK M1 is a holoenzyme; PK M2 is an apoenzyme

B. PK M1 is an apoenzyme; PK M2 is a holoenzyme

C. PK M1 and PK M2 are isozymes

D. PK M1 is the proenzyme of PK M2

E. PK M1 and PK M2 are coenzymes

16. γ-aminobutyrate (GABA) is the primary inhibitory neurotransmitter found in humans. Some diseases, including epilepsy, can be linked to lower-than-normal levels of GABA. These diseases may be successfully treated with inhibitors of an enzyme that catalyzes the degradation of GABA, as shown in the figure below. Which of the following coenzymes is most likely required for the activity of this GABA-degrading enzyme?

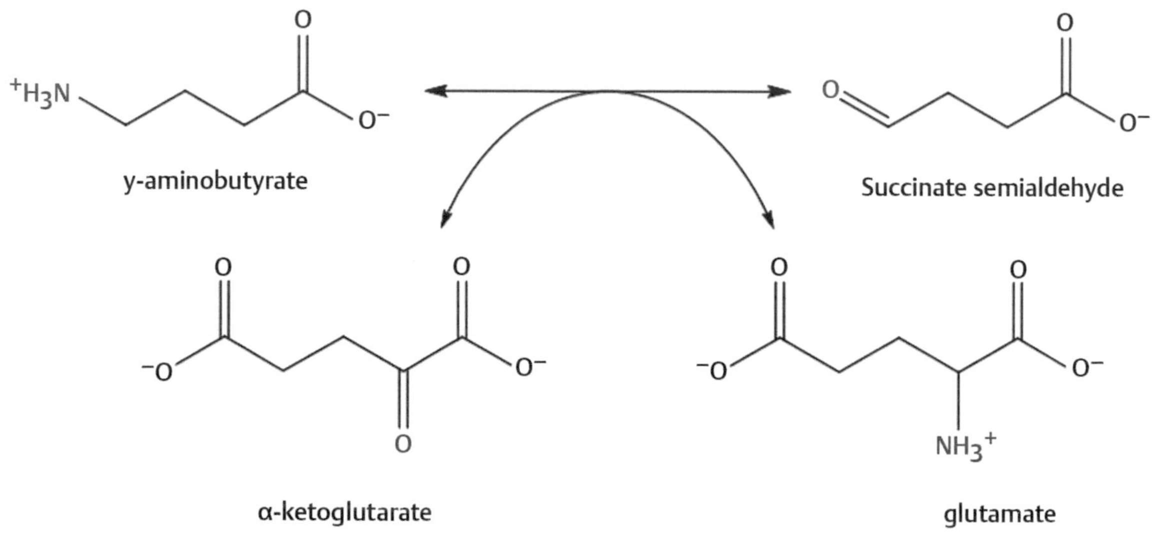

y-aminobutyrate

Succinate semialdehyde

α-ketoglutarate

glutamate

A. Biotin
B. Tetrahydrofolate
C. NAD+
D. Pyridoxal phosphate
E. Thiamine pyrophosphate

17. Methylmalonyl-CoA mutase was isolated from fibroblasts of an infant girl recently diagnosed with methylmalonic aciduria. In order to more thoroughly characterize her disease, the kinetic properties of the enzyme were determined at varying concentrations of methymalonyl-CoA in the presence and absence of cobalamin. When cobalamin was added, the rate of the enzyme-catalyzed reaction increased, but the affinity of the enzyme for methylmalonyl-CoA was unchanged. If the black dashed line in the plot shown in the graph below represents data obtained with the patient's enzyme in the absence of added cobalamin, which of the other lines most likely represents the data obtained in the presence of added cobalamin?

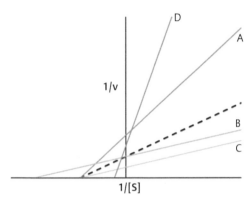

A. Line A

B. Line B

C. Line C

D. Line D

18. A 60-year-old woman with a recently diagnosed peptic ulcer is prescribed omeprazole. Once activated by acidic conditions, omeprazole forms a disulfide bond with either cysteine 813 or cysteine 892 on K^+/H^+ ATPase, an integral membrane protein responsible for gastric acid secretion. Upon treatment with omeprazole, the V_{max} for K^+/H^+ ATPase decreases, but the K_m values for its substrates remain unchanged. Which of the following most accurately describes the nature of inhibition K^+/H^+ ATPase by omeprazole?

A. Competitive

B. Uncompetitive

C. Noncompetitive

D. Irreversible

E. Mixed

19. The enzyme-catalyzed reaction shown in the figure below is a key step in the synthesis of essential metabolites in several pathogenic bacteria. Because there is not an analogous enzyme in mammals, significant efforts have been directed toward developing inhibitors of this enzyme that could be used clinically as antibiotics. Which of the following cofactors or coenzymes is most likely required for the activity of this enzyme?

A. Biotin

B. NADPH

C. Thiamine pyrophosphate

D. Tetrahydrofolate

E. Pyridoxal phosphate

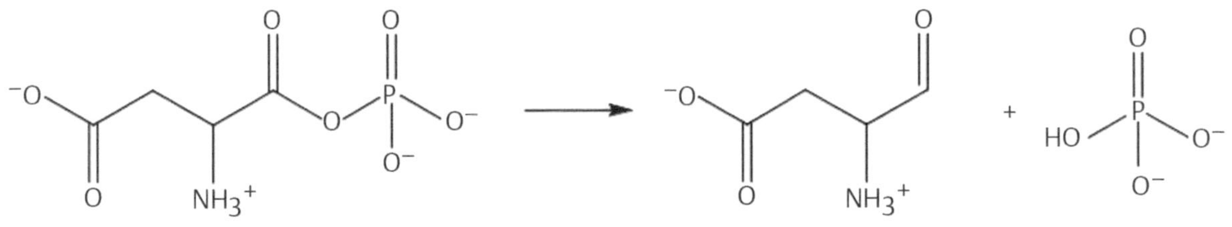

20. Ethylene glycol, the major component in anti-freeze, is itself relatively nontoxic but is metabolized, initially by alcohol dehydrogenase, to toxic substances. Treatment of ethylene glycol poisoning generally involves administration of an inhibitor of alcohol dehydrogenase, either ethanol or fomepizole. Although treatment with these competitive inhibitors is often effective, there is interest in developing a noncompetitive inhibitor of alcohol dehydrogenase for use in treating ethylene glycol poisoning. Why would treatment of ethylene glycol poisoning with a noncompetitive inhibitor be more advantageous than treatment with ethanol or fomepizole?

A. Its effectiveness would be independent of the amount of ethylene glycol ingested

B. It would not affect the Km value of alcohol dehydrogenase for ethylene glycol

C. It would decrease both the Vmax and the Km values of alcohol dehydrogenase

D. It would irreversibly inhibit alcohol dehydrogenase

E. Its effectiveness would be independent of the concentration of alcohol dehydrogenase

3.2 Answers and Explanations

Easy	Medium	Hard

1. Correct: B. Curve B.

Captopril is a competitive inhibitor of ACE; therefore, curve B represents the kinetic data obtained in the presence of captopril. For a review of the graphical representations of competitive inhibition, see the figure below. Competitive inhibitors form a reversible complex with an enzyme and thus prevent subsequent binding of substrate to the enzyme. In the presence of a competitive inhibitor, the enzyme will still reach its maximal velocity (V_{max}), but will only be able to do so at higher substrate concentrations than are required to reach V_{max} in the absence of inhibitor. This means that the K_m, the substrate concentration

at which the enzyme functions at ½ V_{max}, will necessarily increase. Graphically, this results in a shift of the Michaelis–Menten (v_o vs. [substrate]) curve to the right relative to the curve obtained without inhibitor present. The curve reaches the same asymptote, or V_{max}.

A is incorrect. This curve represents data obtained in the absence of inhibitor.

C is incorrect. This curve represents data obtained in the presence of either an uncompetitive or a noncompetitive inhibitor. Both uncompetitive and noncompetitive inhibitors form reversible complexes with the enzyme–substrate complex that result in decreased catalytic function. An uncompetitive inhibitor binds only to the enzyme–substrate complex, while a noncompetitive inhibitor may bind to either the free enzyme or the enzyme–substrate complex. In either case, the enzyme's catalytic function is impaired when the inhibitor is bound. This results in a decrease in V_{max} (i.e., a lower asymptote on the Michaelis–Menten curve), as observed in curve C. In the presence of an uncompetitive inhibitor, the enzyme K_m value decreases. In the presence of a noncompetitive inhibitor, the enzyme K_m value increases or does not change.

D is incorrect. This curve does not display saturation kinetics, and is thus not representative of typical Michaelis–Menten kinetic behavior.

2. Correct: C. PDAT binds with equal affinity to both free and substrate-bound enzyme.

This double-reciprocal plot (also known as a Lineweaver–Burk plot) shows the characteristic pattern observed with pure noncompetitive inhibitors, which bind with equal affinity to both free and substrate-bound enzyme. For a review of graphical representations of noncompetitive inhibition, see the figure on the next page. In pure noncompetitive inhibition, V_{max} decreases in the presence of the inhibitor, but K_m remains unchanged, thus the Lineweaver–Burk plot will show in an increase in $1/V_{max}$ (Y-intercept) and no change in $-1/K_m$ (X-intercept) for the line representing kinetics in the presence of inhibitor.

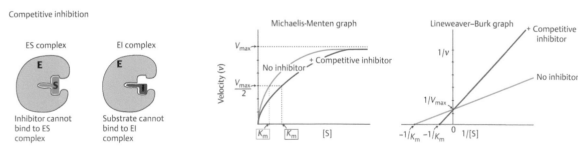

Source: Panini S. Medical Biochemistry - An Illustrated Review. 1st Edition. Thieme; 2013.

Noncompetitive inhibition

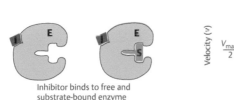

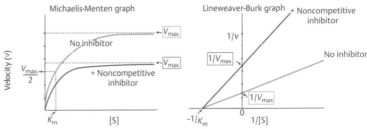

Inhibitor binds to free and
substrate-bound enzyme

Source: Panini S. Medical Biochemistry - An Illustrated Review. 1st Edition. Thieme; 2013.

A is incorrect. An inhibitor that binds only to the substrate binding site of the free enzyme is classified as a competitive inhibitor. The Lineweaver–Burk plot for competitive inhibition characteristically has lines that intersect on the Y-axis. In competitive inhibition, the substrate K_m increases when inhibitor is present, but V_{max} remains unchanged. Converting these V_{max} and K_m values to their reciprocals for the Lineweaver–Burk plot predicts no change in $1/V_{max}$ (Y-intercept) for the line representing kinetics in the presence of inhibitor, and a decrease in $-1/K_m$ (X-intercept).

B is incorrect. An inhibitor that binds only to the enzyme–substrate complex is classified as uncompetitive. The Lineweaver–Burk plot for uncompetitive inhibition characteristically has parallel lines. In uncompetitive inhibition, the substrate K_m decreases when inhibitor is present, as does V_{max}. Converting these V_{max} and K_m values to their reciprocals determines that the Lineweaver–Burk plot will result in an increase in $1/V_{max}$ (Y-intercept) for the line representing kinetics in the presence of inhibitor, and a decrease in $-1/K_m$ (X-intercept).

D is incorrect. An inhibitor that binds only to free enzyme, but at a site different than the active site, is generally an allosteric regulator. In allosteric enzyme systems, the kinetics do not follow the Michaelis–Menten model and Lineweaver–Burk plots are not used in data analysis.

3. Correct: E. Isoleucine (I).

The substrate with the highest K_m value, GPRSIL, will have the lowest binding affinity for gingipain HRgpA. Recall that K_m, the Michaelis constant, reflects the enzyme's affinity for its substrate; a low K_m indicates tight binding, while a high K_m indicates weak binding.

A, B, C, and D are incorrect. The V_{max} values provided in the table do not provide any information regarding substrate binding affinity; V_{max} is the velocity of the enzyme-catalyzed reaction when

the substrate concentration is high enough that the enzyme is saturated with substrate. Analysis of K_m values provides information regarding substrate binding affinity. The substrate with the lowest K_m value has the highest affinity for substrate, while the substrate with the highest K_m has the lowest affinity for substrate.

4. Correct: D. 8.4 nmol/min.

This problem is solved using the Michaelis–Menten equation:

$$v_o = \frac{V_{max}\,[S]}{K_M + [S]}$$

v_o = initial reaction velocity

V_{max} = maximal reaction velocity = 10 nmol/min

K_m = Michaelis constant = 130 mmol/L

[S] = substrate concentration = 700 mmol/L

Plugging the values provided in the question into the Michaelis–Menten equation yields 8.4 nmol/min.

5. Correct: G. G. Maximal rate = Decrease; Substrate affinity = No change.

The mutation decreases the maximal rate of catalysis by the enzyme but has no effect on substrate binding affinity. The kinetic results are shown in the form of a double-reciprocal, or Lineweaver–Burk, plot. In this linear form, the Y-intercepts indicate $1/V_{max}$, the slopes represent K_m/V_{max}, and the X-intercepts indicate $-1/K_m$. In the data shown here, the Y-intercept of the mutant enzyme is increased relative to that of the wild-type, and the X-intercept is unchanged. An increase in $1/V_{max}$ means that V_{max}, the maximal rate at which the enzyme functions when it is saturated with substrate, has decreased. The lack of change in the X-intercept indicates that K_m, which represents the binding affinity of the substrate for the enzyme, has not changed.

A is incorrect. An increase in V_{max} would show up as an increase in the Y-intercept on the Lineweaver–Burk plot, and an increase in substrate affinity would shift the X-intercept to a more negative value.

B is incorrect. An increase in V_{max} would show up as an increase in the Y-intercept on the Lineweaver–Burk plot, and a decrease in substrate affinity would shift the X-intercept to a less negative value.

C is incorrect. An increase in substrate affinity would shift the X-intercept on the Lineweaver–Burk plot to a more negative value.

D is incorrect. A decrease in substrate affinity would shift the X-intercept on the Lineweaver–Burk plot to a less negative value.

E is incorrect. If there were no change in maximal rate, the Y-intercept on the Lineweaver–Burk plot would be identical for wild-type and mutant enzymes. Furthermore, a decrease in substrate affinity would shift the X-intercept to a less negative value.

F is incorrect. If there were no change in maximal rate, the Y-intercept on the Lineweaver–Burk plot would be identical for wild-type and mutant enzymes. Furthermore, an increase in substrate affinity would shift the X-intercept to a more negative value.

H is incorrect. An increase in V_{max} would show up as an increase in the Y-intercept on the Lineweaver–Burk plot.

6. Correct: C. Hydrolase.

This enzyme, glutaminase, is a member of the hydrolase class of enzymes. Hydrolases catalyze the cleavage of bonds via the addition of water. In the reaction shown, the amide bond between the carbonyl carbon and nitrogen in the glutamine side chain is cleaved by water to generate a carboxylic acid (glutamate) and free ammonia. For a review of enzyme classes, see the table below.

Class	Reaction type	Important subclasses
1 Oxidoreductases Transfer electrons from a donor (reducing agent) to an acceptor (oxidizing agent)	○ = Reduction equivalent A (Reduced) + B (Oxidized) ⇌ A (Oxidized) + B (Reduced)	Dehydrogenases Oxidases, peroxidases Reductases Monooxygenases Dioxygenases
2 Transferases Transfer a functional group (e.g., amino, phosphate) between molecules	A (Func. grp) + C ⇌ A + C (Func. grp)	C_1–Transferases Glycosyltransferases Aminotransferases Phosphotransferases
3 Isomerases Rearrange/isomerize molecules	A ⇌ A (isomerized)	Epimerases *cis trans* Isomerases Intramolecular transferases
4 Lyases ("synthases") Add or remove atoms (e.g., elements of water, ammonia, or CO_2) to or from a double bond	A + B ⇌ A–B	C–C–Lyases C–O–Lyases C–N–Lyases C–S–Lyases
5 Ligases ("synthetases") Form (C–O, C–S, C–N, or C–C) bonds with the hydrolysis of ATP	A, B + ATP ⇌ A–B + ADP + P_i	C–C–Ligases C–O–Ligases C–N–Ligases C–S–Ligases
6 Hydrolases Cleave bonds via the addition of water	A–B + H_2O ⇌ A–H + B–OH	Esterases Glycosidases Peptidases Amidases

Source: Panini S. Medical Biochemistry - An Illustrated Review. 1st Edition. Thieme; 2013.

A is incorrect. Oxidoreductases catalyze oxidation-reduction reactions, in which electrons are transferred from one substrate to another. Electrons are not transferred in this reaction.

B is incorrect. Transferases catalyze the transfer of a functional group between molecules *not* hydrolysis, as shown here.

D is incorrect. Isomerases catalyze the rearrangement or isomerization of bonds within a molecule.

E is incorrect. Lyases catalyzed the cleavage of a C–C, C–N, or C–O bond by means other than hydrolysis or oxidation.

F is incorrect. Ligases form C–O, C–S, C–N or C–C bonds with the concomitant hydrolysis of ATP.

7. Correct: E. Lyase.

This reaction is catalyzed by a lyase. Lyases catalyze the cleavage of a C–C, C–N, or C–O bonds by means other than hydrolysis or oxidation. In the reaction shown, the α-amino nitrogen is broken, and a double bond is created between the α and β carbons of histidine. The reaction does not involve hydrolysis, and electrons are not transferred (i.e., there is no oxidation/reduction). For a review of enzyme classes, see table corresponding to Answer 6.

A is incorrect. Oxidoreductases catalyze oxidation-reduction reactions, in which electrons are transferred from one substrate to another. There is no change in oxidation states of the reactants during the reaction shown.

B is incorrect. Transferases catalyze the transfer of a functional group between molecules. There is no such transfer in the reaction shown.

C is incorrect. Hydrolases catalyze the cleavage of bonds via the addition of water. Water is not a reactant in the reaction shown.

D is incorrect. Isomerases catalyze the rearrangement or isomerization of bonds within a molecule.

F is incorrect. Ligases form C–O, C–S, C–N or C–C bonds with the concomitant hydrolysis of ATP.

8. Correct: B. Competitive.

GPN is a competitive inhibitor. The inhibitor increases the K_m value (i.e., the glutamine concentration at which the transport velocity is half of the maximal velocity) for the transporter, but does not alter the maximal velocity. In other words, the curve shifts to the right, but the asymptote remains unchanged. (Although the measured velocity at 1000 µM glutamine is not the same on all three of these curves, the three curves extrapolate to the same maximal velocity.) This is characteristic behavior for a competitive inhibitor. For a review of competitive enzyme inhibitors and their effects on enzyme kinetics, see the figure under Answer 1.

A is incorrect. Irreversible inhibitors decrease V_{max}, as they cannot be displaced from the enzyme by increasing the substrate concentration. GPN does not alter V_{max}.

C is incorrect. Uncompetitive inhibitors decrease V_{max}, as they cannot be displaced from the enzyme by increasing the substrate concentration. GPN does not alter V_{max}.

D is incorrect. Noncompetitive inhibitors decrease V_{max}, as they cannot be displaced from the enzyme by increasing the substrate concentration. GPN does not alter V_{max}.

9. Correct: E. Transferase.

By definition, all kinases are transferases. They catalyze the transfer of a phosphate group from ATP to a second enzyme substrate, forming a phosphorylated product and ADP, or from a phosphorylated substrate to ADP, forming ATP and an unphosphorylated product. In the case of pyruvate kinase under physiological conditions, a phosphate is transferred from phosphoenolpyruvate to ADP, forming pyruvate and ATP.

A, B, C, and D are incorrect. By definition, all kinases are members of the transferase enzyme class.

10. Correct: B. Role of FBP = Allosteric activator; Effect of R532W = Loss of FBP responsiveness.

FBP is an allosteric activator of pyruvate kinase, and the R532W mutation results in loss of FBP responsiveness. The sigmoidal shape of the initial velocity versus [substrate] curve for the wild-type enzyme indicates that pyruvate kinase is an allosteric enzyme. When FBP is added to the enzyme, the curve shifts significantly to the left. This shows that FBP is an allosteric activator of the enzyme; binding of FBP to the enzyme significantly increases its affinity for substrate. Analysis of the two curves for the R532W mutant show that FBP no longer has an effect on pyruvate kinase activity; the enzyme has lost the ability to respond to FBP. The mutation also decreases the enzyme V_{max} and increases phosphoenolpyruvate binding affinity (as shown by the left-shift in the curve). For a review of enzyme allostery, see the figure on the next page.

A is incorrect. Although the curves for the wild-type enzyme do indicate that FBP is an allosteric activator, the data for the R532W mutant do not indicate that binding affinity for phosphoenolpyruvate is decreased. A reasonable estimate for the $K_{0.5}$ (i.e., the substrate concentration at which the reaction velocity is half of the maximal reaction velocity) of WT enzyme in the absence of FBP is 1 mM phosphoenolpyruvate, based on the curves shown

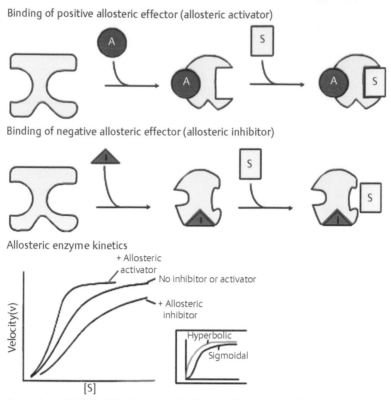

Binding of positive allosteric effector (allosteric activator)

Binding of negative allosteric effector (allosteric inhibitor)

Allosteric enzyme kinetics

Source: Panini S. Medical Biochemistry - An Illustrated Review. 1st Edition. Thieme; 2013.

here. A reasonable estimate for the R532W mutant in the absence of FBP is 0.5 mM; the mutant actually has a slightly higher binding affinity for phosphoenolpyruvate.

C and D are incorrect. If FBP were an allosteric inhibitor of pyruvate kinase, addition of FBP to the enzyme-catalyzed reaction would result in a right-shift of the curve, indicating that the enzyme binding affinity for phosphoenolpyruvate was reduced. An allosteric inhibitor could also cause a decrease in the maximal velocity, which does not occur here.

E is incorrect. If FBP were a cosubstrate in the reaction, there would be no enzyme activity observed in the experiments performed in the absence of FBP.

F is incorrect. If FBP were a cosubstrate in the reaction, there would be no enzyme activity observed in the experiments performed in the absence of FBP.

11. Correct: C. Increased pancreatic zymogen activation.

The mutation in *PRSS1* increases activation of pancreatic zymogens. This patient has hereditary pancreatitis. Several different mutations in *PRSS1* have been linked to hereditary pancreatitis. Although the various mutations result in different biochemical deficiencies in the processing of pancreatic trypsinogen (a zymogen), they all result in increased interpancreatic

levels of active trypsin. Active interpancreatic trypsin causes proteolysis of cellular proteins, resulting in cellular injury. As a result, calcification of damaged pancreatic tissue is sometimes observed, as illustrated in this patient's CT scan. The damaged pancreatic tissue releases digestive enzymes, including lipase and amylase, into the serum, resulting in the elevated serum enzyme levels observed in this patient.

A is incorrect. While some mutations in trypsinogen might result in increased trypsin activity in the small intestine, this is not consistent with this patient's laboratory and imaging results which are indicative of pancreatitis resulting from intrapancreatic activation of trypsinogen.

B is incorrect. Pancreatitis does sometimes result in decreased pancreatic lipase secretion. However, decrease lipase secretion does not contribute to the symptoms or laboratory and imaging results observed in this patient. Decreased lipase secretion causes steatorrhea, which is observed in some individuals with pancreatitis.

D is incorrect. Trypsinogen is a zymogen, and thus has almost negligible enzyme activity. What little activity it has would be *decreased* by an increase in K_m and would not initiate pancreatitis.

E is incorrect. Trypsinogen is a zymogen, and thus has almost negligible enzyme activity. What little activity it has would be *decreased* by a decrease in V_{max} and would not initiate pancreatitis.

12.   Correct: B. Isozyme expressed = B; Effectiveness of codeine for pain relief = weak.

A poor metabolizer would have a very low rate of conversion of codeine to morphine and would express isozyme B. Codeine would be only weakly effective, if at all, in relieving pain. Of the two listed CYP2D6 isozymes, the one having the lowest activity at hepatic concentrations of codeine, and thus corresponding to the weak metabolizer phenotype, is isozyme B. The isozyme B K_m value is 8.5 mM; close to a thousand times higher than the micromolar concentrations of codeine found in hepatocytes. Thus, even though isozyme B has a faster V_{max} value than isozyme A, it will not bind substrate well, and thus will have extremely low activity. The activities of both isozymes can be estimated using the Michaelis–Menten equation:

$$v_0 = \frac{V_{max}\,[S]}{K_M + [S]}$$

Assuming a hepatic codeine concentration of 10 µM, the initial reaction velocities of isozymes A and B would be 0.11 nmol/h/mg protein and 0.008 nmol/h/mg protein, respectively. Alternatively, the V_{max}/K_m values for the two isozyme can be compared. The V_{max}/K_m value is a second-order rate constant that describes the reaction velocity at very low, nonsaturating substrate concentrations. V_{max}/K_m for isozyme A is 15.4 nmol/h/mg protein/mM substrate, and V_{max}/K_m for isozyme B is 0.75 nmol/h/mg protein/mM substrate; isozyme B is clearly the less active enzyme at low substrate concentrations.

A is incorrect. Although this choice correctly indicates weak effectiveness of codeine in relieving pain for poor metabolizers, it incorrectly identifies isozyme A as the less active CYP2D6 isozyme. See explanation for the correct response to understand why isozyme B is the less active form.

C and D are incorrect. Both of these options indicate that codeine will be strongly effective for reducing pain in weak metabolizers. However, weak metabolizers will not be able to effectively convert codeine to morphine. Therefore, codeine will be weakly effective, if at all, in reducing pain.

13.   Correct: E. V_{max} = Increased; Km = No change.

V_{max} will increase and K_m will remain unchanged. V_{max} is a function of enzyme concentration, but K_m is not; thus, when the expression level of an enzyme is altered, its V_{max} will be altered proportionately but the K_m will remain unchanged. In this case, SRCA expression levels increase, so V_{max} would increase.

A is incorrect. In individuals with central core disease, SRCA pump expression is increased; therefore, V_{max} will also increase.

B is incorrect. In individuals with central core disease, SRCA pump expression is increased; therefore, V_{max} will also increase.

C is incorrect. Although this response correctly indicates that an increase in SRCA pump expression will result in an increased V_{max}, it incorrectly indicates that K_m will decrease. K_m is an intrinsic property of an enzyme; that is, the substrate concentration at which the enzyme-catalyzed reaction velocity is half of V_{max}. The K_m does not depend on enzyme concentration.

D is incorrect. In individuals with central core disease, SRCA pump expression is increased; therefore V_{max} will also increase.

F is incorrect. Although this response correctly indicates that an increase in SRCA pump expression will result in an increased V_{max}, it incorrectly indicates that K_m will increase.

14.   Correct: D. It is an allosteric activator of GDH.

Leucine is an allosteric activator of GDH. In the absence of leucine, GDH functions at half-maximal velocity when the glutamate concentration is 3 mM, that is, the $K_{0.5}$ is 3 mM. In the presence of leucine, the V_{max} for GDH remains unchanged, but the $K_{0.5}$ decreases; the velocity versus [substrate] curve shifts to the left. For a review of velocity versus [substrate] curves for allosteric enzymes, see the graph on the next page. This is characteristic of allosteric activators, which typically allow enzymes to catalyze reaction rates more quickly at lower substrate concentrations.

A is incorrect. An allosteric inhibitor would cause the GDH-catalyzed reaction rate to decrease by either decreasing V_{max} or shifting the velocity versus [substrate] curve to the right, which would result in a lower rate of catalysis at 3 mM glutamate.

C is incorrect. Although a competitive inhibitor would have no effect on V_{max}, as we see here, it would shift the velocity versus [substrate] curve to the right, resulting in a decrease in the reaction velocity at 3 mM glutamate.

E is incorrect. Competitive activators do not exist.

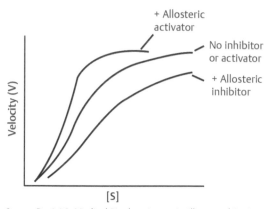

Source: Panini S. Medical Biochemistry - An Illustrated Review. 1st Edition. Thieme; 2013.

15. Correct: C. PK M1 and PK M2 are isozymes.

PK M1 and PK M2 isozymes; enzymes that catalyze the same reaction, but have different amino acid sequences, kinetic properties and/or regulatory mechanisms.

A and B are incorrect. A holoenzyme is an active complex formed between an enzyme and its coenzyme or cofactor. An apoenzyme is an enzyme that is inactive because it is not complexed with a required coenzyme or cofactor. The information provided in this description of PK gives no indication that either PK M1 or PK M2 is missing a required cofactor or coenzyme.

D is incorrect. A proenzyme is an inactive form of an enzyme that is activated by proteolytic cleavage. The difference between PK M1 and PK M2 is due to alternative splicing, and not to proteolytic modification.

E is incorrect. Coenzymes are small organic molecules, mostly derived from vitamins. Some enzymes are only catalytically active when they are associated with a required coenzyme. Coenzymes are not actually enzymes, as suggested by this response.

16. Correct: D. Pyridoxal phosphate.

This enzyme will require pyridoxal phosphate. This is a transamination reaction; the amino group on GABA is transferred to α-ketoglutarate, leading to the formation of glutamate and the keto-form of GABA, succinate semialdehyde. Enzymes that catalyze transamination reactions require pyridoxal phosphate as a coenzyme. Other enzymes that require pyridoxal phosphate, which is derived from vitamin B_6, include amino acid decarboxylases (and decarboxylases of amino acid derivatives), glycogen phosphorylase, and δ-aminolevulinic acid synthase.

A is incorrect. Biotin, which is derived from vitamin B_7, is required for carboxylase enzymes, including pyruvate carboxylase and acetyl CoA carboxylase.

B is incorrect. Tetrahydrofolate, derived from vitamin B_9, is required for enzymes that catalyze the addition of a single carbon atom (which is donated to the tetrahydrofolate coenzyme by a donor molecule) to a substrate. The reaction shown here does not involve transfer of carbon atoms.

C is incorrect. NAD$^+$ which, like NADP$^+$, is derived from either vitamin B_3 or tryptophan, is a coenzyme that is required by some enzymes that catalyze redox reactions.

E is incorrect. Thiamine pyrophosphate is derived from vitamin B_1. It is a required coenzyme for enzymes that catalyze oxidative decarboxylation reactions, such as pyruvate dehydrogenase and α-ketoglutarate dehydrogenase.

17. Correct: C. Line C.

Addition of cobalamin to the mutant enzyme resulted in an increase in the enzyme's V_{max} value, and no change in K_m. The plot shown here is a double-reciprocal, or Lineweaver–Burk, plot; an increase in V_{max} will produce a decrease in $1/V_{max}$, the Y-intercept on the Lineweaver–Burk plot. The X-intercept corresponds to $-1/K_m$, which remains unchanged on line C. There are two possible explanations for the experimental findings with this patient's methylmalonyl CoA mutase enzyme. The first is that her methylmalonic aciduria is caused by a defect in intracellular cobalamin metabolism; her ability to convert methylmalonyl CoA to succinyl CoA is due to low intracellular cobalamin levels, and the enzyme isolated from her fibroblasts is able to regain full function when supplemented with cobalamin. The second possibility is that the patient harbors a mutation in methylmalonyl CoA mutase that decreases its affinity for cobalamin; the normal cytosolic concentration of cobalamin is not adequate to saturate the enzyme with this required cofactor.

A is incorrect. This line is indicative of a decrease in V_{max}, and no change in K_m.

B is incorrect. This line is indicative of a decrease in K_m, and no change in V_{max}.

D is incorrect. This line is indicative of a decrease in V_{max}, and a decrease in K_m.

18. Correct: D. Irreversible.

Omeprazole is an irreversible inhibitor of K$^+$/H$^+$ ATPase. Irreversible inhibitors either covalently modify residues in or near the active site, thus inhibiting catalysis, or bind so tightly to the active site that dissociation is insignificant. In either case, the net effect is similar to what would be observed if the enzyme were degraded; the V_{max} decreases, but there is no effect on K_m. In the case described here, omeprazole covalently modifies the K$^+$/H$^+$ ATPase, forming a disulfide adduct that inhibits the catalytic cycle. For a review of irreversible enzyme inhibition, see the figure on the next page.

A is incorrect. Competitive inhibitors do not form covalent adducts with enzymes. Furthermore, V_{max} is not affected by competitive inhibitors.

B is incorrect. Uncompetitive inhibitors do not form covalent adducts with enzymes. Furthermore, K_m values *increase* in the presence of uncompetitive inhibitors.

C is incorrect. Although pure noncompetitive inhibitors do decrease V_{max}, and leave K_m unaffected, as described in this case, they do not form covalent adducts with their target enzymes.

E is incorrect. Mixed inhibitors do not form covalent adducts with enzymes. Although they do decrease V_{max}, as is the case with omeprazole, their effect on K_m varies.

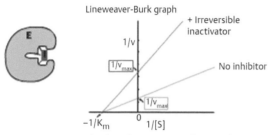

Lineweaver-Burk graph

Source: Panini S. Medical Biochemistry - An Illustrated Review. 1st Edition. Thieme; 2013.

19. Correct: B. NADPH.

This enzyme most likely requires NADPH as a cofactor. This reaction, catalyzed by aspartate semialdehyde dehydrogenase, involves the reduction of the carbonyl carbon in the phosphoester bond; the carbonyl carbon goes from a carboxyl to an aldehyde oxidation state. The enzyme requires NADPH, which provides the reducing equivalents for the reaction.

A is incorrect. Biotin is a cofactor used by enzymes, such as pyruvate carboxylase and acetyl-CoA carboxylase, that catalyze carboxylation reactions.

C is incorrect. Thiamine pyrophosphate is a cofactor used by enzymes that catalyze reductive decarboxylation reactions (e.g., pyruvate dehydrogenase). It is also used by transketolase.

D is incorrect. Tetrahydrofolate is used as a source of one-carbon groups, at various oxidation states, for enzymes that transfer carbons between molecules.

E is incorrect. Pyridoxal phosphate is a cofactor for enzymes that catalyze transamination reactions as well as decarboxylation of amino acids. It is also used by glycogen phosphorylase and δ-aminolevulinic acid synthase.

20. Correct: A. Its effectiveness would be independent of the amount of ethylene glycol ingested.

Noncompetitive inhibitors generally function better as therapeutic drugs than competitive inhibitors because they are effective at all substrate concentrations. (The same can be said of uncompetitive inhibitors.) Competitive inhibitors are less effective at high substrate concentrations, where the substrate can displace the inhibitor.

B is incorrect. While it is true that a pure noncompetitive inhibitor would not affect the affinity of alcohol dehydrogenase for ethylene glycol (i.e., the K_m value), this would provide no advantage for inhibition of enzyme activity.

C is incorrect. A pure noncompetitive inhibitor would not affect the K_m value. Furthermore, a decrease in the ethylene glycol K_m value, which could occur with mixed inhibitor (i.e., a noncompetitive inhibitor that is not "pure"), would not improve the drug's inhibitory effectiveness.

D is incorrect. Noncompetitive inhibitors are, by definition, reversible, as are competitive inhibitors.

E is incorrect. Although the rates of enzyme-catalyzed reactions are dependent on enzyme concentration, the equilibrium constants associated with substrate binding (i.e., K_m) and reversible inhibitor binding (i.e., K_i) are not. Thus, the effectiveness of a reversible inhibitor, whether competitive, uncompetitive, or noncompetitive, is not dependent on enzyme concentration.

Chapter 4

Protein Structure and Function

Primary structure	–Ala–Gln–Val–Lys–Gly–His–Gly– Lys–Lys–Val–Ala–Asp–Ala–Leu– Thr–Asn–Ala–Val–Ala–His–Val–
Secondary structure	Helix 53-74
Tertiary structure	Hemoglobin-α_1-subunit
Quaternary structure	Hemoglobin tetramer

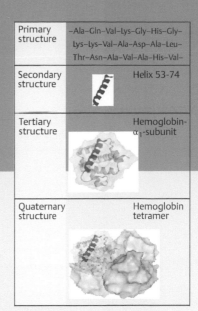

LEARNING OBJECTIVES

▶ Discuss how changes in primary amino acid sequence can lead to changes in protein structure and function.

▶ Describe the basic secondary structures found in proteins including α-helices and β-sheets.

▶ Define primary, secondary, tertiary, and quaternary structures of proteins and list the chemical bonds that maintain them.

▶ Compare and contrast the different physical and chemical properties of classes of amino acids.

▶ Describe the function of specific, critical proteins in human health and disease.

▶ Explain the formation of coiled-coils and protein fibrils and compare and contrast structure-function of fibrillar proteins to globular proteins.

▶ Describe the structural features of secreted and integral membrane proteins.

▶ Describe how accumulation of unfolded protein and the failure cellular machinery to maintain protein homeostasis (e.g., chaperones and proteasome) can cause disease.

4.1 Questions

Easy	Medium	Hard

1. A vial of regular insulin (Humulin R) was stored improperly and when analyzed the insulin molecule was found to have dissociated into two specific peptides. Which of the following chemical bonds were most likely broken to produce the two peptides?

A. Disulfide

B. Hydrogen

C. Hydrophobic

D. Ionic

E. Peptide

2. A 51-year-old homeless man with an active history of alcoholism and a chief complaint of loose teeth, bleeding gums, and "strange markings on his arms" is brought to a community clinic by his social caseworker (as shown in the figure below).[1] On physical examination, you observe evidence of skin hemorrhage on his arms and legs and confirm the problems with his teeth and gums. With the assistance of the caseworker, you take a thorough history including the man's diet, which is primarily snack foods and fast food hamburgers. You confirm he eats essentially no fruits or vegetables. The patient also reports some shortness of breath and aching joints. Absence of a key vitamin results in the loss of structure of which of the following proteins, leading to at least some of the patient's presenting symptoms?

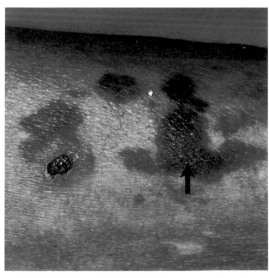

A. Albumin

B. Collagen

C. Hemoglobin

D. Immunoglobulin

E. Tubulin

[1] (Reproduced from Riede U-N, Werner M. Color Atlas of Pathology: Pathologic Principles, Associated Diseases, Sequela. 1st ed. New York, NY: Thieme; 2004.20, Panel C.)

3. A 19-year-old girl, who is a college student, comes to the student health clinic with the chief complaint of a leg ulcer she had for almost 3 months above the right medial malleolus. Her history reveals recurrent joint pain, primarily in the knees and elbows, and mild exertional dyspnea. Starting in the second grade, she has had episodes of severe abdominal pain, which were cramp-like, unrelated to meals or posture, and only partially relieved by over-the-counter pain medication. Her father (deceased) was an immigrant from North Africa, her mother is African American, and she has two younger siblings, one of which has similar symptoms. If your diagnosis is correct, the substitution of valine for glutamic acid in her hemoglobin β-chain results in which of the following events, leading to her disease?

A. Creation of a proteolytic site resulting in inappropriate cleavage of her β-chain protein

B. Disruption of proper folding which results in proteasomal degradation of her β-chain protein

C. Formation of long chains of β-globin molecules, stabilized by hydrophobic interactions

D. Loss of a phosphorylation site which leads to altered carbon dioxide/oxygen affinity

E. An overall protein structure change that dramatically lowers the affinity of hemoglobin for oxygen

Consider the figure below, that shows the b2 adrenergic receptor, for questions 4 and 5.

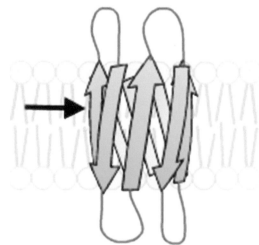

Source: Koolman J, Röhm K. Color Atlas of Biochemistry. 3rd Edition. 2012.

4. Which of the following amino acid residue is most likely to present at the location indicated by the arrow?

A. Aspartate

B. Glutamate

C. Lysine

D. Leucine

E. Serine

5. A DNA mutation results in a substitution of the wild-type amino acid at the position indicated by the arrow. This substitution results in a disruption of receptor function. Which of the following amino acids is most likely the substitution causing the functional defect in the mutant receptor?

A. Arginine

B. Glycine

C. Methionine

D. Phenylalanine

E. Valine

6. A 56-year-old woman who has a history of renal failure and a 12-year duration of biweekly dialysis treatments presents with a chief complaint of intense pain in her wrists that has resulted in the inability of her to work as an administrative assistant. After appropriate workup, she is diagnosed with renal failure associated amyloidosis. The insoluble b2 microglobulin protein aggregates that are causing her wrist pain are typically characterized by which of the following secondary structures?

A. Anti-parallel α-helices

B. Anti-parallel β-pleated sheets

C. β-sheets

D. Coiled-coils

E. Random coils

7. A 13-year-old boy presents with a history of three bone fractures over the past 2 years that were the result of relatively modest initiating trauma. You immediately notice a striking feature in the boy's eyes. A social history taken from his mother reveals that no other family members, through both sets of grandparents, have a history of excessive bone fracture, early deafness, or this eye feature. A gene coding for which of the following proteins is most likely mutated in this 13-year-old boy?

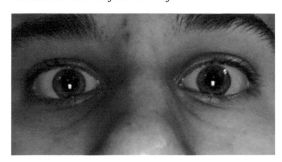

A. Collagen, type I

B. Elastin

C. Fibrillin

D. Keratin

E. Lysyl hydroxylase

8. A change to which of the following structural components explains the cooperative binding of oxygen to hemoglobin?

A. Primary

B. Secondary

C. Tertiary

D. Quaternary

9. The oxygen saturation curves of hemoglobin in muscles during active exercise and muscles at rest are shown in the figure given below. Which of the following explains the difference between the two curves?

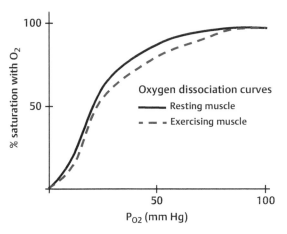

A. Binding of carbon monoxide by hemoglobin

B. Oxidation of iron in hemoglobin

C. Proteolysis of α- and β-subunits of hemoglobin

D. Protonation of specific amino acid side chains in hemoglobin

E. Unfolding of β-sheets in hemoglobin

10. A 61-year-old woman with long-standing, poorly controlled type II diabetes dies from complications of her disease. Panel B of the figure given below shows the accumulation of amyloid deposits in the islet cells of her pancreas (normal islet cells are shown in panel A)[2]. Which of the following cellular mechanisms of protein homeostasis might have been overwhelmed, contributing to this pathologic feature?

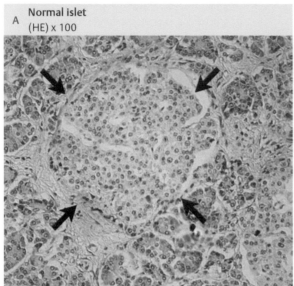

A Normal islet (HE) x 100

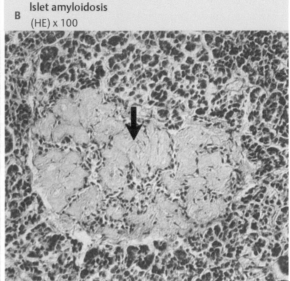

B Islet amyloidosis (HE) x 100

A. tRNA charging by amino acyl tRNA synthetases
B. Nuclear import mechanisms
C. Protein translation by ribosomes
D. Post-translational processing in the Golgi apparatus
E. Ubiquitin-proteasome system

11. A recent report in a leading medical journal describes a nonsense mutation in the gene coding for the thyroid hormone receptor, which results in a truncated protein missing a "C-terminal α-helix." Which of the following terms best describes the structure absent from the receptor protein produced by the mutated gene?

A. Amyloid
B. Primary
C. Secondary
D. Tertiary
E. Quaternary

12. In the third year, away-rotation through an exchange program, a medical student was assigned to a hematology clinical in New Delhi, India. At the clinic, the student sees a 57-year-old man with a 2-year history of gastrointestinal bleeding. His medical record indicates he had been treated by multiple, periodic blood transfusions that did not provide lasting improvement. He denies of any family history of bleeding disorders. On screening, he had normal platelet count, prolonged bleeding time, and decreased collagen-bound VWF: VWF antigen ratio. In consultation with the attending physicians, the student arrives at a diagnosis of acquired von Willebrand syndrome (AVWS). Which of the following describes the biochemical defect underlying the pathophysiology of AVWS?

A. Failure of N-glycosylation of the VWF protein in the endoplasmic reticulum
B. Formation of disulfide bonds between VWF proteins
C. Mutation resulting in substitution of a critical amino acid in the VWF protein
D. Unfolding of VWF protein and loss of multimer formation

---

[2] (Reproduced from Riede U-N, Werner M. Color Atlas of Pathology: Pathologic Principles, Associated Diseases, Sequela. 1st ed. New York, NY: Thieme; 2004:51.)

13. A 70-year-old man with a history of hypertension, hypercholesterolemia, and sleep apnea complains to his physician that he's been experiencing unusual weakness in the last 4 weeks and that it's becoming increasingly difficult for him to climb stairs without becoming fatigued. He also mentions that he sometimes feels as if his heart is fluttering. The physician orders an electrocardiogram, which provides results consistent with atrial fibrillation. Initial pharmaceutical treatment to restore normal rhythm is not successful, and the patient elects to undergo electrical cardioversion. In order to decrease the risk of stroke during or after the cardioversion procedure, the patient is started on warfarin therapy. To maximize the effectiveness of warfarin therapy, which of the following foods should this patient avoid?

A. Citrus fruits

B. Leafy greens

C. Dairy products

D. Beef and lamb

E. Sweets

14. A 22-year-old woman presents to the urgent care clinic complaining of pain in her right leg. She reports having just returned, via a 13-hour flight, from a semester-long study-abroad program in Bolivia. Examination reveals pitting edema in the right leg, as well as swollen superficial veins. Family history includes an aunt who died at the age of 28 as a result of a pulmonary embolism, and further testing including an ultrasonography is consistent with a deep vein thrombosis in the right common femoral vein. Proteolysis of which of the following proteins contributed to this patient's thrombosis?

A. Factor III

B. Protein C

C. Fibrin

D. Antithrombin III

E. Factor IX

15. A 4-year-old boy was brought to his pediatrician after the boy's dentist expressed concern that his gums bled excessively during a routine dental examination and cleaning. The boy's mother reported that the boy had always bruised easily. Subsequent bloodwork and genetic testing resulted in a diagnosis of hemophilia A. Which of the following most accurately describes the role of the protein that is deficient in this patient?

A. It is a cofactor that facilitates activation of Factor X

B. It is a cofactor that facilitates activation of Factor IX

C. It is a protease that activates Factor X

D. It is a protease that activates Factor VIII

E. It catalyzes the formation of covalent cross-links between aggregated fibrin monomers

16. A 12-year-old boy with a chief complaint of "long-term stomach ache" is brought to your clinic by his father. Taking his history, you find that the pain began 2 weeks prior, with no apparent imitating trauma or event. It intensified over several days and subsequently became a chronic dull ache. Physical examination revealed pain in his upper abdomen in the epigastric region bilaterally. On closer questioning, you discover the ache seems to radiate to his back. Radiologic exam was unremarkable except for pancreatic calcifications. The child ultimately is seen by a medical geneticist who determines that he has a heterozygous missense mutation in the *SPINK1* gene that encodes a serine protease inhibitor. Which of the following accounts for the child's abdominal pain?

A. Autoimmune destruction of pancreatic islet cells

B. Damage to pancreatic tissue by digestive enzymes

C. Diminished protein synthesis from low levels of serine production

D. Excessive activation of apoptotic protease enzymes

E. Lack of activation of enzymes in the exocrine pancreas

17. A 39-year-old man is referred to your neurology clinic with a chief complaint of increasing clumsiness in the past 6 months, tiring more easily when active and occasional slurring of words. During your social history, you discover that he is adopted but had some contact with his biological mother when he was a teenager. At that time, his mother was very ill with "...some muscle disease...," which she had told him ran in her family. She died 2 years after they first spoke, with little contact during the interim. Following extensive testing over a period of a month, you conclude he most likely has amyotrophic lateral sclerosis (ALS) that may be familial in nature. Genetic testing for common genetic mutations associated with ALS confirms your suspicions, when you discover he has a mutation in his *superoxide dismutase 1 (SOD1)* gene, which encodes a globular protein consisting of a single polypeptide chain. The mutation results in a single amino acid substitution, from glycine to alanine. Of the following general protein structure, which can you be certain is altered by the gene mutation?

A. Primary

B. Secondary

C. Tertiary

D. Quaternary

18. You are a coinvestigator in a clinical trial of a novel drug that may slow the progression of Alzheimer's disease. The drug has been engineered to disrupt the activity of the unfolded protein response/endoplasmic reticulum stress response. Which of the following best describes the mechanistic rationale for such a drug?

A. Prevent aggregation of specific neuronal proteins

B. Prevent apoptosis of neurons

C. Prevent global inhibition of protein translation

D. Prevent induction of protein chaperones

E. Prevent neuro-inflammation

19. G-protein coupled receptor 5 phosphorylates (GRK5) β_1-adrenergic receptors. Multiple alleles of the GRK5 exist in human populations, with different distributions dependent on race. At amino acid position 41, ~25% of African Americans have leucine (GRK5-Leu41) while the remainder have glutamine (GRK5-Gln41). In contrast, only ~1.5% of European Americans have GRK5-Leu41. The GRK5-Leu41 and GRK-Gln41 enzymes have different properties. This might be explained by which of the following?

A. Only one of the amino acids can be phosphorylated

B. Only one of the amino acids contains sulfur

C. Only one of the amino acids is polar

D. Only one of the amino acids is aromatic

E. Only one of the amino acids is charged

20. Panobinostat (Farydak) is currently approved by the FDA for the treatment of multiple myeloma. Treatment of cells with panobinostat results in reduced lysine acetylation of multiple proteins, including histones present in chromatin-associated nucleosomes. This leads to a higher affinity interaction between the nucleosomes and DNA within the chromatin. Based on these observations, which one of the following types of bonds between nucleosomes and DNA is most likely decreased by the drug panobinostat?

A. Covalent

B. Electrostatic

C. Hydrophobic

D. Van der Waals

4.2 Answers and Explanations

Easy	Medium	Hard

1. Correct: A. Disulfide.

Mature, processed insulin is two peptides held together by intermolecular disulfide bonds between cysteine residues. Under reducing conditions these bonds can be broken, resulting in two free peptides that are not biologically active.

B is incorrect. Hydrogen bonds play an important role in maintaining three-dimensional protein folding but are not involved in holding the insulin molecule together.

C is incorrect. Hydrophobic bonds do not participate in holding the insulin molecule together.

D is incorrect. Ionic bonds play an important role in maintaining three-dimensional protein folding but are not involved in holding the insulin molecule together.

E is incorrect. Adjacent amino acids in protein are joined by peptide bonds between amino and carboxyl groups, but the bonds between the two components of insulin are not peptide bonds.

2. Correct: B. Collagen.

The patient's history, symptoms, and signs are consistent with vitamin C deficiency (scurvy). During collagen synthesis, ascorbic acid is required for the hydroxylation of proline and lysine in the collagen molecule. Hydroxyproline and hydroxylysine form cross-links that stabilize the triple helix of collagen. In humans, the only structural proteins that require hydroxyproline are collagen and elastin.

A is incorrect. Albumin does not require hydroxyproline or hydroxylysine for synthesis, nor could its reduced synthesis account for the symptoms.

C is incorrect. Hemoglobin does not require hydroxyproline or hydroxylysine for synthesis, nor could its reduced synthesis account for the symptoms.

D is incorrect. Immunoglobulin does not require hydroxyproline or hydroxylysine for synthesis, nor could its reduced synthesis account for the symptoms.

E is incorrect. Tubulin does not require hydroxyproline or hydroxylysine for synthesis, nor could its reduced synthesis account for the symptoms.

3. Correct: C. Formation of long chains of β-globin molecules, stabilized by hydrophobic interactions.

Sickle cell anemia is the result of substitution of valine for glutamate at position six of the β-chain of hemoglobin. The hydrophobic valine binds a hydrophobic pocket on other β-molecules (only occurs in deoxy-hemoglobin), resulting in the formation of long polymers. These rigid polymers produce the characteristic "sickling" of erythrocytes that gives the disease its name. Occlusion of capillaries and the resulting inflammation produces the symptoms she reports.

A is incorrect. This mechanism is incorrect; no identified sickle cell anemia mutations create a new proteolysis site.

B is incorrect. Some amino acid substitutions can produce this result, but it is not the case for the mutation that results in sickle cell anemia.

D is incorrect. This mechanism is incorrect; no identified sickle cell anemia mutations lead to the loss of a phosphorylation site.

E is incorrect. This mechanism is incorrect; no identified sickle cell anemia mutations lead to changes in the overall structure of the β-globin protein.

4. Correct: D. Leucine.

The portion of transmembrane receptors buried in the plasma membrane bilayer contains hydrophobic amino acids that interact with the membrane lipids. Leucine is one of nine hydrophobic amino acids: methionine, alanine, leucine, isoleucine, valine, proline, phenylalanine, glycine, and tryptophan.

A is incorrect. Aspartate (aspartic acid) is negatively charged at physiological pH and hydrophilic, which is not amenable to the lipophilic nature of the plasma membrane interior.

B is incorrect. Glutamate (glutamic acid) is negatively charged at physiological pH and hydrophilic, which is not amenable to the lipophilic nature of the plasma membrane interior.

C is incorrect. Lysine is positively charged at physiological pH and hydrophilic, which is not amenable to the lipophilic nature of the plasma membrane interior.

E is incorrect. Serine has a hydroxyl group and is polar in nature, which is not amenable to the lipophilic nature of the plasma membrane interior.

5. Correct: A. Arginine.

Both charge and size of the amino acid side chain should be taken into account in assessing whether a given amino acid might disrupt protein structure and therefore function. However, given the fact that this location is within the lipid bilayer, charge is a critical issue since the repulsion between the charge side chain and the lipid tails would have a prominent effect on the protein's ability to correctly integrate into the membrane. Arginine is positively charged at physiological pH and therefore would most likely result in a receptor with reduced function.

B is incorrect. Glycine has a much smaller side chain than leucine, the amino acid present in the wild-type protein. However, it is hydrophobic and therefore is less likely to be detrimental to the protein's integration into the membrane and its function.

C is incorrect. Methionine is only slightly larger than leucine, the amino acid present in the wild-type protein. In addition, it is also hydrophobic. Taken together, methionine is not likely to be detrimental to the protein's integration into the membrane and its function.

D is incorrect. Phenylalanine has a larger side chain than leucine, the amino acid present in the wild-type protein. However, it is hydrophobic and therefore is less likely to be detrimental to the protein's integration into the membrane and its function.

E is incorrect. Isoleucine is about the same size as leucine, the amino acid present in the wild-type protein. In addition, it is also hydrophobic. Taken together, leucine is not likely to be detrimental to the protein's integration into the membrane and its function.

6. Correct: B. Anti-parallel β-pleated sheets.

The generally extracellular protein aggregates in essentially all types of amyloidosis take on a common antiparallel, β-pleated sheet conformation and form into higher order oligomers and then fibrils characteristic of these diseases.

A, C, D, and E are incorrect. Protein aggregates associated with amyloidosis are not characterized by these structures.

7. Correct: A. Collagen, type I.

About 90% of all cases of the autosomal dominant congenital disease osteogenesis imperfecta cause mutations in the type I collagen genes COL1A1 or COL1A2. The severity and onset of this disease varies depending on the defect in type I collagen produced by the mutation, but can include brittle bones, deafness, loose joints, and blue sclera.

B is incorrect. Mutations in the elastin gene are associated with a range of connective tissue diseases, including Marfan's syndrome, congenital supravalvular aortic stenosis, and cutis laxa.

C is incorrect. There are four fibrillin genes producing fibrillin protein that forms microfibrils that surround the elastin. Mutations in the fibrillin genes *FBN1* or *FBN2* can cause adolescent idiopathic scoliosis. Mutations in *FBN1* can also cause Marfan's syndrome.

D is incorrect. There are 54 known keratin genes in humans, mutations of many result in different congenital disorders of connective tissues.

E is incorrect. Lysyl hydroxlase is a critical enzyme for collagen synthesis, which catalyzes oxidative deamination of lysine, necessary to form cross-links between collagen fibrils in mature collagen. Mutation of the gene encoding lysyl hydroxylase (*PLOD1*) can result in Ehlers–Danlos syndrome.

8. Correct: D. Quaternary.

Quaternary structure refers to the structural association of multiple peptide subunits into a functional complex. Hemoglobin is a pair of identical αβ dimers that combine to make the hemoglobin tetramer—its quaternary structure is shown in the figure below. On binding of the first oxygen, the iron ion bound to the porphyrin, which leads to movement of an associated α-helix that lies in the interface between the two αβ dimers. Note that the α-helix itself does not change in structure, it just moves in space. The movement of the α-helix in the αβ dimer interface causes the dimers to rotate with respect to one another. The rearrangement allows communication between subunits facilitating the cooperative binding of oxygen.

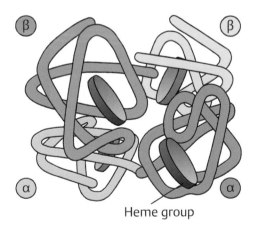

Heme group

Source: Panini S. Medical Biochemistry - An Illustrated Review. 1st Edition. Thieme; 2013.

A is incorrect. Primary structure refers to the sequence of amino acids in a peptide chain. This is not altered upon binding of oxygen.

B is incorrect. Secondary structure refers to the coiling and/or pleating of peptide chains into specific structural components (α-helices, β-sheets, etc.). There are no significant changes in these structures following oxygen binding to hemoglobin.

C is incorrect. Tertiary structure is the overall, three-dimensional structure of a protein (e.g., globular, fibrillary, etc.). There are no significant changes in these structures following oxygen binding to hemoglobin.

9. Correct: D. Protonation of specific amino acid side chains in hemoglobin.

Increased carbon dioxide and acidity in muscles under exercise results in the Bohr effect, decreasing the affinity of oxygen for hemoglobin. Protonation of two specific histidine residues, one each in α- and β-globin, are responsible for changes in the quaternary structure of hemoglobin, producing the change in oxygen affinity.

A is incorrect. Carbon monoxide is not present normally in muscles during exercise and in any case would not account for the changes in oxygen affinity shown in the figure given in the question.

B is incorrect. An alteration of the oxidation state of iron is not responsible for the change in oxygen affinity in muscle during exercise.

C is incorrect. The α- and β-chains of hemoglobin do not undergo proteolysis in muscle during exercise and in any case would not account for the change in oxygen affinity shown in the figure given in the question.

E is incorrect. β-sheets in hemoglobin do not denature in muscle during exercise and in any case would not account for the change in oxygen affinity shown in the figure given in the question.

10.   Correct: E. Ubiquitin-proteasome system.

One cellular system responsible for removal of proteins that are damaged or unfolded is the ubiquitin-proteasome system. Proteins ubiquitinated by ubiquitin ligases are marked for destruction by the proteasome, a large, barrel-shaped complex in the cytoplasm that has proteolytic activity. While the mechanisms leading to the creation of unfolded protein aggregates (amyloids) are not fully characterized, their accumulation might be due to the ubiquitin-proteasome system becoming overwhelmed and unable to quantitatively degrade the aggregates.

A is incorrect. tRNA charging could not be "overwhelmed" in any manner that would lead to aggregate formation.

B is incorrect. Protein aggregates would not be imported into the nucleus; this system being overwhelmed would not be responsible for the pathologic feature shown.

C is incorrect. New protein synthesis could not be "overwhelmed" in any manner that would lead to aggregate formation.

D is incorrect. Post-translational processing in the Golgi could not be "overwhelmed" in any manner that would lead to aggregate formation.

11. Correct: C. Secondary.

Secondary structure refers to common, discrete protein structures that are components of the overall, three-dimensional (tertiary) structure of the protein. Common secondary structures include α-helices and β-sheets.

A is incorrect. Amyloid structures are denatured, unfolded protein aggregates that can result in various pathologies.

B is incorrect. Primary structure refers to the amino acid sequence of a protein.

D is incorrect. Tertiary structure refers to the overall, three-dimensional structure of the protein.

E is incorrect. Quaternary structure refers to the multipeptide components of a protein complex, such as the α- and β-globin subunits of hemoglobin.

12. Correct: D. Unfolding of VWF protein and loss of multimer formation.

Each monomer of von Willebrand factor (VWF) is a relatively large protein that contains several functional domains. VWF monomers undergo N-glycosylation in the endoplasmic reticulum, which results in the formation of VWF dimers. The dimers form higher order quaternary structures (multimers) via disulfide bond formation between cysteine residues. Under appropriate conditions, the VWF multimers interact with platelets and initiated hemostasis. VWF multimers bind to subendothelial collagen exposed from vascular injury. The interaction results in the unfolding of some of the tertiary structure of VWF that exposes a platelet-binding domain. AVWS results from the loss of VWF multimers in the blood. This can be due to multiple mechanisms, including increased shear stress on the blood (e.g., during mitral valve regurgitation) due to turbulent blood flow. The shear converts multimers into an elongated structure that exposes residues that are cleaved by specific serum proteases, resulting in the defect in hemostasis mechanisms. A decrease in collagen-bound VWF:VWF antigen ratio, along with the history of bleeding indicates a high likelihood of loss or decrease in HMW VWF multimers.

A is incorrect. Failure of N-glycosylation of the VWF protein in the endoplasmic reticulum would affect the structure and function of the VWF protein. However, it is not a mechanism of AVWS.

B is incorrect. Formation of disulfide bonds between VWF proteins occurs to stabilize the formation of high-order complexes of dimers (multimers). As such, it is necessary for the function of VWF in hemostasis and not a cause AVWS.

C is incorrect. AVWS can have multiple underlying causes that result in the loss of higher order VWF protein complexes. It is not a congenital disease and therefore is not caused by a mutation.

13. Correct: B. Leafy greens.

Warfarin is an inhibitor of vitamin K reductase and vitamin K epoxide reductase, two enzymes involved in the recycling of vitamin K after it is oxidized during the vitamin K-dependent carboxylation of several clotting factors. Warfarin effectively decreases the amount of vitamin K available for carboxylation of clotting factors, and thus decreases the efficiency of the clotting process. Patients who are on warfarin therapy should avoid consumption of vitamin K-rich foods, such as leafy greens and cruciferous vegetables; these foods may decrease the efficacy of warfarin and its related anticoagulant drugs.

A is incorrect. Citrus fruits do not provide a significant amount of vitamin K.

C is incorrect. Dairy products are not considered a significant source of vitamin K.

D is incorrect. Beef and lamb do not contain significant amounts of vitamin K.

E is incorrect. Sweet foods do not contain significant amounts of vitamin K.

14. Correct: E. Factor IX.

Development of a thrombus involves enzymatic proteolysis of Factors XI, IX, and X in the intrinsic pathway, and Factors VII and X in the extrinsic pathway. Factors II (prothrombin) and I (fibrinogen) in the joint final pathway are also activated by proteolysis during clot formation. This patient most likely has a genetic hypercoagulative condition that either stimulates the activation of clotting factors or impairs normal inhibition of the clotting process.

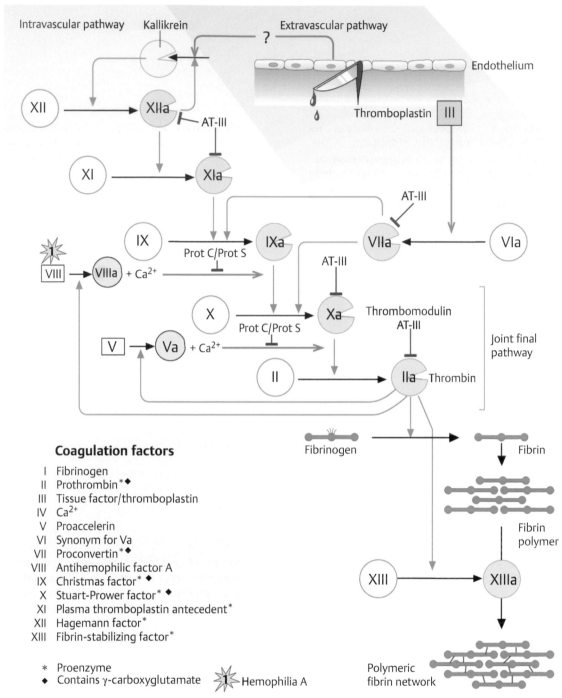

Coagulation factors

I   Fibrinogen
II   Prothrombin*◆
III Tissue factor/thromboplastin
IV   Ca²⁺
V   Proaccelerin
VI   Synonym for Va
VII Proconvertin*◆
VIII Antihemophilic factor A
IX   Christmas factor* ◆
X   Stuart-Prower factor* ◆
XI   Plasma thromboplastin antecedent*
XII Hagemann factor*
XIII Fibrin-stabilizing factor*

* Proenzyme
◆ Contains γ-carboxyglutamate
1 Hemophilia A

Source: Koolman J, Röhm K. Color Atlas of Biochemistry. 3rd Edition. 2012.

A is incorrect. Factor III, also known as tissue factor, is a protein cofactor that forms a complex with Factor VII to facilitate autoproteolysis of Factor VII and subsequent proteolysis of Factor X. Damaged tissues present Factor III to the blood at the site of injury, thus stimulating the activity of Factor VII. Factor III is not proteolyzed in this process.

B is incorrect. Proteolysis of Factor C activates the Factor C/S complex, which in turn *inhibits* the clotting process by proteolyzing and inactivating, Factors V and VIII, which are activating cofactors that enhance the activities of Factors X and IX, respectively.

C is incorrect. Fibrin is the end product of the coagulation cascade and is produced by proteolysis of fibrinogen (Factor I). Proteolysis of fibrin results in dissolution of a clot (i.e., fibrinolysis).

D is incorrect. Antithrombin III does not undergo proteolytic regulation.

15. Correct: A. It is a cofactor that facilitates activation of Factor X.

Hemophilia A is caused by inactivating mutations in Factor VIII. Factor VIII circulates in the serum, associated with VWF. On proteolytic activation by thrombin, Factor VIIIa associates with activated Factor IXa, and enhances the proteolytic activity of Factor IXa toward Factor X (prothrombin). A deficiency in Factor VIII, then, impairs the ability of Factor IXa to activate thrombin, and thus results in hypocoagulation.

B is incorrect. Factor VIII does not participate in the activation of Factor IX.

C is incorrect. The proteases that activate Factor X (prothrombin) are Factors IXa and VIIa. This response would be correct if the patient was afflicted with hemophilia B (deficiency in Factor IX) rather than hemophilia A.

D is incorrect. Factor Xa (thrombin) is the protease that activates Factor VIII.

E is incorrect. The role described here is that of Factor XIII, transglutaminase.

16. Correct: B. Damage to pancreatic tissue by digestive enzymes.

The serine protease inhibitor encoded by the *SPINK1* gene binds to and inhibits pancreatic digestive enzymes prior to their entry into the duodenum. The nonsense mutation (a mutation that results in the introduction of a premature stop codon in the protein-coding sequence of the gene) in one copy of the *SPINK1* gene results in lower levels of the protease inhibitor, leading to activity of proteases within the pancreas and damage of cells by autodigestion. This specific SPINK1 mutation is low-penetrance for pancreatitis by itself but is a significant modifier gene for cystic fibrosis associated pancreatitis for those with homozygous pathogenic mutations in cystic fibrosis transmembrane conductance regulator (CFTR) genes.

A is incorrect. Type I diabetes mellitus is the result of autoimmune destruction of β-islet cells of the pancreas and is unrelated to mutations in the *SPINK1* gene.

C is incorrect. The SPINK1 serine protease inhibitor has nothing to do with the synthesis of the amino acid serine. Serine proteases are a class of proteolytic enzymes that have a serine residue in their active site and SPINK1 inhibits enzymes in this class.

D is incorrect. The SPINK1 serine protease inhibitor does not directly activate apoptotic protease enzymes.

E is incorrect. SPINK1 inhibits serine protease enzymes in the exocrine pancreas. Loss of SPINK1 leads to premature, inappropriate activity of proteases in the exocrine pancreas, not the lack of these enzymes.

17. Correct: A. Primary.

The primary structure of a protein is simply its amino acid sequence. In this instance, since a single amino acid substitution occurred and no additional information is provided regarding the outcome on protein structure or function, the only thing certain is that the primary structure is altered.

B is incorrect. Secondary structure refers to the coiling and/or pleating of peptide chains into specific structural components (α-helices, β-sheets, etc.). While a single amino acid change can potentially disrupt these structures, it is impossible to predict based upon the information given. In addition, the amino acid change is relatively conservative; that is, the side chains of alanine (–CH$_3$) and glycine (–H) are both small, with relatively modest differences in physical properties. This also argues against changes in secondary structure.

C is incorrect. Tertiary structure is the overall, three-dimensional structure of a protein (e.g., globular, fibrillary, etc.). While a single amino acid change can potentially disrupt the tertiary structure of a protein, it is impossible to predict based on the information given. In addition, the amino acid change is relatively conservative; that is, the side chains of alanine (–CH$_3$) and glycine (–H) are both small, with relatively modest differences in physical properties. This also argues against changes in tertiary structure.

D is incorrect. Quaternary structure refers to the structural association of multiple peptide subunits into a functional complex. Since *SOD1* is a single polypeptide chain, it does not have quaternary structure.

18. Correct: B. Prevent apoptosis of neurons.

Formation of amyloid beta (Aβ) aggregates in Alzheimer's disease is hypothesized to activate the cellular unfolded protein response/endoplasmic reticulum stress response in neurons. Activation of this pathway leads to the cell ceasing global protein translation, while increasing translation of proteins that (1) can refold proteins, for example, chaperones and (2) initiate apoptosis. However, for the unfolded protein response/endoplasmic reticulum stress response to initiate apoptosis, the pathway must be activated at a high intensity and/or for an extended duration. Thus, the mechanistic rationale of the novel drug is to dampen the unfolded protein response/endoplasmic reticulum stress and prevent apoptosis of CNS neurons.

A is incorrect. While aggregation of the Aβ protein is thought to at least contribute to the pathogenesis of Alzheimer's disease, the inhibition of the unfolded protein response/endoplasmic reticulum stress response would not have a beneficial effect on the improper folding of Aβ.

C is incorrect. Activation of the unfolded protein response/endoplasmic reticulum stress response leads to global inhibition of protein synthesis secondary to modification of a key factor required for protein translation. While this is part of the mechanism of the unfolded protein response/endoplasmic reticulum stress response, it is the inhibition of apoptosis by the investigational drug that is the therapeutic goal (i.e., preventing neuronal death).

D is incorrect. Activation of the unfolded protein response/endoplasmic reticulum stress response leads induction/activation of protein chaperones that can refold incorrectly or unfolded proteins. While this is part of the mechanism of the unfolded protein response/endoplasmic reticulum stress response, it is the inhibition of apoptosis by the investigational drug that is the therapeutic goal (i.e., preventing neuronal death).

E is incorrect. The unfolded protein response/endoplasmic reticulum stress response is not directly related to inflammation in the brain or other tissues, so this cannot be the mechanism responsible.

19.   Correct: C. Only one of the amino acids is polar.

Protein function is determined by structure and structure is determined by primary amino acid sequence. Amino acid substitutions in a protein generally have little effect on function if the physicochemical properties of the amino acid substitution are similar to the original amino acid (e.g., valine substituted by leucine). When the substitution is very different from the original (e.g., negatively charge glutamate for positively charged lysine), the effect on protein structure/function is more likely to be pronounced.

Source: Panini S. Medical Biochemistry - An Illustrated Review. 1st Edition. Thieme; 2013.

A is incorrect. Only serine, threonine, and tyrosine can be phosphorylated.

B is incorrect. Only methionine and cysteine contain sulfur.

C is correct. Leucine is nonpolar whereas glutamine is polar, which is consistent with altering protein function.

D is incorrect. Only phenylalanine, tyrosine, and tryptophan are aromatic.

E is incorrect. Only aspartate, glutamate, lysine, arginine, and histidine are charged.

20.   Correct: B. Electrostatic.

The N-terminal "tails" of histone proteins have a net positive charge, due to numerous lysine and arginine residues. These positively charged residues form electrostatic interactions with the negative charged phosphate backbone of DNA, helping in the efficient packaging of chromatin. The amino acid lysine has an epsilon amino group that has a net positive charge at physiological pH. Acetylation results in loss of the net positive charge of lysine, reducing the affinity of nucleosomes for the negatively charged backbone of DNA and is responsible, in part, for the "loosening" of chromatin upon histone acetylation.

A is incorrect. The bonds between nucleosomes and DNA are all noncovalent.

C is incorrect. Hydrophobic bonds may contribute to the interaction between nucleosomes and DNA but are not influenced by histone acetylation.

D is incorrect. Van der Waals bonds may contribute to the interaction between nucleosomes and DNA but are not influenced by histone acetylation.

Chapter 5

The TCA Cycle and Oxidative Phosphorylation

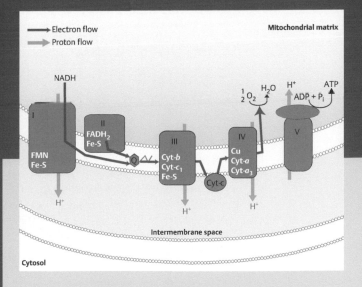

LEARNING OBJECTIVES

▶ Describe the purpose and regulation of the pyruvate dehydrogenase complex (and related complexes), as well as its required cofactors/vitamins.

▶ Describe both the catabolic and anabolic purposes of the tricarboxylic acid (TCA) cycle, as well as its regulation.

▶ Describe the roles of thiamine, niacin, riboflavin, and biotin in the TCA cycle and the common causes and clinical results of deficiencies in these micronutrients.

▶ Describe the effects of electron transport chain (ETC) inhibitors, adenosine triphosphate (ATP) synthase inhibitors, and uncouplers of oxidative phosphorylation, knowing specific examples of each type of drug.

▶ Explain how electron transport and ATP synthase are functionally coupled, and how the coupled process is regulated.

▶ Explain the roles of creatine, creatine kinase, and phosphocreatine in intracellular energy maintenance.

▶ Describe the common manifestations of mitochondrial diseases, and why some show maternal inheritance while others are inherited in an X-linked or autosomal recessive pattern.

5.1 Questions

Easy	Medium	Hard

1. In the fall of 2003, several infants in Israel were hospitalized with encephalopathy. Two of the patients died of cardiomyopathy. The cases were all eventually tied to a vitamin deficiency in a new formulation of a popular nondairy soy-based infant formula. Metabolic profiles, when obtained, revealed elevated serum lactate and pyruvate levels. There was no evidence of fasting hypoglycemia in the patients. As a result of the vitamin deficiency, which of the following metabolites would also be elevated in these infants?[1]

A. Acetoacetate

B. α-Ketoglutarate

C. Methylmalonic acid

D. Homocysteine

E. Propionic acid

2. Leigh syndrome is a rare neurodegenerative disorder caused by genetic deficiencies in any of the four complexes involved in the ETC. Researchers who study Leigh syndrome have developed model systems in which they simulate deficiencies in any of the four ETC complexes by adding specific drugs to actively respiring mitochondria or whole cells. Which of the following correctly describes which drug would simulate a deficiency in each of the four ETC complexes?

	Complex I	Complex II	Complex III	Complex IV
A	Rotenone	Malonate	Antimycin	Cyanide
B.	Cyanide	Antimycin	Malonate	Rotenone
C.	Malonate	Antimycin	Rotenone	Cyanide
D.	Antimycin	Rotenone	Cyanide	Malonate
E.	Rotenone	Cyanide	Malonate	Antimycin

3. A researcher who studies both genetic and acquired defects in oxidative phosphorylation regularly conducts experiments in which she incubates intact mitochondria isolated from diseased tissues with succinate, adenosine diphosphate (ADP), inorganic phosphate, and oxygen (O_2). She measures the rate of oxygen consumption in the reaction mixtures before and after adding potassium cyanide, 2,4-dinitrophenol, or oligomycin. The graphs shown below depict typical results obtained while adding these drugs to control (i.e., non-diseased) mitochondria. Which graph, A, or B, most accurately represents data that would be obtained in the presence of each of the three drugs?

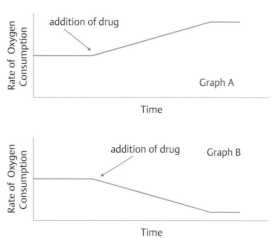

Source: Koolman J, Röhm K. Color Atlas of Biochemistry. 3rd Edition. 2012.

Drug Added		
Potassium cyanide	**2,4-Dinitrophenol**	**Oligomycin**
A Graph A	Graph B	Graph B
B Graph A	Graph A	Graph B
C Graph A	Graph B	Graph A
D Graph B	Graph A	Graph A
E Graph B	Graph B	Graph A
F Graph B	Graph A	Graph B

1 (Case based on Fattal-Valevski A. Outbreak of life-threatening thiamine deficiency in infants in Israel caused by a defective soy-based formula. Pediatrics. 2005;115(2). doi:10.1542/peds.2004-1255.)

4. A 35-year-old female who has worked at a facility that produces semi-conductors for the last 15 years developed symptoms of arsenic poisoning, including painful peripheral neuropathy and hyperpigmentation. Many of the toxic effects of arsenic are linked to its trivalent form, arsenite, which has a very high affinity for sulfhydryl groups, especially vicinal sulfhydryl groups. Which of the following *direct* effects would arsenite have on the citric acid cycle?

A. Inhibition of the phosphorylation of guanosine diphosphate (GDP) by succinyl-CoA synthase

B. Inhibition of the anaplerotic generation of oxaloacetate

C. Stimulation of the activity of succinate dehydrogenase

D. Inhibition of the activities of pyruvate, isocitrate, α-ketoglutarate, and malate dehydrogenases

E. Inhibition of the generation of acetyl-CoA from carbohydrates

5. A 24-year-old woman suffering from a severe head cold had a very poor appetite and had not eaten more than 300 calories per day for the last 3 days. By the third day, which of the following enzymes is playing a key role in the synthesis of her plasma glucose?

A. Citrate synthase

B. Glycogen phosphorylase

C. Malic enzyme

D. Propionyl-CoA carboxylase

E. Pyruvate dehydrogenase

Consider the following vignette for questions 6 and 7.

A 24-year-old male was diagnosed with mitochondrial myopathy, encephalomyopathy, lactic acidosis, and stroke-like episodes (MELAS) after a 10-year history of progressive neurological and muscular degeneration and loss of vision.

6. When genetic testing was done to diagnose this patient, it was noted that the particular mutation in transfer ribonucleic acid (tRNA)^{Leu} that he harbors was found in a muscle biopsy sample, but not in buccal samples. Which of the following is the most likely explanation for this laboratory observation?

A. Buccal cells do not contain mitochondria

B. Heteroplasmy

C. Spontaneous somatic mutation

D. Trinucleotide repeats

E. Variable expressivity

7. Regarding energy production, which of the following situations would be expected in this patient's mitochondria?

A. An abnormally high proton motive force

B. A high ATP:ADP ratio

C. A high NADH:NAD+ ratio

D. Uncoupled oxidative phosphorylation

8. Guanidinoacetate methyltransferase deficiency is a rare autosomal recessive inborn error in creatine biosynthesis. Symptoms of the disorder include global developmental delay and intellectual disability. Some individuals with the disorder develop epilepsy. The neurological pathology of this disease is partially attributed to the toxicity of guanidinoacetate, which accumulates in the serum. Which of the following biochemical changes most likely also contributes to the neurological pathology?

A. Alterations in enzyme regulation

B. Decreased creatinine production

C. Elevation of creatine kinase in the serum

D. Increased oxidative stress

E. Inhibition of fatty acid transport into mitochondria

9. As a result of biochemical and genetic testing, a 9-month-old boy with a history of neurodevelopmental delay, hypotonia, and several hospitalizations for severe lactic acidosis was diagnosed with an inherited disorder in energy metabolism. Fasting hypoglycemia was not noted during these hospitalizations. Following the diagnosis, his pediatric specialist prescribed a very low-carbohydrate, high-fat diet, and the boy's clinical course showed some improvement. Which of the following enzymes or proteins is most likely deficient in this patient?

A. Fumarase

B. Glucose 6-phosphatase

C. Mitochondrial tRNA

D. Pyruvate carboxylase

E. Pyruvate dehydrogenase

10. A 15-year-old boy was admitted to an emergency department after he was found unconscious in his bedroom by his parents, who had just returned home and heard their household carbon monoxide detector beeping. Blood tests were indicative of elevated levels of carboxyhemoglobin and lactate. Which of the following substances is the primary regulator of the TCA cycle in this patient's tissues at the time of his hospital admission?

A. Acetyl-CoA

B. ADP

C. Citrate

D. Insulin

E. NADH

11. Individuals with biotinidase deficiency frequently present with organic acidemia and mild hyperammonemia. Which of the following organic acids will be elevated in these individuals?

	β-Hydroxybutyric	Lactic	Methylmalonic	Propionic
A	X	X	X	X
B	X	X	X	
C	X	X		X
D	X		X	X
E		X	X	X

5.2 Answers and Explanations

Easy	Medium	Hard

1. Correct: B. α-Ketoglutarate.

α-Ketoglutarate levels would also be elevated in these infants. Elevated serum lactate and pyruvate levels, as well as the development of encephalopathy, are consistent with a deficiency in thiamine (vitamin B1), the precursor for thiamine pyrophosphate (TPP), which is a cofactor for the pyruvate dehydrogenase complex. TPP is also a cofactor for the α-ketoglutarate dehydrogenase complex; therefore, a thiamine deficiency will additionally impair conversion of α-ketoglutarate to succinyl-coenzyme A (CoA) in the TCA cycle. For a review of the regulation and coenzyme requirements of the pyruvate dehydrogenase complex, see the figure below. The pyruvate and α-ketoglutarate dehydrogenase complexes,

as well as the dehydrogenase complexes involved in metabolism of branched chain amino acids, are all structurally similar and utilize the coenzymes TPP, lipoic acid, CoA, flavin adenine dinucleotide (FAD), and nicotinamide adenine dinucleotide oxidized (NAD+) (Tender Loving Care For Nancy is a helpful mnemonic).

A is incorrect. Acetoacetate, along with β-hydroxybutyrate and acetone, is a ketone body. Accumulation of ketone bodies occurs when oxaloacetate is unavailable for condensation, via citrate synthase, with acetyl-CoA in mitochondria. The fact that fasting hypoglycemia is not observed in these patients indicates that the gluconeogenic pathway is functioning well and that pyruvate carboxylase, which generates oxaloacetate from pyruvate, is not affected by the vitamin deficiency. Therefore, we would not expect accumulation of ketone bodies above their normal levels.

C is incorrect. Methylmalonyl-CoA is the substrate for methylmalonyl-CoA mutase, an enzyme involved in the catabolism of odd-chain fatty acids and branched-chain amino acids. Methylmalonyl-CoA mutase is one of only two enzymes in the human body that utilize cobalamin (vitamin B_{12}) as a cofactor—the other is methionine synthase. A deficiency in vitamin B_{12} results in accumulation of methylmalonic acid in the serum but does not result in accumulation of lactate or pyruvate.

D is incorrect. Homocysteine is a substrate for cystathionine β-synthase, a pyridoxal phosphate (PLP)-dependent enzyme, and for methionine synthase, a cobalamin-dependent enzyme. Deficiencies in either pyridoxine (vitamin B_6) or cobalamin (vitamin B_{12}) can lead to hyperhomocysteinemia but will not lead to serum accumulation of pyruvate and lactate.

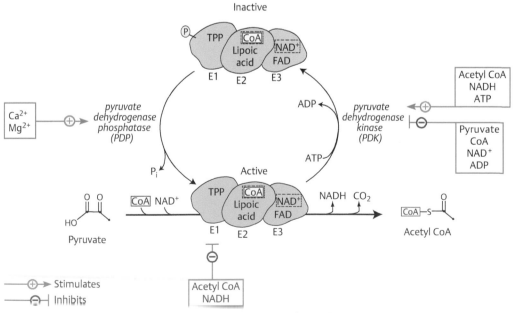

Source: Panini S. Medical Biochemistry - An Illustrated Review. 1st Edition. Thieme; 2013.

E is incorrect. Propionyl-CoA is the substrate for propionyl-CoA carboxylase, an enzyme involved in the catabolism of odd-chain fatty acids and branched-chain amino acids. It requires biotin (vitamin B_7) as a cofactor. A deficiency in biotin would result in elevated serum propionic acid levels, as well as elevated pyruvate and lactate as biotin is also a cofactor for pyruvate carboxylase. However, we can rule out a biotin deficiency in this case, due to the fact that fasting hypoglycemia is not observed; pyruvate carboxylase activity is not affected by the vitamin deficiency in the infant formula.

2. **Correct: A. Complex I = Rotenone; Complex II = Malonate; Complex III = Antimycin; Complex IV = Cyanide.**

This choice correctly identifies well established inhibitors of the various complexes in the ETC. As illustrated in the figure below, rotenone inhibits Complex I, malonate inhibits Complex II, antimycin inhibits Complex III, and cyanide inhibits Complex IV.

B in incorrect. This option does not correctly correlate the various ETC inhibitors with the specific complexes that they inhibit.

C in incorrect. This option does not correctly correlate the various ETC inhibitors with the specific complexes that they inhibit.

D in incorrect. This option does not correctly correlate the various ETC inhibitors with the specific complexes that they inhibit.

E in incorrect. This option does not correctly correlate the various ETC inhibitors with the specific complexes that they inhibit.

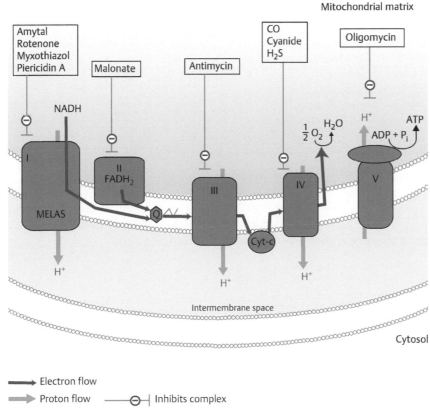

Source: Panini S. Medical Biochemistry - An Illustrated Review. 1st Edition. Thieme; 2013.

3. **Correct: F. Graph B Graph A Graph B.**

Graph A represents the expected results upon addition of an uncoupler of oxidative phosphorylation, while Graph B represents the expected results upon addition of an inhibitor of oxidative phosphorylation. Cyanide binds tightly to a cytochrome in Complex IV, thus inhibiting movement of electrons through complex IV. This disruption in the ETC will result in decreased reduction of O_2, and thus also a decreased rate of O_2 consumption (Graph B). 2,4-Dinitrophenol is an uncoupler of oxidative phosphorylation; it is a lipophilic weak acid that binds protons in the intermembrane space, carries them across the inner mitochondrial membrane, and releases them into the matrix. The dissipation of the proton gradient generated by the ETC disrupts mitochondrial ATP synthesis and simultaneously stimulates oxidation of nicotinamide adenine dinucleotide reduced (NADH) and flavin adenine dinucleotide reduced

(FADH$_2$) by the ETC in an attempt to re-generate the proton gradient. Thus, more O$_2$ will be reduced in the ETC, and the rate of mitochondrial O$_2$ consumption will increase (Graph A). Oligomycin is an inhibitor of ATP synthase; it inhibits transport of protons from the intermembrane space to the mitochondrial matrix via the ATP synthase channel. This causes the proton gradient to increase to such an extent that it becomes energetically unfeasible for the ETC to run. Thus, less O$_2$ will be reduced by the ETC, and the rate of O$_2$ consumption will decrease (Graph B).

A is incorrect. This set of assignments does not accurately reflect the predicted effects of the three drugs on oxygen consumption in treated mitochondria.

B is incorrect. This set of assignments does not accurately reflect the predicted effects of the three drugs on oxygen consumption in treated mitochondria.

C is incorrect. This set of assignments does not accurately reflect the predicted effects of the three drugs on oxygen consumption in treated mitochondria.

D is incorrect. This set of assignments does not accurately reflect the predicted effects of the three drugs on oxygen consumption in treated mitochondria.

E is incorrect. This set of assignments does not accurately reflect the predicted effects of the three drugs on oxygen consumption in treated mitochondria.

4. Correct: E. Inhibition of the generation of acetyl-CoA from carbohydrates.

Arsenite inhibits the generation of acetyl-CoA from carbohydrates, as arsenite binds tightly to the vicinal sulfhydryl groups of lipoic acid and thus inhibits pyruvate dehydrogenase. Lipoic acid is a cofactor for the various dehydrogenases that catalyze α-decarboxylation reactions; the pyruvate, α-ketoglutarate, and branched chain α-keto acid dehydrogenase complexes. For a review of the catalytic cycle of the pyruvate dehydrogenase complex and the roles of the cofactors involved, see the figure below. The pyruvate and α-ketoglutarate dehydrogenase complexes, as well as the dehydrogenase complexes involved in metabolism of branched chain amino acids, are all structurally similar and utilize the coenzymes **T**PP, **L**ipoic acid, **C**oA, **F**AD, and **N**AD$_+$ (**T**ender **L**oving **C**are **F**or **N**ancy is a helpful mnemonic).

A is incorrect. Lipoic acid is not a cofactor for succinyl-CoA synthase.

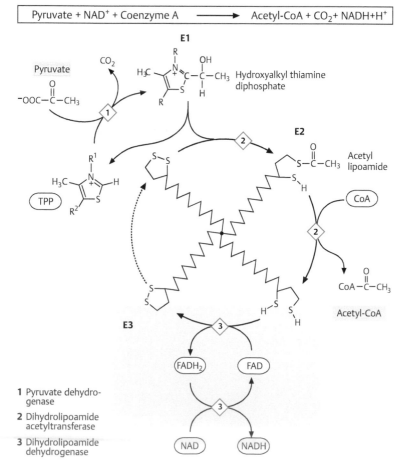

Pyruvate + NAD$^+$ + Coenzyme A $\longrightarrow$ Acetyl-CoA + CO$_2$+ NADH+H$^+$

1 Pyruvate dehydrogenase
2 Dihydrolipoamide acetyltransferase
3 Dihydrolipoamide dehydrogenase

Source: Panini S. Medical Biochemistry - An Illustrated Review. 1st Edition. Thieme; 2013.

B is incorrect. Anaplerotic generation of oxaloacetate is accomplished largely by the activities of pyruvate carboxylase and aspartate transaminase. Neither of these enzymes require lipoic acid as a cofactor.

C is incorrect. Succinate dehydrogenase does not require lipoic acid as a cofactor.

D is incorrect. Of the dehydrogenases listed here, only pyruvate dehydrogenase complex and α-ketoglutarate dehydrogenase complex utilize lipoic acid as a cofactor.

5. Correct: D. Propionyl-CoA carboxylase.

By the third day of this woman's fast, propionyl-CoA carboxylase will be contributing significantly to the generation of her plasma glucose. Her liver glycogen store will be depleted, and her liver will be utilizing gluconeogenesis to provide plasma glucose. Anaplerotic reactions will provide TCA cycle intermediates that can be converted to malate, which is pulled from the cycle for use in gluconeogenesis. Propionyl-CoA carboxylase catalyzes the first step in the anaplerotic conversion of propionyl-CoA to succinyl-CoA (see the figure below). Propionyl-CoA is the product of catabolism of valine, isoleucine, methionine, and threonine, as well as odd-chain fatty acids.

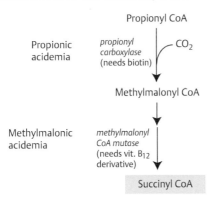

A is incorrect. Citrate synthase catalyzes the condensation of oxaloacetate and acetyl-CoA to form citrate. The citrate thus formed could be converted to malate for gluconeogenesis. However, under fasting conditions, oxaloacetate will preferentially be directly reduced to malate, via malate dehydrogenase, thus bypassing the rest of the TCA cycle. The reasons for this are that (1) mitochondrial NADH levels are elevated due to significant β-oxidation of fatty acids; this inhibits the activities of isocitrate dehydrogenase and α-ketoglutarate dehydrogenase and causes malate dehydrogenase to favor reduction of oxaloacetate to malate, and (2) the activity of citrate synthase is low due to lack of activation by insulin and oxaloacetate and inhibition by NADH and ATP.

B is incorrect. This woman's fast has persisted long enough (i.e., more than 24 h) that her liver glycogen stores have been depleted, and her liver is relying on gluconeogenesis for serum glucose generation. Hence, glycogen phosphorylase, which catalyzes the release of glucose from glycogen, will be inactive.

C is incorrect. Malic enzyme catalyzes the cytosolic oxidative decarboxylation of malate to pyruvate and plays an important role in the generation of NADPH for fatty acid synthesis. This reaction would be wasteful under conditions where gluconeogenesis is needed; conversion of cytosolic malate to pyruvate would create a futile cycle in which the pyruvate would have to be converted to oxaloacetate, via pyruvate carboxylase, and then oxaloacetate would be converted back to malate. Under gluconeogenic conditions, cytosolic malate is preferentially oxidized to oxaloacetate, which is then converted to phosphoenolpyruvate (PEP) by PEP carboxykinase. PEP then enters the glucogenic pathway.

D is incorrect. Pyruvate dehydrogenase is active under conditions where carbons generated in glycolysis are being oxidized in the TCA cycle. This will not occur in the liver under fasting conditions, where the liver's function is to generate glucose for transport in the serum to other tissues.

6. Correct: B. Heteroplasmy.

The most likely explanation for the differential expression of this mutation is heteroplasmy. As indicated by its name, MELAS is a mitochondrial disease. Genetic mitochondrial disorders can be caused by mutations in either mitochondrial or nuclear deoxyribonucleic acid (DNA); MELAS results from mutation in a mitochondrial gene that encodes tRNA^{Leu}. (Recall that all tRNAs for synthesis of mitochondrial DNA-encoded proteins are themselves encoded in the mitochondrial DNA.) Mitochondrial gene mutations are maternally inherited, as mitochondria from the sperm are rapidly destroyed upon fertilization of the egg. During subsequent cell division, mitochondria and their DNA molecules are apportioned by chance, as illustrated in the figure below. Thus, in the developed fetus, some tissues will have higher numbers of mitochondria that carry mutated DNA, while others will have lower numbers or even no mitochondria that carry the mutation. The presence of varying mitochondrial genomes in different cells is referred to as heteroplasmy.

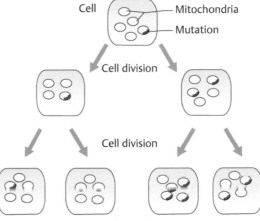

Source: Passarge E. Color Atlas of Genetics. 4th Edition. 2012.

75

A in incorrect. Buccal cells do contain mitochondria. The only cells in the human body that contain no mitochondria are erythrocytes.

C is incorrect. Spontaneous somatic mutation, depending on the life-cycle stage during which it occurs, does result in different genetic profiles indifferent tissues (cancer is a good example of spontaneous somatic mutation). However, MELAS, like several other mitochondrial diseases, is maternally inherited.

D is incorrect. Genetic disorders, such as Huntington disease, that involve expanded trinucleotide repeats are inherited in an autosomal dominant pattern and involve nuclear DNA mutations that will be detected in all cell types.

E is incorrect. Variable expressivity refers to the phenomenon of differing phenotype or clinical features among individuals that carry the same genotype.

7.   Correct: C. A high NADH:NAD+ ratio.

There will most likely be a high NADH:NAD$^+$ ratio in this patient's mitochondria. In MELAS and other mitochondrial disorders of energy production, ETC function is compromised. In this case, the deficiency in mitochondrial tRNA^{Leu} impairs synthesis of all of the 13 mitochondrial-encoded proteins that function as subunits for complexes in the respiratory chain and ATP synthase. This results in an inability to effectively transfer electrons from NADH to O$_2$. Because all TCA cycle enzymes are encoded on nuclear DNA, the TCA cycle will function normally and generate NADH. Thus, the NADH:NAD$^+$ ratio will be elevated. The elevated NADH:NAD$^+$ ratio inhibits some enzymes in the TCA cycle, as well as the pyruvate dehydrogenase complex. Inhibition of the pyruvate dehydrogenase complex is the cause of the lactic acidosis that is commonly observed in individuals with MELAS and other disorders of oxidative phosphorylation.

A is incorrect. An abnormally high proton motive force is generated under conditions where the respiratory chain is functioning adequately, thus generating an electrochemical gradient, but the ATP synthase is not functioning at an adequate level to dissipate the gradient. In MELAS, the respiratory chain is not functioning well, and the proton motive force will most likely be lower than normal.

B is incorrect. The ATP:ADP ratio will be low. The inability to effectively translate the mitochondrial enzymes encoded in mtDNA results in impaired function of the ETC. Thus, mitochondrial ATP synthesis via oxidative phosphorylation is inhibited.

D is incorrect. Oxidative phosphorylation is uncoupled in the presence of proton ionophores or uncoupling proteins that dissipate the proton gradient generated by the respiratory chain.

8.   Correct: A. Alterations in enzyme regulation.

Alterations in enzyme regulation by ATP most likely also contribute to neurological pathology in individuals who are unable to synthesize creatine due to this enzyme deficiency. Phosphocreatine is present in millimolar concentrations primarily in the brain, heart, and skeletal muscle, where it functions as a reservoir of high-energy phosphate that can swiftly regenerate ATP from ADP. As illustrated in the figure below, when ATP concentrations are high, creatine kinase utilizes ATP to phosphorylate creatine. This reaction is catalyzed primarily by a mitochondrial isozyme of creatine kinase located in the intermembrane space; thus, ATP produced by oxidative phosphorylation is rapidly used to generate phosphocreatine when free creatine levels are high. In the cytosol, another isoform of creatine kinase (CK-BB in the brain and CK-MM and CK-MB in skeletal muscle and heart) associates with various ATP-utilizing enzymes. Phosphocreatine produced by the mitochondrial creatine kinase acts as a cytosolic energy reserve that can quickly provide ATP for use by these ATP-dependent enzymes in situations where cytosolic ATP concentrations suddenly drop. Storing high energy phosphate in the phosphocreatine reservoir is preferable over utilizing ATP itself as the energy reservoir (i.e., maintaining a very high ATP concentration in the cytosol), as many transporters and metabolic enzymes are allosterically activated or inhibited by cytosolic ATP concentrations. Storing reserve energy in the form of phosphocreatine allows cells to operate well with a broader range of ATP concentrations, and thus more effectively regulate various enzymes and transporters in response to changes in cellular energy levels. This ability to regulate enzymes and transporters according to changes in cellular ATP levels is fundamental to effective cell function.

B is incorrect. Individuals with guanidinoacetate methyltransferase deficiency do have decreased serum creatinine levels. (Recall that creatinine is generated by spontaneous cyclization of creatine.)

Creatine   ATP   ADP   Creatine kinase   Phosphocreatine

However, serum creatinine has no known physiological function or effect on neurological tissues. Serum creatinine levels are measured in order to assess renal function.

C is incorrect. Serum creatine kinase is a biomarker frequently used to detect myocardial infarction and is unrelated to the disease process described here.

D in incorrect. There is little reason to expect elevated levels of oxidative stress in individuals with guanidinoacetate methyltransferase deficiency. Mitochondrial function should not be impaired in such a way as to increase the release of reactive oxygen species. The deficiency in creatine will, if anything, decrease flux through the ETC, as cellular ATP concentrations will be a bit higher than normal due to impaired ability to transfer phosphate to creatine.

E is incorrect. Transport of fatty acids into mitochondria depends on carnitine, not on creatine.

9. Correct: E. Pyruvate dehydrogenase.

This child most likely has a deficiency in pyruvate dehydrogenase. His symptoms and episodes of severe lactic acidosis are consistent with a defect in either the TCA cycle or oxidative phosphorylation. The effective treatment with a low-carbohydrate, high-fat diet indicates that metabolism of carbohydrates, but not fatty acids, is a key contributing factor. Thus, it is reasonable to conclude that the deficiency is in pyruvate dehydrogenase, which converts pyruvate

generated primarily by carbohydrate catabolism (but also from glycine and alanine) to acetyl-CoA for entry into the TCA cycle. (Recall also that pyruvate dehydrogenase deficiency is an X-linked disorder.) See the figure below for a review of sources of acetyl-CoA.

A is incorrect. A deficiency in fumarase would not be partially alleviated by a low-carbohydrate, high-fat diet. (Homozygous fumarase deficiency has been observed and results in severe neuronal dysfunction and early death. Heterozygosity for fumarase deficiency followed by loss of function mutation in the normal fumarase allele is associated with the development of benign skin and uterine tumors as well as aggressive metastatic renal cell carcinoma.)

B is incorrect. Glucose 6-phosphatase deficiency impairs both glycogenolysis and gluconeogenesis, resulting in lactic acidosis in the fasting state. However, the lactic acidosis is accompanied by hypoglycemia. Furthermore, effective treatment of glucose 6-phosphatase deficiency involves frequent feeding and infusion of glucose via a nasogastric tube at night.

C is incorrect. A deficiency in mitochondrial tRNA, could present as described. However the deficiency would not be alleviated by a low-carbohydrate, high-fat diet. Furthermore, mitochondrial diseases generally do not present until later in childhood or early adulthood and have a more gradual onset.

D is incorrect. While a pyruvate carboxylase deficiency would cause lactic acidosis, it also causes

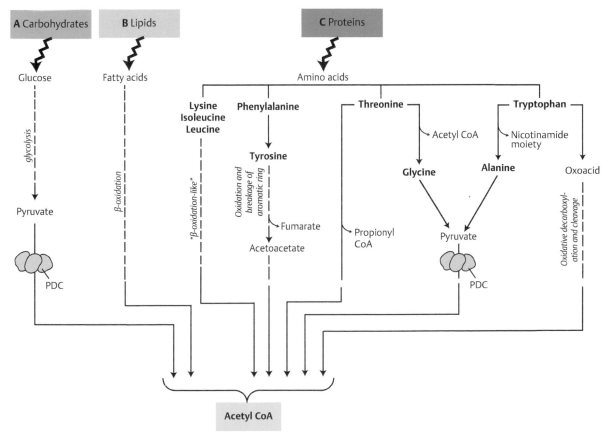

Source: Panini S. Medical Biochemistry - An Illustrated Review. 1st Edition. Thieme; 2013.

fasting hypoglycemia. Furthermore, treatment with a low-carbohydrate, high-fat diet will not alleviate symptoms; it would more likely cause ketoacidosis, as the TCA cycle lacks adequate oxaloacetate to process acetyl-CoA generated by fatty acid metabolism.

10.   Correct: E. NADH.

NADH will be inhibiting the TCA cycle in this patient. Carbon monoxide has a high-binding affinity for hemoglobin, forming carboxyhemoglobin. This effectively decreases the delivery of oxygen to tissues and produces systemic hypoxia. In the absence of adequate oxygen, the rate of electron flux through the respiratory chain will decrease, resulting in increased mitochondrial concentrations of NADH. Several enzymes

in the TCA cycle, as well as the pyruvate dehydrogenase complex, are inhibited by NADH (see the figure below). Thus, TCA cycle function will decrease, and pyruvate will accumulate and be converted to lactate.

A is incorrect. Acetyl-CoA typically accumulates under conditions, such as fasting and poorly controlled diabetes, when β-oxidation yields high amounts of acetyl-CoA and malate is being removed from the TCA cycle for gluconeogenesis. Under these conditions, acetyl-CoA inhibits the pyruvate dehydrogenase complex in order to prevent wasteful entry of glucose-derived carbon into the TCA cycle. Acetyl-CoA is also a weak feedforward activator of citrate synthase. Carbon monoxide poisoning will not stimulate formation of acetyl-CoA; thus, acetyl-CoA will not be regulating the TCA cycle.

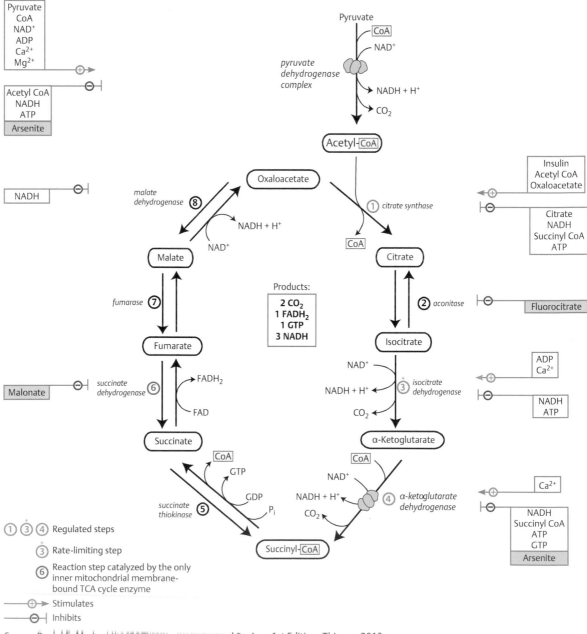

Source: Panini S. Medical Biochemistry - An Illustrated Review 1st Edition. Thieme; 2013

B is incorrect. ADP allosterically activates isocitrate dehydrogenase and the pyruvate dehydrogenase complex. This patient will be relying significantly on anaerobic glycolysis and glycogenolysis for ATP production in his tissues. As that capacity declines, ADP levels will rise. However the high NADH:NAD$_+$ ratio, which inhibits TCA cycle enzymes, will dominate the regulation.

C is incorrect. Citrate is a feedback inhibitor of citrate synthase. Inhibition of citrate synthase by citrate in this individual will be a consequence the initial inhibition of isocitrate dehydrogenase and α-ketoglutarate dehydrogenase by the high mitochondrial NADH:NAD$^+$ ratio, which is the key regulator of the TCA cycle.

D is incorrect. Insulin levels increase in the fed state and stimulate pyruvate dehydrogenase activity. In this patient's case, insulin is not a primary regulator of TCA cycle activity.

11. Correct: C. β-Hydroxybutyric; Lactic; Propionic.

β-Hydroxybutyric, lactic, and propionic acids will be elevated in these individuals, who will have impaired carboxylase activities. Biotin is covalently attached to lysine in the active sites of the carboxylases that utilize it as a cofactor. Biotinidase catalyzes the hydrolysis of biotin from lysine; it plays a key role in recycling biotin in the human body, as well as in releasing dietary biotin from the proteins to which it is attached. Individuals with biotinidase deficiency, which is inherited in an autosomal recessive manner, become deficient in biotin. (Other causes of biotin deficiency are mutations in holocarboxylase synthetase, which catalyzes the covalent linkage of biotin to lysine, and consumption of raw egg whites. Raw egg whites contain the protein avidin, which has a very strong affinity for biotin, thus preventing its uptake in the intestine. Dietary deficiency in biotin is extremely unusual, as biotin is present in most foods.) The four biotin-dependent enzymes in the human body are pyruvate carboxylase, propionyl-CoA carboxylase, acetyl-CoA carboxylase, and β-methylcrotonyl-CoA carboxylase. Pyruvate carboxylase catalyzes the formation of oxaloacetate from pyruvate, a key anaplerotic reaction. Deficiency in the activity of this enzyme results in ketosis (elevation of β-hydroxybutyrate and acetoacetate) due to the build-up of acetyl-CoA resulting from inadequate TCA cycle function. The elevated acetyl-CoA level inactivates pyruvate dehydrogenase, thus contributing to hyperlactatemia due to elevated pyruvate levels. Propionyl-CoA carboxylase participates in the catabolism of odd-chain fatty acids and the amino acids, leucine and valine. Deficiency in its activity results in accumulation of propionate. β-Methylcrotonate also would be present at higher concentrations due to insufficient β-methylcrotonyl-CoA carboxylase activity in the catabolic pathway for leucine but is not one of the answer choices.

A is incorrect. Methylmalonate levels are elevated in cases of methylmalonyl-CoA mutase deficiency. Methylmalonyl-CoA mutase utilizes cobalamin as a cofactor, so elevated levels of methylmalonate are also observed in individuals with a dietary cobalamin deficiency or an inherited deficiency in cobalamin metabolism.

B is incorrect. Biotin deficiency results in elevation of propionate, and methylmalonate levels are elevated in cases of methylmalonyl-CoA mutase or cobalamin deficiency.

D is incorrect. Biotin deficiency results in elevation of lactate, and methylmalonate levels are elevated in cases of methylmalonyl-CoA mutase or cobalamin deficiency.

E is incorrect. Biotin deficiency results in elevation of ketones, and methylmalonate levels are elevated in cases of methylmalonyl-CoA mutase or cobalamin deficiency.

Chapter 6

Carbohydrate Digestion and Metabolism

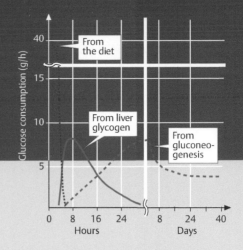

LEARNING OBJECTIVES

▶ Describe the digestion of starch, lactose, and sucrose, knowing the names, functions, and locations of the relevant digestive enzymes.

▶ Describe the overall purpose of glycolysis, its reactants and products, key enzymes, regulation, cellular location, and tissue distribution.

▶ Explain how fructose and galactose feed into the glycolytic pathway, focusing on the biochemical basis for symptoms seen in fructokinase, aldolase B, galactokinase, and galactose-1-phosphate uridyl transferase deficiencies.

▶ Describe the overall purpose of gluconeogenesis, its reactants and products, key enzymes, regulation, cellular location, and tissue distribution.

▶ Describe the overall purpose of glycogenesis and glycogenolysis, their reactants and products, key enzymes, regulation, cellular location, and tissue distribution.

▶ Describe the commonly used treatments for diseases associated with deficiencies in fasting metabolism, and the biochemical basis for their efficacy.

▶ Describe the purpose of the pentose phosphate pathway, its reactants, products of the oxidative and nonoxidative branches, and the biochemical basis for the physiological consequences of glucose 6-phosphate dehydrogenase deficiency.

▶ Describe the functions and structures of the glycosaminoglycans, the process for degradation of proteoglycans, and clinical disorders resulting from deficiencies in that process.

▶ Describe the locations and functions of key glucose transporters.

▶ Explain the role of the polyol pathway in the etiology of metabolically induced disease.

6.1 Questions

Easy	Medium	Hard

1. An 18-month-old boy is brought to the emergency department after a severe episode of vomiting. He is lethargic and his blood sugar is extremely low. The boy's mother reports that his pediatrician has expressed concerned about prior episodes of vomiting and lethargy, as well as his failure to thrive, and has recently ordered various medical tests for which they are awaiting results. You observe, after taking a careful history, that the boy's episodes of vomiting and lethargy occur after ingestion of fruits, pastries, and candy. Which of the following is the most likely cause of his symptoms?

A. Undigested lactose in the intestine

B. High levels of galactose in all tissues

C. Low serum insulin levels

D. Depletion of hepatic phosphate

E. Inability to phosphorylate fructose

2. A 5-year-old girl who is visiting from another state is brought to the emergency room in a hypoglycemic coma. Her parents provide a note from her pediatrician stating that the girl was diagnosed with von Gierke disease shortly after birth. Which one of the following events would most likely have triggered her hypoglycemia?

A. Administration of too much insulin

B. A severe bout of gastroenteritis

C. Consumption of a sugary drink

D. Consumption of milk

E. Exposure to nitrates in drinking water

3. A 55-year-old woman who was recently diagnosed with type II diabetes is prescribed acarbose, an FDA-approved drug that inhibits pancreatic α-amylase. Which of the following statements best describes the mechanism by which acarbose reduces serum glucose levels?

A. It inhibits gluconcogenesis

B. It inhibits glycogenolysis

C. It inhibits the digestion of dietary carbohydrates

D. It stimulates uptake of glucose by myocytes

E. It stimulates pancreatic insulin secretion

4. A teenaged boy becomes disoriented while hiking alone in the mountains and fails to return home. His family reports him missing and 5 days later he is rescued. He reports that the last thing he ate was a granola bar, shortly before leaving home for his hike. Initial examination reveals that although he is dehydrated and fatigued, the boy is healthy and should make a complete recovery from this trauma. At the time of his rescue, which of the following substances was the boy's body using to generate fuel for his erythrocytes?

A. Fatty acids released from adipocytes

B. Glycogen released from hepatocytes

C. Glycogen released from skeletal myocytes

D. Amino acids released from skeletal myocytes

E. Ketone bodies released from hepatocytes

Consider the following scenario and lab results for the questions 5 to 7.

A 6-month-old girl is brought to the emergency department by her parents after she had a seizure. The child seemed to be developing a severe cold in the days prior to the seizure, but otherwise has had no history of illness to date. The mother reports that 3 weeks ago she began weaning the child from on-demand breast feeding, which included at least one night-time feeding, to a more scheduled feeding routine that includes breast feeding and solid foods. Since then, the child has seemed irritable and is sometimes very lethargic in the mornings after she sleeps through the night without feeding. Physical exam shows that the child is febrile, with elevated heart and breathing rates. Otoscopy indicates otitis media. Slight hepatomegaly is also observed. Laboratory results are as follows:

	Patient	Normal
Arterial blood pH	6.9	7.4
Plasma glucose	30 mg/dL	65-100 mg/dL
Plasma lactate	67.5 mM	0.5-2 mM
Plasma β-hydroxybutyrate	5 mM	< 0.2 mM

5. A deficiency in which of the following hepatic enzymes would best account for this patient's symptoms?

A. Glycogen phosphorylase

B. Phosphofructokinase-1

C. Fructose 1,6-bisphosphatase

D. Fructokinase

E. Galactokinase

6. In addition to lactate and β-hydroxybutyrate, which of the following substances would you expect to be elevated in this patient's plasma and/or urine?

A. Ammonia

B. Glycerol

C. Acetyl CoA

D. Galactose

7. Which of the following dietary therapies would be most beneficial for this patient?

A. A high protein, low carbohydrate diet

B. Dietary supplementation with alanine

C. A high carbohydrate diet with frequent feedings

D. A low fat, low calorie diet

E. A high fat diet with infrequent feedings

8. A 5-year-old boy undergoes a regularly scheduled 6-month examination by a pediatric specialist. The pediatrician's physical exam indicates development of corneal clouding in the last 6 months. The boy is short in stature, has experienced significant hearing loss in the last 2 years, has mild mental retardation, and has reached the developmental stage of a typical 3-year-old. What is the most likely cause of corneal clouding in this patient?

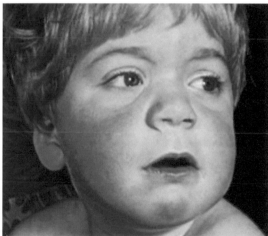

Source: Riede U, Werner M. Color Atlas of Pathology: Pathologic Principles · Associated Diseases · Sequela. 1st Edition. 2004.

A. Vitamin A deficiency

B. Accumulation of uric acid

C. Accumulation of dermatan sulfate

D. Amyloidosis

E. Deposition of lysosomal glycogen

9. A 4-year-old boy's guardian indicated, after being presented at the urgent care center, that the boy had been quite lethargic and complained of a headache and sore throat for the last 5 days. The nurse reported an oral temperature of 101.5°F. The figure below is an image of what the physician observed on viewing the boy's throat. During the last few days, how has the pentose phosphate pathway in the phagocytic white blood cells present in this boy's pharyngeal tissues been utilized?

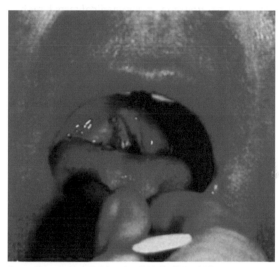

Source: Kayser F, Bienz K, Eckert J et al. Medical Microbiology. 1st Edition. 2004.

	Oxidative phase	Nonoxidative/Regenerative phase
A.	Active	Inactive
B.	Inactive	Favors formation of fructose 6-phosphate and glyceraldehyde 3-phosphate
C.	Inactive	Favors formation of ribulose 5-phosphate
D.	Active	Favors formation of fructose 6-phosphate and glyceraldehyde 3-phosphate
E.	Active	Favors formation of ribulose 5-phosphate
F.	Inactive	Inactive

10. A 3-year-old boy is brought to his pediatrician with complaints of fatigue and intermittent abdominal pain. The boy is in the lower 10th percentile on growth charts and has lost 5 pounds in the last 6 months. Physical examination shows hepatomegaly. Blood tests are ordered, followed by a liver biopsy and molecular testing. The results of these tests are indicative of a deficiency in phosphorylase kinase. Which of the following laboratory or biopsy results were most likely observed in this patient?

A. Hepatocellular lysosomal accumulation of glycogen

B. Fasting hypoglycemia

C. Hypercholesterolemia

D. Hepatocellular cytoplasmic decreased glycogen content

E. Fasting hypoketosis

83

11. Tumor lysis syndrome (TLS) is a serious condition that can occur when cancer cells rapidly lyse, either spontaneously or in response to therapy. It characteristically results in elevated serum levels of potassium, phosphate, uric acid, and cytokines. In order to prevent nephrolithiasis and subsequent renal complications, patients with TLS are often injected with rasburicase, a preparation of recombinant urate oxidase. Urate oxidase catalyzes the reaction shown in the figure below, converting serum uric acid to allantoin, a soluble substance that is readily eliminated in the urine. Treatment with rasburicase would be contraindicated in patients with a genetic deficiency in which of the following enzymes?

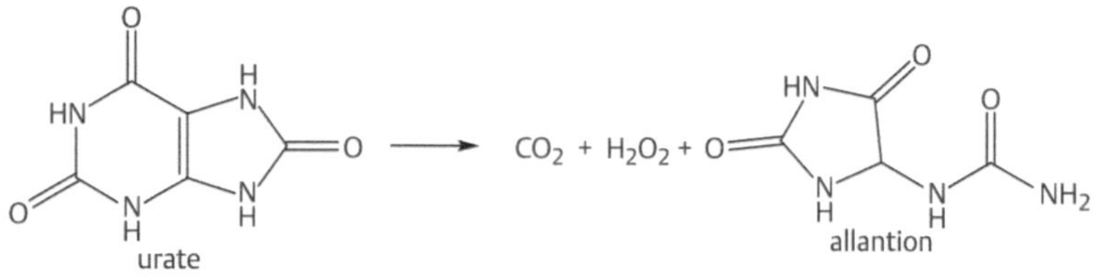

urate

$CO_2 + H_2O_2 + $ allantion

A. Glucose 6-phosphate dehydrogenase

B. Xanthine oxidase

C. Urate oxidase

D. Hypoxanthine-guanine phosphoribosyltransferase

E. Glucose 6-phosphatase

12. A pharmaceutical company is developing a drug, LX4211, for possible use in the treatment of type II diabetes. During phase II trials, they administered either the drug or a placebo to healthy individuals, half an hour before feeding them a 500-calorie meal consisting of 20% protein, 50% carbohydrate, and 30% fat. Serum glucose levels were measured 2 hours before the meal, at the time of the meal, and every half-hour after the meal. The results are shown below. Which of the following enzymes or transporters does this drug *most likely* inhibit?

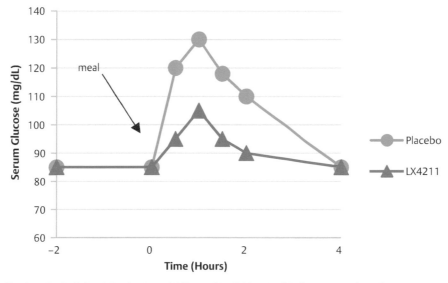

Source: Zambrowicz B, Ogbaa I, Frazier K, et al. Effects of LX4211, a Dual Sodium-Dependent Glucose Cotransporters 1 and 2 Inhibitor, on Postprandial Glucose, Insulin, Glucagon-like Peptide 1, and Peptide Tyrosine Tyrosine in a Dose-Timing Study in Healthy Subjects. Clinical Therapeutics. 2013.

A. Lactase
B. Sodium-dependent glucose transporter 1
C. Glucose transporter 4
D. Sucrase
E. Glucose transporter 3

13. A 3-day-old infant boy began vomiting after feeding. By his fourth day of life, he was jaundiced and began having seizures. After receiving the results of the boy's newborn screening tests, the infant's pediatrician promptly instructed the mother to stop breastfeeding and switch to a lactose-free formula. Which of the following will most likely develop in this infant if he ingests lactose in the future?

A. Diarrhea, due to fermentation of lactose by gut microbes
B. Cataracts, due to accumulation of galactitol in the eye
C. Hepatomegaly, due to incorporation of galactose into glycogen
D. Neurodegradation, due to accumulation of galactose-rich glycolipids in lysosomes

14. An Olympic weightlifter completes a snatch lift of 160 kg. Activation of which of the following enzymes contributes most significantly to the stimulation of ATP production in the weightlifter's biceps during the lift?

A. Phosphofructokinase-2
B. Glucokinase
C. Triose phosphate isomerase
D. Glycogen phosphorylase
E. GLUT4

15. A 50-year-old man with a history of type II diabetes presents with complaints of blurred vision and increased sensitivity to light glare, which his physician suspects is due to the development of cataracts. Which of the following is a significant contributor to the development of these symptoms in this patient?

A. Increased activity of phosphofructokinase-2
B. Increased activity of aldose reductase
C. Increased intracellular galactitol concentrations
D. Decreased activity of glucose 6-phosphate dehydrogenase
E. Decreased neuronal ATP levels

85

16. A researcher who studies insulin receptor substrate-1(IRS-1) performed several experiments with the G972R mutant protein (glycine at position 972 replaced with arginine), a polymorphism found in ~5% of the population. In separate experiments, she incubated WT (wild-type) and G972R IRS-1 proteins with active insulin receptor and ATP for various amounts of time. She then ran SDS-PAGE gels of the reaction mixtures and stained the gels with an antiphosphotyrosine antibody. The results are shown in the figure below, where the bands migrating closer to the top of the gel are phosphorylated IRS-1 proteins. Based on these results, which of the following would you most likely observe in individuals with the G972R IRS-1 polymorphism?

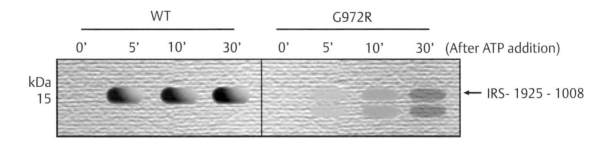

A. Hepatomegaly with increased glycogen stores

B. Decreased pancreatic insulin secretion

C. Increased risk for development of type II diabetes

D. Increased risk of severe fasting hypoglycemia

17. A 55-year-old woman has a fasting serum glucose level of 180 mg/dL and her HbA1c is 8.2%. What is the mechanism by which glucose uptake into her myocytes is contributing to her condition?

A. Glucose transporter 4 (GLUT4) is allosterically inactivated

B. Glucose transporter 1 (GLUT1) is allosterically activated

C. Glucose transporter 4 (GLUT4) is sequestered in microvesicles

D. Glucose transporter 2 (GLUT2) is sequestered in the nucleus

E. Glucose transporter 1 (GLUT1) is phosphorylated

18. A 35-year-old woman who has recently completed chemotherapy for treatment of breast cancer complains that although the nausea she experienced during treatment has subsided, she now experiences bloating, flatulence, and watery diarrhea. Her symptoms are most likely caused by decreased activity of which of the following enzymes?

A. Pepsin

B. α-Amylase

C. Pancreatic lipase

D. Galactokinase

E. Lactase

19. A laboratory researcher incubated rat hepatocytes in media that contained both glucose and alanine. She then added forskolin, an activator of adenylate cyclase. How would the concentrations of glucose and alanine in the media, and fructose 2,6-bisphosphate in the hepatocytes, change on addition of forskolin?

	Glucose	Alanine	Fructose 2,6-bisphosphate
A.	Increase	Increase	Increase
B.	Decrease	Decrease	Decrease
C.	Increase	Decrease	Increase
D.	Decrease	Increase	Increase
E.	Increase	Decrease	Decrease
F.	Decrease	Decrease	Increase

20. A 74-year-old man recently received prostate biopsy results indicative of prostate cancer. In order to determine whether the cancer had metastasized, he was injected with a dose of 2-18F-deoxyglucose (FDG) and then subjected to a positron emission tomography (PET) scan. His PET scan is shown in the figure below. Increased activity of which of the following enzymes most significantly contributes to the appearance of the dark spots indicated by the arrows on this scan?

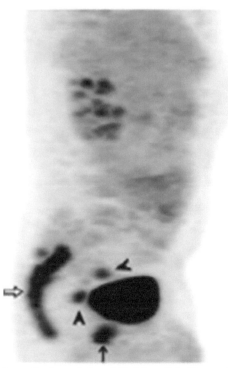

Source: Gunderman R. Essential Radiology. Clinical Presentation, Pathophysiology, Imaging. 3rd Edition. Thieme; 2014.

A. Hexokinase

B. Glucose transporter 4 (GLUT4)

C. Glycogen synthase

D. Pyruvate dehydrogenase

E. Phosphoglucomutase

6.2 Answers and Explanations

Easy	Medium	Hard

1. Correct: D. Depletion of hepatic phosphate.

This child's symptoms most likely can be attributed to depletion of hepatic phosphate. The boy's illness is exacerbated by ingestion of foods such as fruits, pastries, and candy, all of which contain large amounts of fructose. This suggests that he has a deficiency in fructose metabolism. The two possibilities are essential benign fructosuria and hereditary fructose intolerance. As illustrated in the figure on the following page, hereditary fructose intolerance is caused by hepatic deficiency in aldolase B, which catalyzes the splitting of fructose 1-phosphate into glyceraldehyde and dihydroxyacetone phosphate. When aldolase B activity is low, fructose 1-phosphate accumulates and is toxic to the liver. The cell's supply of phosphate is tied up in fructose 1-phosphate, thus inhibiting glycogen phosphorolysis and ATP synthesis, two processes that require phosphate. The reduction in glycogenolysis results in hypoglycemia, as observed in this patient, and inhibition of ATP synthesis prevents the maintenance of normal hepatocyte function. Benign essential fructosuria is caused by a deficiency in fructokinase and is discussed in the explanation for answer choice E.

87

A

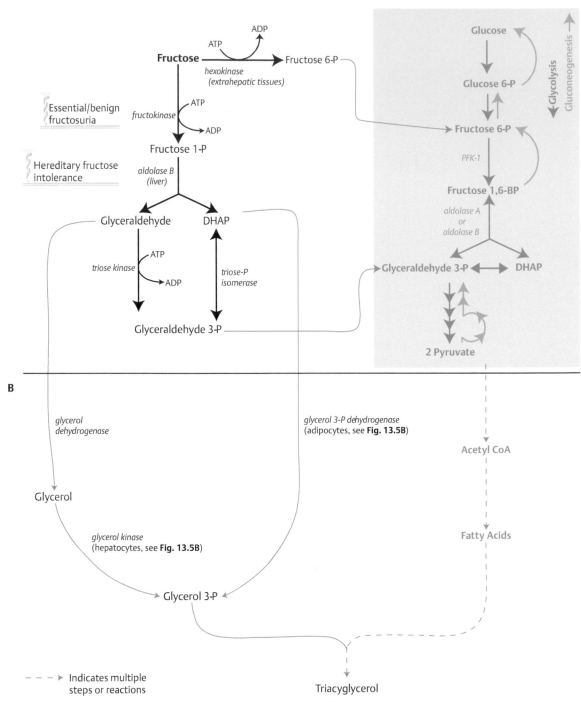

B

- - - ► Indicates multiple
        steps or reactions

Source: Panini S. Medical Biochemistry - An Illustrated Review. 1st Edition. Thieme; 2013.

A is incorrect. The boy is sensitive to fructose rather than lactose, which is found in milk.

B is incorrect. Problems with galactose metabolism would result in difficulties associated with consumption of lactose or other galactose-containing foods.

C is incorrect. Low insulin levels would result in hyperglycemia rather than hypoglycemia.

E is incorrect. Essential benign fructosuria is caused by a deficiency in fructokinase, which catalyzes the phosphorylation of fructose to fructose 1-phosphate, trapping fructose in hepatocytes for further metabolism. The inability to phosphorylate fructose results in accumulation of fructose in the urine and is asymptomatic.

2.   Correct: B. A severe bout of gastroenteritis.

This patient's hypoglycemia was most likely triggered by an event, such as gastroenteritis, that caused her to enter a fasting metabolic state. von Gierke disease is one of several glycogen storage diseases. In this patient, a deficiency in glucose 6-phosphatase impairs the liver's ability to release glucose produced by both glycogenolysis and gluconeogenesis to the serum. A bout of gastroenteritis, or anything else that causes this patient to enter the fasting state, will cause her to become severely hypoglycemic, as her liver's ability to release glucose to the serum is impaired. See the following two figures (second on the next page) for a review of gluconeogenesis and glycogenolysis.

(i) **Gluconeogenesis**
(read from bottom to top)

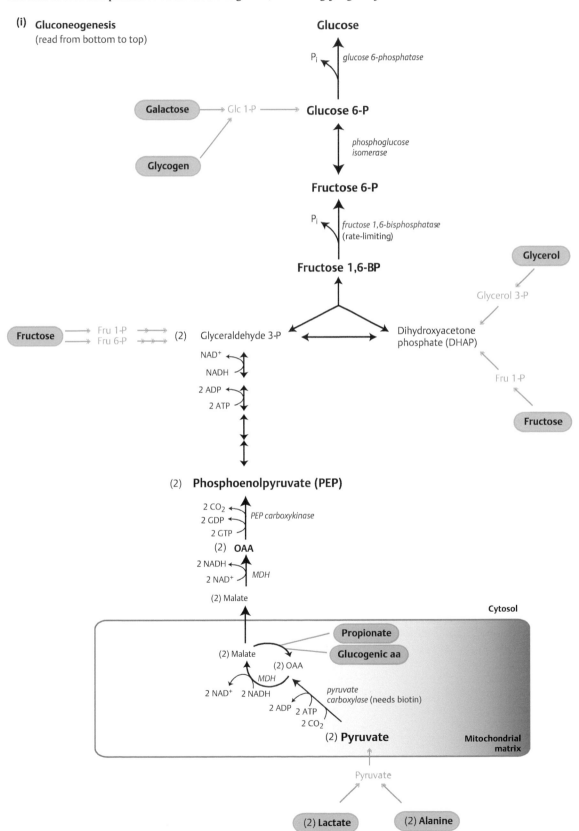

Source: Panini S. Medical Biochemistry - An Illustrated Review. 1st Edition. Thieme; 2013.

(ii)

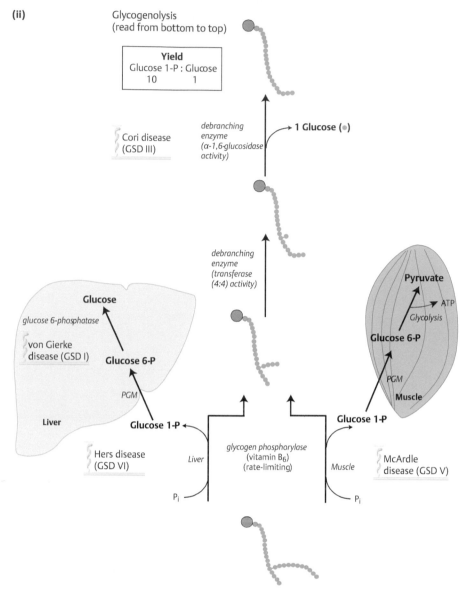

Glycogenolysis
(read from bottom to top)

Yield
Glucose 1-P : Glucose
    10   1

Cori disease
(GSD III)

debranching enzyme (α-1,6-glucosidase activity)

→ 1 Glucose (•)

debranching enzyme (transferase (4:4) activity)

Glucose

glucose 6-phosphatase

von Gierke disease (GSD I)   **Glucose 6-P**

PGM

Liver

Glucose 1-P ←

Hers disease (GSD VI)

Liver

glycogen phosphorylase (vitamin B$_6$) (rate-limiting)

P_i

Pyruvate

→ ATP

Glycolysis

Glucose 6-P

PGM

Muscle

Glucose 1-P

Muscle

McArdle disease (GSD V)

P_i

Source: Panini S. Medical Biochemistry - An Illustrated Review. 1st Edition. Thieme; 2013.

A is incorrect. Administration of too much insulin would result in hypoglycemia, but patients with glycogen storage diseases such as von Gierke disease do not require insulin therapy.

C is incorrect. Consumption of sucrose or fructose would cause hypoglycemia in a patient with a deficiency in fructose metabolism (i.e., hereditary fructose intolerance), but not in a von Gierke disease patient. Note that fructose consumption is restricted in the diets of individuals who have von Gierke disease, as fructose can cause hyperlactatemia in these patients.

D is incorrect. Lactose consumption might cause hypoglycemia in a patient with galactosemia, but not in a patient with von Gierke disease. Note that lactose consumption is restricted in the diets of individuals who have von Gierke disease, as galactose can cause hyperlactatemia in these patients.

E is incorrect. Exposure to nitrates may, in some individuals with deficiencies in erythrocyte carbohydrate metabolism, result in methemoglobinemia. It would not result in hypoglycemia.

3.   Correct: C. It inhibits the digestion of dietary carbohydrates.

Acarbose inhibits the digestion of dietary carbohydrates. Pancreatic α-amylase is a digestive enzyme, secreted by the pancreas to the small intestine, that cleaves the α-1,4-glycosidic bonds in dietary starch. Inhibition of α-amylase by acarbose slows the digestion of complex carbohydrates, thus decreasing the amount of glucose absorbed. This effectively helps to maintain postprandial glucose levels at a reasonable level in type II diabetics. (Acarbose also inhibits other α-glucosidases associated with the intestinal brush border, thus further decreasing intestinal glucose absorption.)

A is incorrect. Although inhibiting gluconeogenesis would decrease serum glucose levels in the postabsorptive states, pancreatic α-amylase, the target of acarbose, is not involved in the gluconeogenic pathway.

B is incorrect. Although inhibiting glycogenolysis would decrease serum glucose levels in the postabsorptive states, pancreatic α-amylase, the target of acarbose, is not involved in the glycogenolytic pathway.

D is incorrect. Acarbose would have no effect on glucose uptake by myocytes.

E is incorrect. Acarbose has no direct effect on pancreatic insulin secretion; if anything, administration of acarbose would decrease pancreatic insulin secretion by reducing serum glucose levels.

4. Correct: D. Amino acids released from skeletal myocytes.

The boy's liver was using amino acids released from skeletal myocytes to generate glucose. Erythrocytes lack mitochondria and thus are only able to metabolize glucose. Because he hasn't eaten in 5 days, the boy will be relying on his liver to provide serum glucose. At the beginning of a fast, the liver supplies serum glucose via glycogenolysis. However, hepatic glycogen stores are generally depleted within 24 hours. At this point the liver will use lactate, glycerol, and glucogenic amino acids as precursors for gluconeogenesis. The glucogenic amino acids are provided primarily by proteolysis of skeletal muscle protein.

A is incorrect. Fatty acids cannot be used as fuel for erythrocytes and are not converted to glucose via gluconeogenesis. (Odd chain fatty acids can be used to provide a small amount of glucose, but not enough to maintain glucose homeostasis.)

B is incorrect. Glycogen stores will be depleted by the time the boy is rescued.

C is incorrect. Muscle glycogen stores are not used to supply serum glucose; they only supply glucose for the individual cell in which the glycogen is stored.

E is incorrect. Erythrocytes cannot use ketone bodies for fuel; they only oxidize glucose.

5. Correct: C. Fructose 1,6-bisphosphatase.

A deficiency in fructose 1,6-bisphosphatase will impair the child's ability to generate glucose via gluconeogenesis in the fasting state. For a summary of the gluconeogenic pathway, see the figure placed with Answer 2 (i). This explains her hypoglycemia (initiated by fasting and increased catabolism due to illness) and the mother's observation that the child appears lethargic after an overnight fast. Because of the deficiency in fructose 1-,6-bisphosphatase, lactate cannot be used for gluconeogenesis, resulting in lactic acidosis (high plasma lactate concentration and low plasma pH). Her hepatomegaly is most likely due to steatosis caused by increased flux of fatty acids to the liver during her hypoglycemic episodes; the increased hepatic fatty acid concentration, coupled

with accumulation of glycerol 3-phosphate, results in increased hepatic triglyceride synthesis. Finally, the child's elevated plasma β-hydroxybutyrate is normal for fasting state metabolism and rules out the possibility of a deficiency in fatty acid oxidation.

A is incorrect. Although a deficiency in glycogen phosphorylase results in fasting hypoglycemia, it will not cause lactic acidosis, as hepatic gluconeogenesis is unaffected.

B is incorrect. Phosphofructokinase-1 is involved in glycolysis; a deficiency would not cause fasting hypoglycemia.

D is incorrect. A deficiency in fructokinase will result in illness linked to the consumption of sucrose or other fructose-containing foods. This child's illness seems to be triggered by fasting rather than by consumption of sugary foods.

E is incorrect. A deficiency in galactokinase will result in illness linked to the consumption of lactose or other galactose-containing foods. This child's illness seems to be triggered by fasting rather than by consumption of milk sugar.

6. Correct: B. Glycerol.

This patient will most likely have elevated levels of glycerol in her plasma. A deficiency in fructose 1,6-bisphosphatase impairs the ability of hepatocytes to convert lactate, glucogenic amino acids, glycerol, and fructose to glucose. The result will be accumulation of these substances and some of their metabolites, in the plasma and/or urine.

A is incorrect. Hyperammonemia is generally caused by insufficient hepatic processing of nitrogen in the urea cycle. Impaired gluconeogenesis will not significantly decrease urea cycle function; the liver will still obtain adequate energy, primarily via oxidation of fatty acids, for processing amino acids.

C is incorrect. Acetyl CoA is generally not released by cells and thus does not accumulate in the plasma or urine. Furthermore, a deficiency in fructose 1,6-bisphosphatase would not be expected to cause hepatic intracellular accumulation of acetyl CoA.

D is incorrect. A fructose 1,6-bisphosphatase deficiency will have no effect on plasma galactose levels.

7. Correct: C. A high carbohydrate diet with frequent feedings.

This patient should be placed on a high carbohydrate diet with frequent feedings. In order to prevent future episodes of hypoglycemia, it is important to maintain adequate serum glucose levels without relying on gluconeogenesis. The patient should avoid fasting for longer than a few hours, so that her glycogen stores are not depleted to the point that gluconeogenesis is required. Thus, frequent feedings are desirable. A high carbohydrate diet will help to build her glycogen stores and will prevent the need for gluconeogenesis.

A is incorrect. A high-protein, low-carbohydrate diet will increase the demand for gluconeogenesis, as even in the fed state amino acids will have to be converted to glucose.

B is incorrect. Supplementation with alanine would serve no purpose in this patient. Alanine is converted to glucose via gluconeogenesis, which does not function properly in this patient.

D is incorrect. A low-calorie diet will cause the patient to spend more time in the fasted state and would only exacerbate her condition. The patient's deficiency in fructose 1,6-bisphosphatase impairs gluconeogenesis, so this diet would cause hypoglycemia.

E is incorrect. A high fat diet with infrequent feeding would cause an increased demand for glucose synthesis in the liver. The diet might not even provide adequate glucose to maintain glucose homeostasis in the fed state. Furthermore, glycogen stores would not be built up to adequate levels in the fed state because fatty acids cannot be converted to glucose. So, the overall demand for gluconeogenesis will increase in the patient if fed a high fat diet. The patient's deficiency in fructose 1,6-bisphosphatase impairs gluconeogenesis, so this diet would cause hypoglycemia.

8. Correct: C. Accumulation of dermatan sulfate.

The most likely cause of corneal clouding is accumulation of dermatan sulfate. This patient exhibits many of the classical signs of some of the mucopolysaccharidoses (deficiencies in lysosomal hydrolases involved in the degradation of glycosaminoglycans): coarse facial features, dwarfism, and mental retardation. Clouding of the corneas is more specifically found in Hurler syndrome, a mucopolysaccharidosis resulting from a deficiency in α-L-iduronidase. In all mucopolysaccharidoses, the patient's symptoms can be traced to the accumulation of undegraded glycosaminoglycans in various tissues. In the case of Hurler syndrome, the glycosaminoglycans that accumulate are heparin sulfate and dermatan sulfate.

A is incorrect. While deficiency in vitamin A can cause corneal clouding due to keratinization, vitamin A deficiency is not associated with the other symptoms presented by this patient.

B is incorrect. Muccopolysaccharidoses do not result in hyperuricemia. Furthermore, uric acid does not accumulate in the cornea to cause clouding.

D is incorrect. Amyloidosis, or deposition of misfolded protein fibers, is not associated with the dwarfism, coarse facial features, or mental impairment exhibited by this patient.

E is incorrect. Accumulation of lysosomal glycogen occurs in Pompe's disease, when there is a deficiency of lysosomal acid maltase. The key features of Pompe's disease, hypotonia and muscle atrophy, do not include the coarse facial features, skeletal abnormalities, and corneal clouding observed with this patient.

9. Correct: D. Oxidative phase = Active; Nonoxidative/Regenerative phase = Favors formation of fructose 6-phosphate and glyceraldehyde 3-phosphate.

The oxidative phase of the pentose phosphate pathway has been actively generating NADPH and the nonoxidative phase has been generating fructose 6-phosphate and glyceraldehyde 3-phosphate. This boy most likely has diphtheria and his phagocytic white blood cells are fighting the bacterial infection. In order to kill the invading bacteria, the phagocytic white blood cells generate large quantities of hydroxyl and hypochlorite radicals in their phagolysosomes, as illustrated in the figure below.

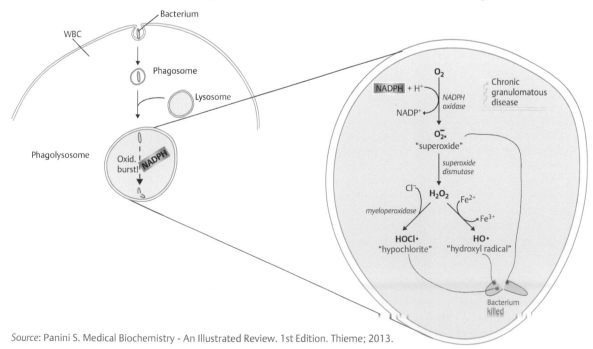

Source: Panini S. Medical Biochemistry - An Illustrated Review. 1st Edition. Thieme; 2013.

Generation of these radicals in the phagolysosomes requires the activity of NADPH oxidase, which utilizes large quantities of NADPH. Furthermore, the cells will use large quantities of NADPH to regenerate reduced glutathione (via the enzyme glutathione reductase), which is needed to neutralize free radicals that leak out of the phagolysosomes into the cytosol. White blood cells generate NADPH using the oxidative phase of the pentose phosphate pathway. For a review of the pentose phosphate pathway, see the figure below. The end products of the oxidative phase are NADPH and ribulose 5-phosphate. Because these cells have minimal need for nucleotides, the ribulose 5-phosphate will be used in the nonoxidative/regenerative phase to produce fructose 6-phosphate (F6P) and glyceraldehyde 3-phosphate (G3P). F6P and G3P can then either undergo gluconeogenesis to generate more glucose for the oxidative phase of the pentose phosphate pathway or undergo glycolysis to generate energy. Recall that the nonoxidative/regenerative phase of the pentose phosphate pathway can be run in "reverse" to generate ribose 5-phosphate from F6P and G3P under conditions where a cell might need to synthesize nucleotides, but not need the NADPH that would be generated by producing ribose 5-phosphate via the oxidative phase of the pentose phosphate pathway.

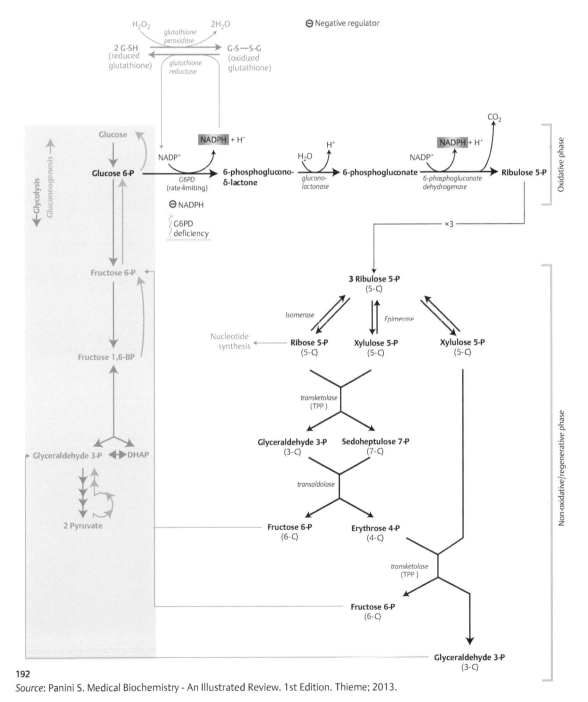

Source: Panini S. Medical Biochemistry - An Illustrated Review. 1st Edition. Thieme; 2013.

A is incorrect. The ribulose 5-phosphate generated in the oxidative phase is not needed for nucleotide synthesis. Therefore, it will become a substrate for the nonoxidative/regenerative phase of the pentose phosphate pathway.

B is incorrect. In order to generate large quantities of NADPH, the oxidative phase of the pentose phosphate pathway will be very active in the white blood cells.

C is incorrect. In order to generate large quantities of NADPH, the oxidative phase of the pentose phosphate pathway will be very active in the white blood cells.

E is incorrect. While it is true that the oxidative phase will be active in order to generate NADPH, the nonoxidative/regenerative phase will be running in the forward and not the reverse, direction. The nonoxidative/regenerative phase is only run in the reverse direction when cells have a high demand for nucleotide biosynthesis, which is not the case here.

F is incorrect. In order to generate large quantities of NADPH, the oxidative phase of the pentose phosphate pathway will be very active in the white blood cells.

10. Correct: B. Fasting hypoglycemia.

The most likely finding of those listed here is fasting hypoglycemia. Phosphorylase kinase catalyzes the phosphorylation of glycogen phosphorylase, thus activating the enzyme. (For a review of the regulation of glycogenolysis, see the figure below.) Deficiency in phosphorylase kinase is known as glycogen storage disease IX (GSD IX). If glycogen phosphorylase is not activated by phosphorylation, hepatocytes are unable to stimulate glycogenoloysis in response to signals generated by epinephrine or glucagon. Thus, less glycogen is hydrolyzed in response to fasting or stimulation of the fight-or-flight response. Notably, the fasting hypoglycemia observed in individuals with hepatic phosphorylase kinase deficiency or glycogen phosphorylase deficiency is generally mild; the liver is most likely able to compensate for these deficiencies utilizing gluconeogenesis. The hepatomegaly observed in these patients is due to accumulation of glycogen.

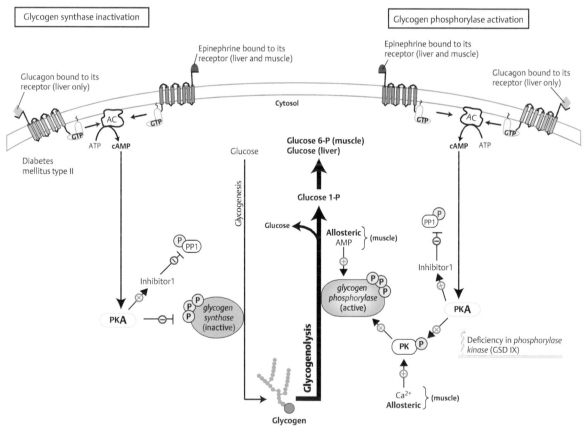

Source: Panini S. Medical Biochemistry - An Illustrated Review. 1st Edition. Thieme; 2013.

A is incorrect. Hepatocellular lysosomal accumulation is observed in Pompe's disease, which results from a deficiency in lysosomal α-glucosidase (also known as acid maltase).

C is incorrect. A defect in glycogenolysis, as occurs in phosphorylase kinase deficiency, will generally have little effect on cholesterol metabolism. The exception is von Gierke's disease (GSD I), where a deficiency in glucose 6-phosphatase results in hepatic accumulation of glucose. The excess glucose can be converted to triglycerides and cholesterol, resulting in hyperlipidemia.

D is incorrect. A deficiency in glycogenolysis, as this patient has, will result in *accumulation* of hepatic glycogen.

E is incorrect. This patient's defect in glycogenolysis will not adversely affect lipid metabolism and the ability to generate ketone bodies on the fasted state.

11. Correct: A. Glucose 6-phosphate dehydrogenase.

Patients with known deficiencies in glucose 6-phosphate dehydrogenase (G6PDH) should not be administered rasburicase. The reaction catalyzed by urate oxidase produces hydrogen peroxide, a free radical generator that induces oxidative stress. Drugs that induce oxidative stress are contraindicated in patients with glucose G6PDH deficiency. In the pentose phosphate pathway, G6PDH catalyzes the oxidation of glucose 6-phosphate, with concomitant reduction of $NADP^+$ to NADPH. Individuals with G6PDH deficiency are not able to generate enough NADPH to protect erythrocytes from abnormal levels of oxidative stress. The increased oxidative stress results in oxidation of hemoglobin, which forms Heinz bodies. Elimination of these damaged erythrocytes in the reticuloendothelial system can result in anemia.

B is incorrect. An individual with a deficiency in xanthine oxidase would have an impaired ability to degrade purine nucleotides to uric acid. They would be less likely to develop TLS and would not be adversely affected by treatment with rasburicase.

C is incorrect. Humans do not express urate oxidase. Urate (i.e., uric acid) is the end product of purine metabolism and is eliminated in the urine.

D is incorrect. Hypoxanthine-guanine phosphoribosyltransferase (HGPRT) participates in the purine salvage pathway. Defects in HGPRT are associated with Lesch–Nyhan and Kelley–Seegmiller syndromes. In these syndromes, purines accumulate that result in hyperuricemia. If anything, these individuals might benefit from rasburicase treatment.

E is incorrect. Individuals with a glucose 6-phosphatase deficiency (aka von Gierke disease) may develop hyperuricemia as a result of the disease and thus would potentially *benefit* from treatment with rasburicase. Recall that accumulation of glucose 6-phosphate in hepatocytes of individuals with glucose 6-phosphatase deficiency may result in depletion of intracellular phosphate. Phosphate depletion, in turn, can cause impaired phosphorylation of ADP, resulting in elevated levels of AMP, which is degraded in to uric acid. Be careful not to confuse glucose 6-phosphatase with glucose 6-phosphate dehydrogenase, the correct answer to this question.

12. Correct: B. Sodium-dependent glucose transporter 1.

This drug most likely inhibits sodium-dependent glucose transporter 1. The data indicate that LX4211 decreases postprandial serum glucose levels. This could be accomplished by inhibiting intestinal uptake of dietary glucose, activating glucose uptake in hepatic and extrahepatic tissues (directly, or by increasing pancreatic insulin secretion), or by stimulating renal secretion of glucose. Of the choices listed here, only inhibition of sodium-dependent glucose transporter 1 will accomplish one of these goals. The rate of intestinal absorption of all sources of dietary glucose will be decreased if LX4211 inhibits the sodium-dependent glucose transporter 1 (SLGT-1), which moves glucose from the intestinal lumen into enterocytes. For a review of the various glucose transporters, see the figure on the following page. Notably, LX4211 also has significant inhibitory activity against the sodium-dependent glucose transporter 2, which is located in renal proximal tubular cells. Inhibition of this transporter impairs renal resorption of glucose, thus further decreasing serum glucose concentrations.

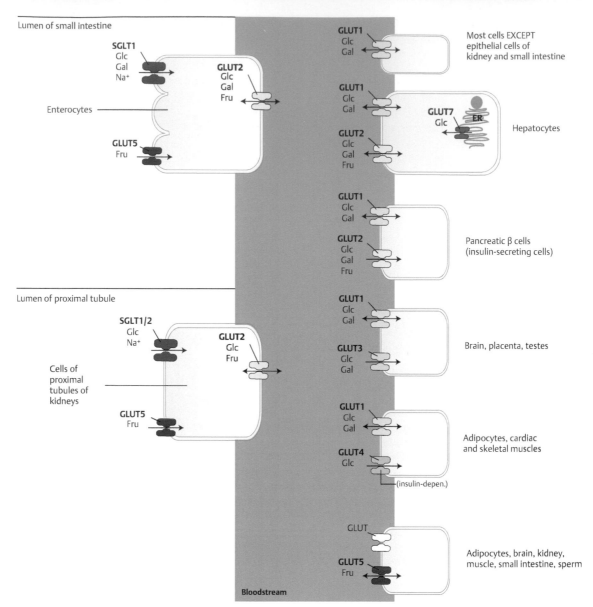

Source: Panini S. Medical Biochemistry - An Illustrated Review. 1st Edition. Thieme; 2013.

A is incorrect. Although inhibition of lactase would decrease absorption of glucose obtained from digestion of dietary lactose, a lactase inhibitor would be a poor choice to treat type II diabetes. The amount of dietary glucose derived from lactose is minor, compared to that obtained from other dietary carbohydrates in most individuals. Furthermore, inhibition of lactase could induce the side effects like those seen in lactose intolerance (i.e., bloating, flatulence, and diarrhea).

C is incorrect. Inhibition of glucose transporter 4 (GLUT4) would have the opposite effect of what is observed with LX2411 treatment, as movement of glucose from the serum into myocytes and adipocytes would be impaired.

D is incorrect. Although inhibition of sucrase would decrease absorption of glucose obtained from digestion of dietary sucrose, a sucrase inhibitor would be a poor choice to treat type II diabetes. The amount of dietary glucose derived from sucrose is minor, compared to that obtained from other dietary carbohydrates in most individuals.

E is incorrect. Glucose transporter 3 (GLUT 3) facilitates diffusion of glucose from the serum into the brain, placenta, and testes. Inhibition of this transporter would, if anything, slightly increase serum glucose concentrations.

13. Correct: B. Cataracts, due to accumulation of galactitol in the eye.

This child is likely to develop cataracts if he ingests lactose. The physician's restriction of lactose metabolism could be in response to a diagnosis of either lactose intolerance or galactosemia. The symptoms of jaundice and seizures are compatible with galactosemia. (Futhermore, lactose intolerance is currently not part of newborn screening panels.) Recall that lactose is digested to galactose and glucose. Galactosemia results from accumulation of galactose in the serum due to an inability to metabolize it. The more severe form of galactosemia is due to a deficiency in galactose 1-phosphate uridyltransferase (GALT) activity. For a review of galactose metabolism and galactosemia, see the figure below. GALT deficiency results in accumulation of galactose 1-phosphate in tissues,

causing damage to the liver and nervous system, particularly. A less severe form of galactosemia results from galactokinase deficiency. In patients with either GALT or galactokinase deficiency, galactose accumulates in the serum and tissues. Accumulated galactose can be reduced to galactitol by aldose reductase. In the lens of the eye, the resulting osmolar imbalance can result in formation of cataracts.

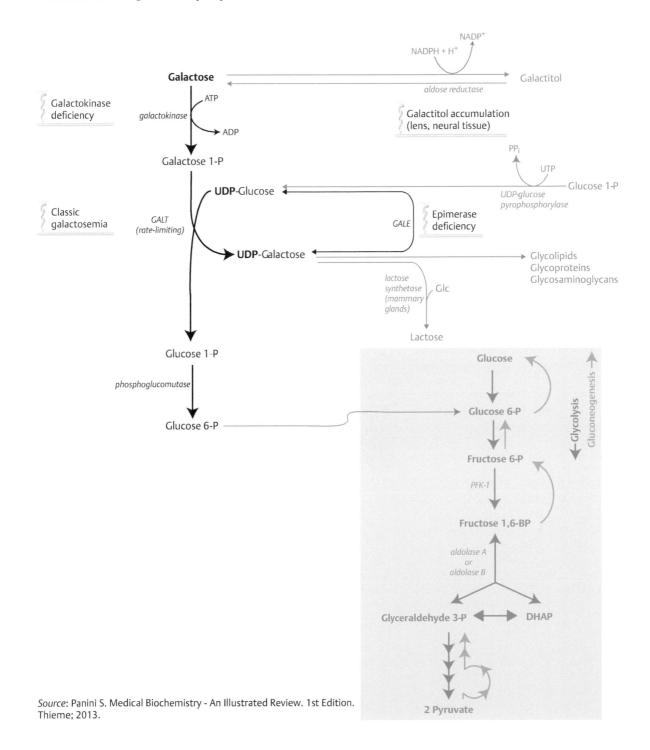

Source: Panini S. Medical Biochemistry - An Illustrated Review. 1st Edition. Thieme; 2013.

A is incorrect. This infant does not have lactose intolerance. His symptoms are too severe and are indicative of a defect in galactose metabolism.

C is incorrect. While galactosemia can cause hepatomegaly, the cause of the hepatomegaly is, in part, due to accumulation of glycogen due to inhibition of glycogen phosphorylase by accumulated galactose 1-phosphate. Galactose is not incorporated into glycogen.

D is incorrect. While untreated galactosemia can result in severe mental retardation, the cause of the neurological damage is linked to osmolar imbalance and accumulation of cytotoxic galactose 1-phosphate. Lysosomal accumulation of undigested glycolipids is not a factor.

14.   Correct: D. Glycogen phosphorylase.

Activation of glycogen phosphorylase stimulates the rapid generation of ATP needed during this lift. During the lift, the athlete's muscle is being stimulated by epinephrine. Furthermore, Ca^{+2} ions are being released from the myosarcoplasmic reticulum and the ATP/ADP ratio in myocytes is decreasing. All of these factors contribute to the activation of glycogen phosphorylase, as illustrated in the figure Answer 10. Binding of epinephrine to its receptor activates protein kinase A, which phosphorylates and activates phosphorylase kinase, which in turn phosphorylates and activates glycogen phosphorylase. Cytosolic Ca^{+2} also activates phosphorylase kinase. In addition, increased cytosolic [AMP] allosterically activates glycogen phosphorylase. Glycogenolysis provides glucose for ATP production in the muscle. At the beginning of the lift, some ATP will be generated from phosphocreatine, but the amount of ATP generated by that mechanism will not be able to power the entire lift.

A is incorrect. Activation of myocyte phosphofructokinase-2 and thus activation of glycolysis, is stimulated by insulin. (Recall that phosphofructokinase-2 catalyzes the formation of fructose 2,6-bisphosphate, an allosteric activator of phosphofructokinase-1.) Insulin regulates glucose metabolism in response to changes in serum glucose levels. It does not stimulate glucose metabolism in response to increased muscular work.

B is incorrect. Glucokinase is the liver isoform of hexokinase. It is stimulated by increased hepatic concentrations of glucose; its function will not influence ATP production in working muscle tissue.

C is incorrect. Triose phosphate isomerase catalyzes an equilibrium reaction in the glycolytic pathway. Its activity is not regulated.

E is incorrect. GLUT4 controls entry of glucose into myocytes. The number of GLUT4 transporters in muscle tissue is regulated largely by insulin, which stimulates the fusion of cytosolic microvesicles that sequester GLUT4 with the plasma membrane, thus enabling the tranporters to facilitate glucose uptake. The number for GLUT4 transporters in the athlete's muscle tissue will not change during the time it take him to lift the weight.

15.   Correct: B. Increased activity of aldose reductase.

The development of cataracts in this diabetic patient is due at least in part to increased activity of aldose reductase, the first enzyme in the polyol pathway. Under hyperglycemic conditions, glucose reaches high concentrations in cells, such as those of the lens, that have unregulated glucose uptake. When glucose levels are high enough, glucose is converted to sorbitol by aldose reductase, which has a very high K_m value for glucose. Because the second enzyme in the pathway, sorbitol dehydrogenase, is not present in the lens, sorbitol increases to high intracellular concentrations. The increased osmolality triggers the influx of water, resulting in swelling and subsequent tissue damage. Increased activity of aldose reductase also depletes cellular NADPH concentrations, thus also potentially increasing levels of oxidative stress. The consequences of increased aldose reductase activity may also contribute significantly to the development of retinopathy, neuropathy, and nephropathy found in diabetic patients.

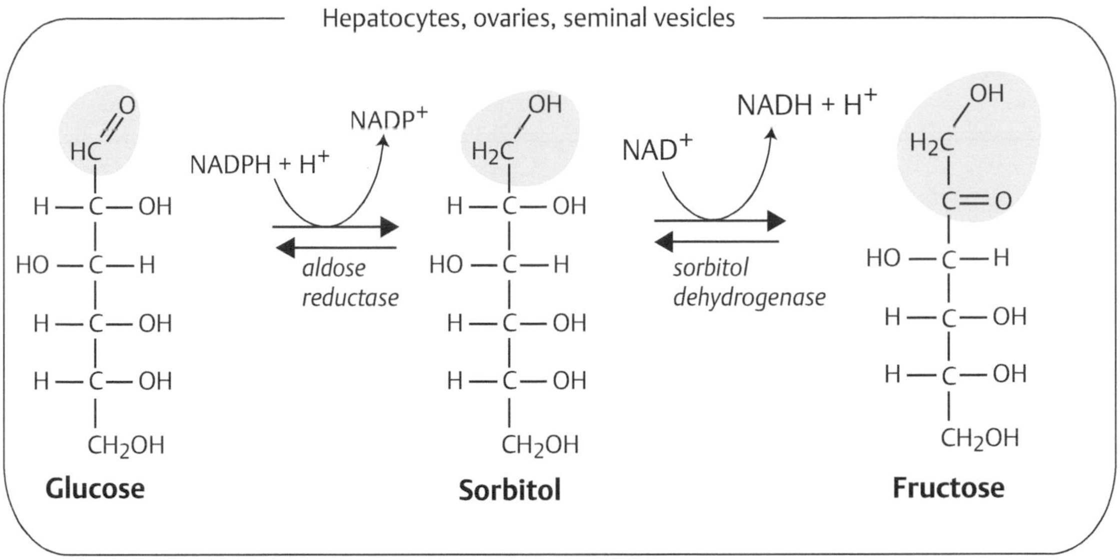

Hepatocytes, ovaries, seminal vesicles

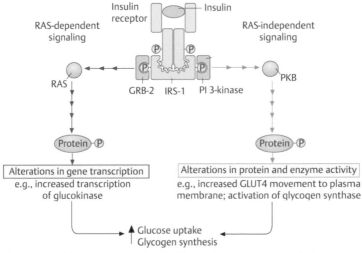

Glucose   **Sorbitol**   **Fructose**

Source: Panini S. Medical Biochemistry - An Illustrated Review. 1st Edition. Thieme; 2013.

A is incorrect. Increased activity of phosphofructokinase-2 results in increased concentrations of fructose 2,6-bisphosphate, an allosteric activator of phosphofructokinase-1. This is one process by which insulin stimulates glycolysis. Stimulation of glycolysis has no bearing on the development of cataracts. Furthermore, patients with type II diabetes have impaired response to insulin.

C is incorrect. Galactitol is the product of reduction of galactose by aldose reductase. It accumulates in the lens of patients with galactosemia and causes cataracts. This patient most likely has developed cataracts as a result of his diabetes, and not galactosemia.

D is incorrect. Decreased activity of glucose 6-phosphate dehydrogenase, the first enzyme in the oxidative phase of the pentose phosphate pathway, results in oxidative stress and Heinz body formation in the erythrocytes of individuals who consume certain oxidizing drugs or fava beans and are deficient in the enzyme and consume certain oxidizing medications or fava beans.

E is incorrect. The development of cataracts is not linked to altered neuronal function.

16. Correct: C. Increased risk for development of type II diabetes.

Individuals with the G972R IRS-1 polymorphism have increased risk for the development of type II diabetes. The staining pattern on the western blot indicates that phosphorylation of tyrosine residues on WT IRS-1 increases over time when IRS-1 is incubated with active insulin receptor and ATP. The extent of phosphorylation is significantly reduced with G972R IRS-1 under the same conditions. Phosphorylation of IRS-1 by activated insulin receptor is a key step in the insulin signaling pathway. (For a review of the insulin signaling pathway, see the figure below.) The G972R mutation impairs this process, thus reducing the cellular response to insulin. Individuals with this polymorphism have decreased sensitivity to insulin and are thus more likely to develop insulin resistance and type II diabetes.

Source: Panini S. Medical Biochemistry - An Illustrated Review. 1st Edition. Thieme; 2013.

A is incorrect. The G972R polymorphism results in decreased activation of IRS-1 and thus a decreased cellular response to insulin. Glycogen synthesis is stimulated by insulin; therefore, this polymorphism would hinder, rather than enhance, glycogen storage.

B is incorrect. Pancreatic insulin secretion will not be affected by this mutation; secretion of insulin is not regulated by binding of insulin to its receptors.

D is incorrect. The G972R polymorphism results in decreased activation of IRS-1 and thus a decreased cellular response to insulin. This would result in decreased hepatic glycogen storage. However, in the fasting state there is little risk of severe hypoglycemia, as gluconeogenesis will be stimulated. Although glycogen stores would be lower than normal, sufficient blood glucose will still be generated.

17.   Correct: C. Glucose transporter 4 (GLUT4) is sequestered in microvesicles.

GLUT4 is sequestered in microvesicles to a greater extent in this patient than in someone with a lower HbA1c level. This individual's elevated fasting serum glucose and HbA1c levels indicate that she has diabetes. Her lack of insulin, if she has type I diabetes, or her insensitivity to insulin, if she has type II diabetes, results in decreased uptake of glucose by myocytes.

GLUT4 is the primary transporter of glucose across myocyte, cardiomyocyte, and adipocyte membranes. It is stored in microvesicles that fuse with the plasma membrane in response to stimulation of the insulin signaling cascade, as illustrated in the figure below. In diabetic individuals, this cascade is not stimulated, so the GLUT4 transporters remain sequestered in microvesicles in the cytosol. The impaired uptake of glucose by myocytes and adipocytes contributes significantly to the elevation of serum glucose in diabetic individuals.

A is incorrect. Although GLUT4 is, indeed, the primary glucose transporter in myocytes, it is not regulated allosterically.

B is incorrect. GLUT1 is a ubiquitous transporter found in most cells except epithelial cells of the kidney and small intestine. Although it is present in myocytes, its function is not regulated allosterically or any other mechanism stimulated by insulin.

D is incorrect. GLUT2 is the main glucose transporter found in the liver. Its activity is independent of glucose.

E is incorrect. GLUT1 is a ubiquitous transporter found in most cells except epithelial cells of the kidney and small intestine. Although it is present in myocytes, its function is not regulated by phosphorylation or any other mechanism stimulated by insulin.

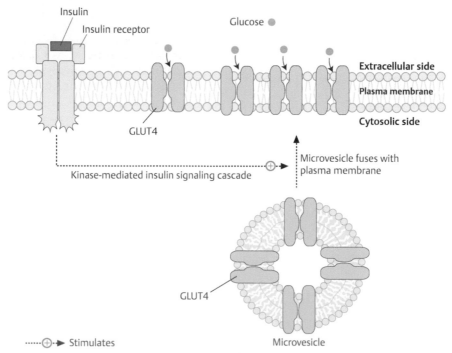

Source: Panini S. Medical Biochemistry - An Illustrated Review. 1st Edition. Thieme; 2013.

18. Correct: E. Lactase.

This patient most likely has decreased lactase activity. Her recent chemotherapy treatment, which can sometimes result in long-term damage to intestinal enterocytes, along with her symptoms of bloating, flatulence, and diarrhea, are consistent with a diagnosis of secondary lactose intolerance. Her damaged enterocytes are not producing enough lactase—a transmembrane protein located on the luminal surface of intestinal enterocytes—to digest the lactose that she is consuming in her diet. The undigested lactose presents an osmotic load in her intestinal lumen, resulting in diarrhea. Bacterial fermentation of the lactose generates methane and hydrogen gases that contribute to her bloating and flatulence.

A is incorrect. Pepsin is a gastric protease. Pepsin deficiency is not a known side effect of cancer chemotherapy. Furthermore, protease deficiencies are not associated with flatulence, bloating, and diarrhea.

B is incorrect. α-Amylase can be produced by either the salivary glands or the pancreas. Its function is to hydrolyze dietary starch, forming oligosaccharides. Treatment with cancer chemotherapeutics is much more likely to damage rapidly dividing intestinal enterocytes than the pancreatic cells that produce α-amylase.

C is incorrect. Pancreatic lipase production is unlikely to be impaired following treatment with cancer chemotherapeutic agents. Furthermore, a deficiency in pancreatic lipase would impair digestion of dietary lipids, resulting in steatorrhea rather than diarrhea.

D is incorrect. Galactokinase catalyzes the intracellular phosphorylation of galactose. A deficiency in this enzyme results in accumulation of galactose and galactitol in the serum and tissues. It does not cause the intestinal symptoms described here.

19. Correct: E. Glucose Alanine = Increase; Fructose = Decrease; 2,6-bisphosphate = Decrease.

Glucose will be generated, alanine will be consumed, and intercellular fructose 2,6-bisphosphate concentrations will decline. Forskolin, an activator of adenylate cyclase, will mimic many of the effects of glucagon on hepatocytes. (Recall that the glucagon receptor is a G-protein coupled receptor that stimulates the activity of adenylate cyclase.) The resulting increase in intracellular cAMP levels activates protein kinase A (PKA) which, among other things, phosphorylates and activates enzymes involved in gluconeogenesis and glycogenolysis. Thus, we would expect that the concentration of glucose in the media would rise, and alanine, a precursor for gluconeogenesis, would fall. The phosphofructokinase-2/fructose bisphosphatase-2 (PFK-2/FBPase-2) bifunctional enzyme is one of the substrates for PKA. (For a review, see the figure on the following page.) The phosphorylated form of PFK-2/FBPase-2 has elevated FBPase activity, thus resulting in increased hydrolysis of fructose 2,6-bisphosphate (F26BP), and subsequently a decrease in

intracellular concentrations of F26BP. F26BP is an allosteric activator of phosphofructokinase-1 and an allosteric inhibitor of fructose 1,6-bisphosphatase. F26BP thus stimulates glycolysis and inhibits gluconeogenesis. When cellular concentrations of F26BP fall, phosphofructokinase-1 activity decreases and fructose 1,6-bisphosphatase activity increases, thus impairing glycolysis and stimulating gluconeogenesis.

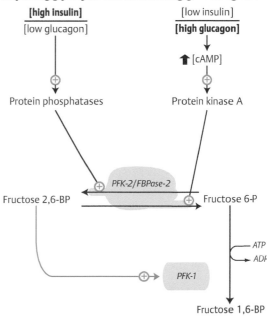

Source: Panini S. Medical Biochemistry - An Illustrated Review. 1st Edition. Thieme; 2013.

A is incorrect. Although an increase in glucose concentration is expected, as gluconeogenesis and glycogenolysis will be stimulated, we would expect a decrease in alanine and fructose 2,6-bisphosphate concentrations.

B, D, and F are incorrect. Because forskolin increases intracellular cAMP concentrations, an increase in gluconeogenesis and glycogenolysis are expected. This would result in increased glucose concentration in the media.

C is incorrect. Although an increase in glucose concentration and a decrease in alanine concentration is expected with stimulation of gluconeogenesis and glycogenolysis by forskolin, we would also expect a decrease in fructose 2,6-bisphosphate concentrations.

20. Correct: A. Hexokinase.

The dark spots indicate accumulation of FDG, which occurs due to increased activity of hexokinase in tumor cells relative to noncancerous cells. FDG enters cells through glucose transporters and mixes with intracellular glucose. It is a substrate for hexokinase, which phosphorylates FDG at a rate proportional to the rate of glycolysis in the cell. FDG 6-phosphate is not significantly metabolized further, as it is not a substrate for the various glucose 6-phosphate-utilizing enzymes. FDG 6-phosphate also cannot be transported across cell membranes and thus accumulates in the cytosol. Tumor cells have significantly higher metabolic flux of glucose through glycolysis than do healthy cells. Thus, their hexokinase activity is elevated and FDG 6-phosphate will accumulate.

B is incorrect. The tissues that accumulate FDG and thus appear dark on the PET scan, do not express GLUT4. Myocytes, cardiomyocytes, and adipocytes are the primary cells that utilize GLUT4. Furthermore, increased activity of GLUT4 would not necessarily result in accumulation of FDG, as the form of FDG that accumulates intracellularly is FDG 6-phosphate.

C is incorrect. Glycogen synthase activity is not elevated in tumor cells relative to normal; tumor cells have increased flux of glucose through glycolysis and do not store excess glycogen. Furthermore, FDG 6-phosphate is not a substrate for phosphoglucomutase, which catalyzes the first step in glycogen synthesis.

D is incorrect. Pyruvate dehydrogenase activity is generally not elevated in tumor cells, which rely on increased flux of glucose through the glycolytic pathway to generate precursors for biosynthetic pathways.

E is incorrect. Phosphoglucomutase activity is not elevated in tumor cells relative to normal; tumor cells have increased flux of glucose through glycolysis and do not store excess glycogen. Furthermore, FDG 6-phosphate is not a substrate for phosphoglucomutase, which catalyzes the first step in glycogen synthesis.

Chapter 7

Fatty Acid Metabolism and Lipid Digestion

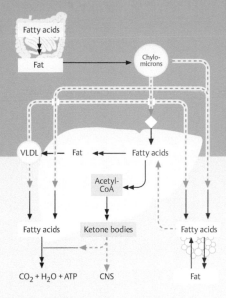

LEARNING OBJECTIVES

▶ Describe the digestion of triglycerides and cholesterol, knowing the names of key digestive enzymes and the general process of chylomicron formation.

▶ Explain the mechanisms and hormonal regulation of adipocyte triglyceride storage and lipolysis.

▶ Describe the mechanism for activation and transport of fatty acids into mitochondria for catabolism.

▶ Outline the sequence of reactions that occur during fatty acid oxidation, and the modifications that occur to accommodate unsaturated, branched-chain, and odd-chain fatty acids.

▶ Explain the mechanism and regulation of ketone body synthesis.

▶ Describe the overall purpose of fatty acid synthesis, its reactants and products, key enzymes, cellular location, and its tissue distribution.

▶ Describe the processes for synthesis of triglycerides and glycerophospholipids.

▶ Identify the composition of different sphingolipids and explain how specific enzyme deficiencies can result in sphingolipidoses.

▶ Describe the roles of dietary ω-3 and ω-6 fatty acids in the synthesis of eicosanoids, knowing the names and functions of key enzymes in the synthesis of prostaglandins, thromboxanes, and leukotrienes, and the actions of steroidal and nonsteroidal anti-inflammatory drugs in these pathways.

▶ Evaluate the metabolic effects and clinical significance of ethanol, methanol, ethylene glycol, and their metabolites.

7.1 Questions

Easy	Medium	Hard

1. Many infant formulas advertise that they are supplemented with ω-3 fatty acids and choline for optimal brain development. Which of the following is the best rationale for including choline in infant formula?

A. It is an important antioxidant

B. It is needed for synthesis of sphingomyelin

C. It is needed for the synthesis of glycoproteins

D. It is used as a methylating agent for synthesis of several neurotransmitters

E. It is a component of several neuropeptides

2. Television personality Dr. Oz claims that extracts of garcinia cambogia, a tamarind-like fruit grown in Southeast Asia, are a "magic" weight loss aid. The active ingredient is hydroxycitrate, which inhibits citrate lyase. Which of the following best explains how the extract might promote weight loss?

A. It inhibits digestion of dietary fats

B. It inhibits uptake and storage of triglycerides in adipocytes

C. It stimulates lipolysis of triglycerides in adipocytes

D. It inhibits conversion of dietary carbohydrates to fatty acids

E. It inhibits carbohydrate metabolism, thus stimulating fatty acid oxidation

3. The 9-year-old son of Nigerian immigrants is brought to the emergency department with severe epigastric pain, vomiting, tachychardia, paresthesia, and in a disturbed mental state. His parents are concerned that the boy may have eaten some of the unripe ackee fruit that they brought home with them from a recent trip to West Africa. Unripe ackee fruit is known to contain a toxin that is metabolized to compounds that irreversibly inhibit carnitine palmitoyltransferase I and acyl-CoA dehydrogenases. If the boy has indeed ingested unripe ackee fruit, which of the following will be observed in his laboratory results?

A. Ketoacidosis

B. Hyperuricemia

C. Hypoglycemia

D. Hyperinsulinemia

E. Dicarboxylic aciduria

4. A 20-year-old girl has a 5-year history of asthma and chronic rhinosinusitis that she successfully treats with corticosteroids and over-the-counter oral decongestants. She complains to her primary care physician that her respiratory symptoms have worsened significantly in the last week. She also mentions that these new symptoms seem to have started around the same time that she experienced a severe ankle sprain while playing tennis. Further questioning by her physician reveals that this patient has been using ibuprofen to treat her ankle pain. An increase in the concentration of which of the following substances is most likely contributing to this patient's worsening symptoms?

A. Thromboxane A_2

B. Prostaglandin I_2

C. Lysophospholipid

D. Prostaglandin H_2

E. Arachidonic acid

5. A 54-year-old homeless veteran is brought to the emergency room after she collapsed on the sidewalk outside of a local bar. Physical examination revealed nystagmus, ataxia, and slurred speech. Initial laboratory results showed an elevated blood ethanol level and metabolic acidosis. Which of the following contributes to metabolic acidosis in this patient?

A. Decreased activity of isocitrate dehydrogenase in hepatocytes

B. Increased activity of lactate dehydrogenase in myocytes

C. Uncoupling of oxidative phosphorylation in all cell types

D. Increased activity of the microsomal ethanol oxidizing system (MEOS)

E. Increased activity of fatty acyl-CoA dehydrogenases in hepatocytes

6. Ingesting alcoholic beverages within hours to days of consuming the mushroom *Coprinus ataramentarius* (commonly known as inky cap) induces symptoms that include heart palpitations, flushing, headache, nausea, and vomiting. The illness has been traced to a molecule in the inky cap mushroom that has been appropriately named coprine. Which of the following enzymes does coprine most likely inhibit?

A. Alcohol dehydrogenase

B. CYP2E1

C. Cytochrome P450 reductase

D. Acetaldehyde dehydrogenase

E. Lactate dehydrogenase

7. A 12-year-old girl of Jewish Eastern European descent is brought to the emergency department after falling off her bicycle. X-rays reveal a broken hip. Given the patient's young age and the relatively benign nature of her accident, the attending physician obtains a thorough history and physical exam, during which he notes normal pediatric growth and development, but discovers that the girl has recently been complaining of fatigue and bone pain in her legs. He also detects significant hepatosplenomegaly, and orders a liver biopsy that provides the image shown in the figure below. Which of the following substances is accumulating in, and causing the unique appearance of, several of the macrophages in the image (see *black arrow*)?

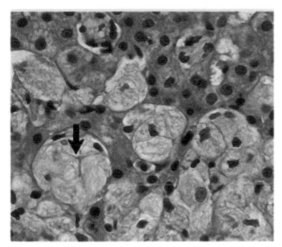

Source: Riede U, Werner M. Color Atlas of Pathology: Pathologic Principles · Associated Diseases · Sequela. 1st Edition. 2004.

A. Glycosaminoglycans
B. Glucocerebrosides
C. Proteoglycans
D. Glycerophospholipids
E. Glycogen

8. A 15-year-old girl with a known allergy to glucocorticoids presented to her physicians with complaints that her short-acting β2 agonist inhaler was no longer sufficient to control her intermittent asthma. Her physician prescribed a medication that would supplement the antibronchoconstrictive activity of the β2 agonist. What is the most likely mechanism by which the new drug acts?

A. It inhibits a cyclooxygenase
B. It stimulates linoleic acid synthesis
C. It inhibits a lipoxygenase
D. It stimulates isoprostane synthesis
E. It inhibits release of arachidonic acid

9. A 55-year-old woman with a history of hyperlipidemia and type II diabetes fasted for 12 hours prior to having blood drawn for a lipid panel. Her laboratory results indicated a serum triglyceride level of 320 mg/dL (normal is < 150 mg/dL). Diabetes-associated inhibition of which lipase activity contributes to her abnormal serum triglyceride level, and which lipoprotein particle most likely carries the majority of this patient's triglycerides?

	Lipase	Lipoprotein
A.	Hormone-sensitive lipase	VLDL
B.	Capillary lipoprotein lipase	VLDL
C.	Pancreatic lipase	VLDL
D.	Hormone-sensitive lipase	Chylomicron
E.	Capillary lipoprotein lipase	Chylomicron
F.	Pancreatic lipase	Chylomicron

10. A 22-year-old boy was referred to a neurologist with complaints of mild intermittent peripheral neuropathy for the last 2 years. In the last month, he had been experiencing difficulty with his balance, as well as a constant ringing sound in his ears and difficulty seeing at night. After analyzing the results of several diagnostic tests, the neurologist told the patient that he should eliminate milk products and fat obtained from cows, sheep, and goats from his diet. Within months, the most of the patient's symptoms were relieved. Which of the following substances was most likely elevated in this patient's serum at the time of diagnosis?

A. Pristanic acid
B. Oleic acid
C. Dicarboxylic acids
D. Cerotic acid
E. Phytanic acid

11. A 3-year-old boy is admitted to the emergency room with complaints of confusion, dizziness, and vomiting. His temperature, blood pressure, and pulse are normal, but he is hyperventilating. His parents report that they suspect that he consumed a toxic household substance approximately 8 hours ago. The following laboratory results were obtained:

	Patient	Normal
Arterial pCO_2	20 mm Hg	40 mm Hg
Arterial pH	7.20	7.35–7.45
Serum bicarbonate	12 mEq/L	19–24 mEq/L
Serum creatinine	1.3 mg/dL	0.5–1.0 mg/dL
BUN	27 mg/dL	5–20 mg/dL

The child has an elevated ion gap, and urinalysis reveals colorless crystals. Which of the following substances did the boy most likely consume?

A. Denatured ethanol

B. Dish soap

C. Ethylene glycol antifreeze

D. Philodendron leaves

E. Wood alcohol

Consider this vignette for questions 12 to 14.

A 15-month-old boy died suddenly of unexplained causes after exhibiting flu-like symptoms for 3 days. He had been born at home and had not been subject to newborn screening. Postmortem genetic testing revealed homozygosity for a mutation in the medium-chain acyl-CoA dehydrogenase (MCAD) gene.

12. If newborn screening had been performed on this child, levels of which of the following substances would have been detected at higher-than-normal levels in his blood sample?

A. β-hydroxybutyrate

B. Free carnitine

C. Octanoylcarnitine

D. Phenyllactate

E. Phytanic acid

13. Which of the following histological or gross anatomical finding would be expected on autopsy of this child?

A. Absence of peroxisomes in all tissues

B. Cardiovascular plaque accumulation

C. Cytoplasmic lysosomal vacuoles in all tissues

D. Demyelination of neurons

E. Fatty infiltration of the liver

14. If this child had been properly diagnosed as a result of newborn screening, which dietary therapy might have prevented his death?

A. A high fat, low carbohydrate diet

B. Avoidance of fasting

C. Elimination of dairy products

D. Elimination of medium-chain fatty acids

E. Supplementation with cobalamin

15. An 8-year-old boy with a history of epilepsy that is not well controlled pharmaceutically is placed on a special diet that is sometimes therapeutic in epileptic patients. After 2 weeks on the diet, the boy's serum ketone levels are about 10 times higher than they were before he started the diet. Which of the following enzyme activities is most likely stimulated in this patient?

A. Hormone sensitive lipase

B. Capillary lipoprotein lipase

C. HMG CoA reductase

D. Acetyl CoA carboxylase

E. Pyruvate dehydrogenase

16. A 55-year-old woman was recently diagnosed with rheumatoid arthritis. Her physician suggested that including at least two servings of salmon or halibut in her weekly diet might be beneficial in reducing her pain. Which of the following is the most likely mechanism of this effect?

A. Inhibition of COX-2

B. Increased production of resolvins and protectins

C. Increased production of prostaglandins

D. Reduction of oxidative stress

E. Inhibition of phospholipase A_2

17. A political prisoner has been on a hunger strike, consuming only water, for 10 days. His breath has developed a fruity odor. Depletion of which of the following metabolites in his hepatocytes contributes to the development of the fruity odor?

A. Acetyl CoA

B. Carnitine

C. Glycerol

D. NADH

E. Oxaloacetate

18. A 15-year-old boy presents at the urgent care center complaining of a sore throat and extreme weakness and muscle pain. His temperature is 101.5 °C. He indicates that his urine has been light brown for the last 18 hours. Further questioning reveals that he experienced a similar episode of muscle weakness and pain 2 years ago after hiking in the mountains for 6 hours. Some of his laboratory results are shown below.

	Patient	Normal
Leukocytes	18×10^9 /L	4.5–11×10^9/L
Creatine kinase	1500 U/L	25–90 U/L
Free carnitine, serum	15 µmol/L	30–50 µmol/L
Total carnitine, serum	80 µmol/L	25–69 µmol/L
Octanoylcarnitine	0.35 µmol/L	< 0.78 µmol/L
Palmitoylcarnitine	1.1 µmol/L	< 0.26 µmol/L

A deficiency in which of the following proteins is most likely the cause of this patient's muscle pain and weakness?

A. Na$^+$-dependent carnitine transporter protein

B. Carnitine palmitoyltransferase I

C. Carnitine palmitoyltransferase II

D. Medium-chain acyl-CoA dehydrogenase

E. Propionyl CoA carboxylase

19. A 15-year-old girl who had been diagnosed with cystic fibrosis at age 8 has recently begun losing weight. She complains of fatigue and large, foul-smelling stools. A deficiency in the activity of which of the following enzymes is most likely the cause of her symptoms?

A. Pancreatic lipase

B. α-amylase

C. Microsomal transfer protein

D. Pepsin

E. 7 α-hydroxylase

20. Several natural inhibitors of fatty acid synthase are being explored as potential chemotherapeutic agents, as increased dependence on fatty acid synthesis is a common feature of many neoplasms. Most of these fatty acid synthase inhibitors are cytotoxic because in addition to inhibiting fatty acid synthesis, they also impair cellular energy production. What is the most likely mechanism by which these inhibitors impair ATP synthesis?

A. They indirectly inhibit glycolysis

B. They indirectly inhibit β-oxidation

C. They indirectly inhibit TCA cycle function

D. They indirectly inhibit the electron transport chain

E. They indirectly inhibit ATP synthase

7.2 Answers and Explanations

Easy	Medium	Hard

1. Correct: B. It is needed for synthesis of sphingomyelin.

Choline is utilized in the synthesis of sphingomyelin. Initially, choline is used to produce phosphatidylcholine, as illustrated in the figure below (iA). (First, CDP-choline is formed, as shown in panel A, and then phosphatidylcholine is generated, as shown in panel B.) Phosphatidylcholine, in turn, provides the choline head group for sphingomyelin, an important neural membrane lipid found in particularly high concentrations in the myelin sheath. For a review of sphingolipid metabolism, see the figure on the following page (ii). In addition to its role in synthesis of phosphatidylcholine and sphingomyelin, choline is used in the synthesis of the neurotransmitter acetylcholine.

(i) **A** CDP-bound substrates

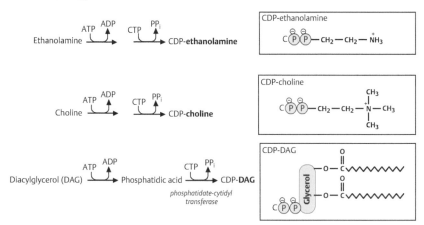

B Glycerophospholipid synthesis

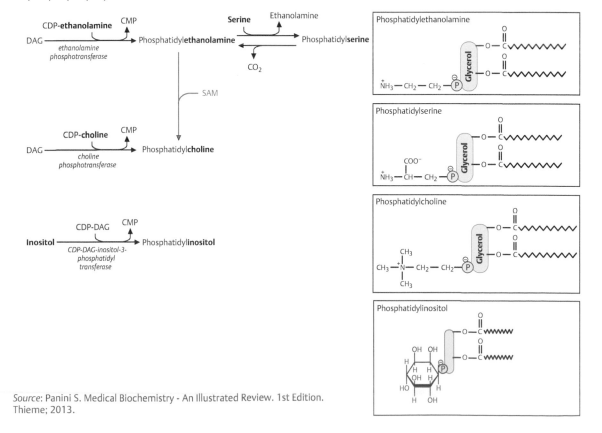

Source: Panini S. Medical Biochemistry - An Illustrated Review. 1st Edition. Thieme; 2013.

(ii) Synthesis/degradation of sphingomyelin and gangliosides

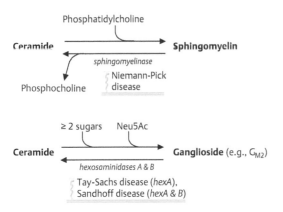

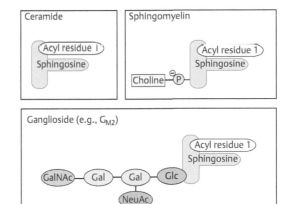

Synthesis/degradation of cerebrosides

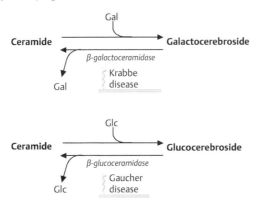

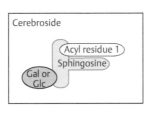

Synthesis/degradation of globosides

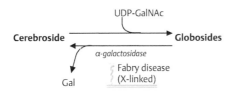

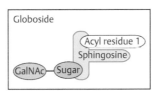

Synthesis/degradation of sulfatides

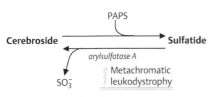

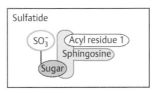

Source: Panini S. Medical Biochemistry - An Illustrated Review. 1st Edition. Thieme; 2013.

A is incorrect. Choline is not an antioxidant.

C is incorrect. Choline is not required for synthesis of glycoproteins.

D is incorrect. Although choline can be converted to betaine, which may be used as a methylating agent, this process occurs primarily in the liver. The predominant methylating agent for synthesis of neurotransmitters is *S*-adenosylmethionine.

E is incorrect. Neuropeptides are composed of amino acids. Choline is not an amino acid.

2. Correct: D. It inhibits conversion of dietary carbohydrates to fatty acids.

Hydroxycitrate potentially inhibits conversion of dietary carbohydrates to fatty acids. Citrate lyase (also known as ATP citrate lyase) catalyzes the cytosolic conversion of citrate to oxaloacetate and acetyl CoA in the citrate shuttle. (For a review of fatty acid synthsis, see the figure on the following page.) In the fed state, excess dietary carbohydrates are converted to acetyl CoA in the liver via glycolysis. The acetyl CoA, initially generated in the mitochondria, is condensed with mitochondrial oxaloacetate to form citrate, which is transported to the cytosol. In the cytosol, citrate lyase converts the citrate back to oxaloacetate and acetyl CoA. Cytosolic acetyl CoA is then used for the synthesis of fatty acid chains, which are incorporated into triglycerides for storage in adipocytes. Inhibiting citrate lyase should, then, decrease the rate of conversion of dietary carbohydrates to fatty acids.

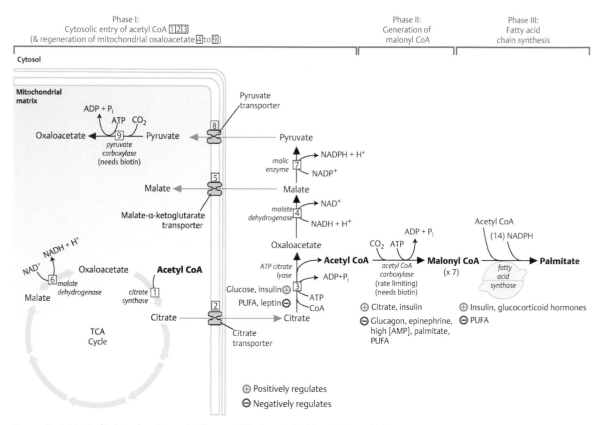

Source: Panini S. Medical Biochemistry - An Illustrated Review. 1st Edition. Thieme; 2013.

A is incorrect. Citrate lyase does not participate in the digestive process.

B is incorrect. Uptake and storage of triglycerides in adipocytes is mediated by several proteins, including Apo-CII and lipoprotein lipase, but not citrate lyase.

C is incorrect. Lipolysis of triglycerides in adipocytes is mediated primarily by hormone sensitive lipase.

E is incorrect. Citrate lyase does not participate in the oxidation of carbohydrates to generate energy; inhibiting its activity will not stimulate oxidation of fatty acids.

3. Correct: C. Hypoglycemia.

This child will be severely hypoglycemic. Carnitine palmitoyltransferase I (CPT I) facilitates the transport of fatty acids into mitochondria, where they are oxidized to acetyl-CoA in the β-oxidation spiral. Acyl-CoA dehydrogenases (there are four types of acyl-CoA dehydrogenases that act on fatty acids of different chain lengths) catalyze the first step in the β-oxidation spiral. For a review of fatty acid activation and transport, see the figure below. Inhibition of CPT I and acyl-CoA dehydrogenases, then, will severely impair the body's ability to generate energy via the oxidation of fatty acids. Furthermore, inhibition of fatty acid oxidation results in decreased ketone body synthesis. Thus, an individual who consumes the toxin found in unripe ackee fruit will rely extensively on glucose for energy production. They will become severely hypoglycemic because body tissues are consuming primarily glucose for energy. Hypoglycemia is further exacerbated by the liver's inability to utilize fatty acids to generate energy for gluconeogenesis.

A is incorrect. Inhibition of CPT I and acyl-CoA dehydrogenases will impair fatty acid oxidation, and thus also *decrease* synthesis of ketone bodies.

B is incorrect. Hyperuricemia is caused by conditions that either increase purine degradation or inhibit renal elimination of uric acid. Neither of these conditions are triggered by the inactivation of fatty acid oxidation, as occurs when the activities of CPT I and acyl-CoA dehydrogenases are inhibited.

D is incorrect. Inhibition of fatty acid oxidation, as occurs when the activities of CPT I and acyl-CoA dehyrogenases are impaired, will result in decreased serum glucose levels. This will, in turn, cause a decrease in pancreatic secretion of insulin, and an increase in glucagon secretion.

E is incorrect. Dicarboxylic acids appear in the urine when ω-oxidation of fatty acids increases. Generally, this occurs when oxidation of medium-chain fatty acids is impaired due to a deficiency in the medium-chain acyl-CoA dehydrogenase and the accumulated medium-chain fatty acids become substrates for ω-oxidation in the endoplasmic reticulum. In the case described here, inhibition of CPT I and all of the acyl-CoA dehydrogenases, will result in a severe *decrease* in intracellular fatty acid levels; ω-oxidation will not be stimulated.

Transport of long-chain fatty acids (13-20 C) into mitochondrial matrix

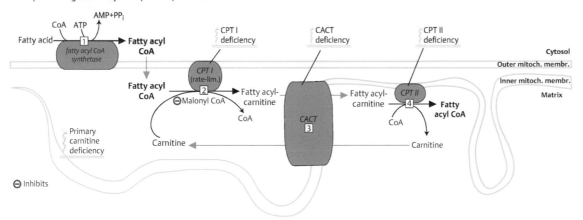

Source: Panini S. Medical Biochemistry - An Illustrated Review. 1st Edition. Thieme; 2013.

4. Correct: E. Arachidonic acid.

This patient's asthmatic symptoms are most likely being exacerbated by an increased arachidonic acid concentration. Nonsteroidal anti-inflammatory drugs (NSAIDS), such as ibuprofen, inhibit the cyclooxygenase (COX) activity of prostaglandin H_2 synthase (PGH synthase). As illustrated in the figure on the following page, inhibition of PGH synthase results in decreased synthesis of various prostaglandins that mediate inflammation and the pain response. Decreased PGH synthase activity, however, also results in accumulation of its substrate, arachidonic acid. In some individuals, the excess arachidonic acid is readily converted by lipoxygenases and leukotriene synthases in myeloid cells to leukotrienes that stimulate constriction of pulmonary airways. Approximately 20% of asthmatics are susceptible to NSAID-induced asthma.

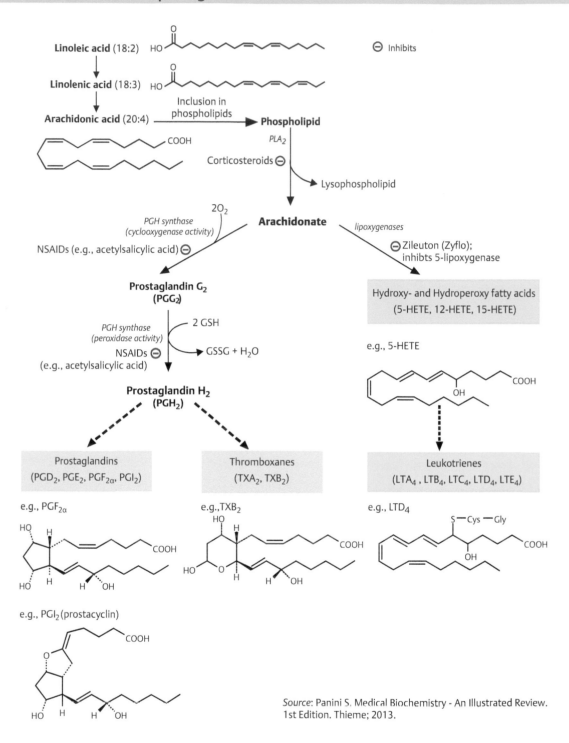

Source: Panini S. Medical Biochemistry - An Illustrated Review. 1st Edition. Thieme; 2013.

A, B, and D are incorrect. NSAIDS inhibit PGH$_2$ synthase, and thus will *decrease* levels of PGH$_2$, the metabolite from which thromboxanes and prostaglandins are derived.

C is incorrect. Lysophospholipid and a free fatty acid chain (usually arachidonic acid) are the two products of the reaction catalyzed by phospholipase A$_2$ (PLA$_2$). Arachidonic acid is the substrate for PGH synthase (the enzyme inhibited by NSAIDS), and the precursor of the series 2 prostaglandins and thromboxanes, as well as many leukotrienes. Lysophospholipids may be converted back to glycerophospholipids, or may play a role in cell signaling. Inhibition of COX activity by the NSAIDS will have little, if any, effect on lysophospholipid levels.

5. Correct: A. Decreased activity of isocitrate dehydrogenase in hepatocytes.

Decreased activity of hepatic isocitrate dehydrogenase is slowing the TCA cycle, thus causing metabolic acidosis in this patient. Ethanol is rapidly oxidized in the liver, via alcohol dehydrogenase and acetaldehyde dehydrogenase, generating a large NADH/NAD$^+$

ratio. (For a review of the acute effects of ethanol, see the figure below.) The large NADH/NAD$^+$ ratio inhibits the NAD$^+$-requiring enzymes, including isocitrate dehydrogenase, in the citric acid cycle. As the citric acid cycle function declines, acetyl CoA begins to accumulate in hepatocytes, and is converted to ketone bodies. Because extrahepatic tissues preferentially utilize the acetate that is generated in the liver by ethanol oxidation, their metabolism of ketone bodies is restricted. This results in alcoholic ketoacidosis. Note that the high NADH/NAD$^+$ ratio also impairs the ability of hepatic lactate dehydrogenase to oxidize lactate to pyruvate, a necessary step in gluconeogenesis. The result of this inability to oxidize lactate to pyruvate in the liver further contributes to acidosis by increasing serum lactate levels. The resulting decrease in flux of lactate/pyruvate through gluconeogenesis contributes to the hypoglycemia observed in individuals who consume alcohol in the fasted metabolic state.

Acute effects of ethanol

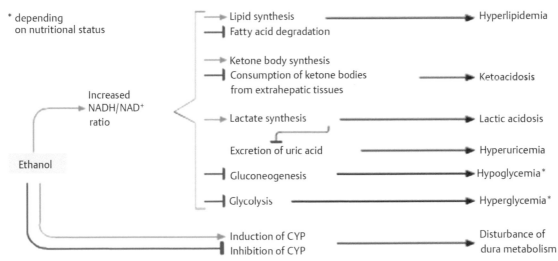

Source: Koolman J, Röhm K. Color Atlas of Biochemistry. 3rd Edition. 2012.

B is incorrect. Ethanol consumption does not affect lactate dehydrogenase activity in myocytes.

C is incorrect. Although hepatic oxidative phosphorylation is sometimes uncoupled as a result of chronic alcoholism, the effects are limited to hepatocytes. Extensive exposure of hepatic mitochondria to acetaldehyde and free radicals generated by the MEOS can result in damage to mitochondrial membranes and uncoupling of oxidative phosphorylation.

D is incorrect. Increased MEOS activity may lead to oxidative damage of mitochondrial membranes and uncoupling of oxidative phosphorylation, but the damage will be limited to hepatocytes, and is not severe enough to result in metabolic acidosis.

E is incorrect. The high NADH/NAD$^+$ ratio resulting from ethanol metabolism *inhibits* hepatic fatty acyl-CoA dehydrogenases. The resulting accumulation of

fatty acids in hepatocytes contributes to the development of alcoholic steatosis.

6. Correct: D. Acetaldehyde dehydrogenase.

Coprine inhibits acetaldehyde dehydrogenase. The symptoms only occur after ingestion of ethanol, so must be linked to a metabolite of ethanol metabolism. As summarized in the figure on the following page, ethanol metabolism is initiated by oxidation of ethanol to acetaldehyde by alcohol dehydrogenase. Acetaldehyde is then further oxidized to acetate by acetaldehyde dehydrogenase. Inhibition of acetaldehyde dehydrogenase results in accumulation of acetaldehyde, which is known to cause the symptoms described above. This is the basis for the administration of Antabuse (disulfiram, an inhibitor of acetaldehyde dehydrogenase) as a deterrent for ethanol consumption.

Ethanol metabolism

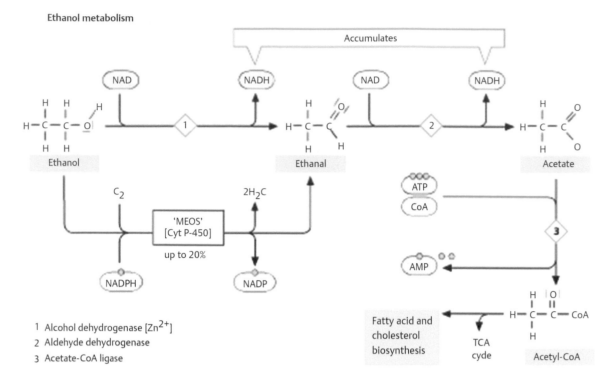

1 Alcohol dehydrogenase [Zn^{2+}]
2 Aldehyde dehydrogenase
3 Acetate-CoA ligase

Source: Koolman J, Röhm K. Color Atlas of Biochemistry. 3rd Edition. 2012.

A is incorrect. Inhibition of alcohol dehydrogenase would result in the accumulation of ethanol in the serum, and cause symptoms of inebriation rather than acetaldehyde toxicity.

B is incorrect. CYP2E1 is a component of the microsomal ethanol oxidizing system (MEOS), which has a lower affinity for alcohol than alcohol dehydrogenase does and is induced by ethanol. The MEOS catalyzes the oxidation of ethanol to acetaldehyde in patients who consume large quantities of alcohol, or who consume alcohol frequently. In these individuals, symptoms of CYP2E1 inhibition would be the same as symptoms of alcohol inebriation.

C is incorrect. Cytochrome P450 reductase catalyzes the transfer of electrons from NADPH to microsomal cytochrome P450 enzymes. It would only play a role in ethanol metabolism in individuals who rely on the MEOS for ethanol metabolism (see comments about CYP2E1 in the explanation for choice B). Inhibition of cytochrome P450 reductase in these individuals would possibly result in increased serum ethanol levels, but not in elevated acetaldehyde.

E is incorrect. Lactate dehydrogenase catalyzes the oxidation of lactate to pyruvate, and conversely the reduction of pyruvate to lactate. The direction of the reaction is determined by the NADH/NAD$^+$ ratio, as well as relative concentrations of pyruvate and lactate. Generally, conditions favor lactate formation in extrahepatic tissues, and pyruvate formation in the liver, especially in the fasted state. Consumption of significant quantities of ethanol, however, results in a higher-than-normal NADH/NAD$^+$ ratio in the liver. This causes the lactate dehydrogenase reaction to disfavor oxidation of lactate to pyruvate, thus decreasing the ability to use lactate as a precursor for gluconeogenesis. While this may contribute to the development of metabolic acidosis, and some of the symptoms described here, the problem is not linked to direct inhibition of lactate dehydrogenase by any particular inhibitory molecule and is thus not a likely result of consumption of coprine.

7. Correct: B. Glucocerebrosides.

Glucocerebrosides are accumulating in this patient's macrophages. The characteristic wrinkled-paper appearance of the enlarged macrophages in the biopsy sample, as well as this patient's bone pain, fatigue, hepatosplenomegaly, and pathological fracture, are all consistent with a diagnosis of Gaucher disease. Gaucher disease is caused by a deficiency in β-glucoceramidase, a lysosomal hydrolase, and results in accumulation of glucocerebrosides in the cells of the macrophage-monocyte system. Recall that sphingolipids are composed of a sphingosine backbone, to which is attached a fatty acid chain and a head group. The head group for sphingomyelin is phosphocholine, and the gangliosides contain sugar polymer head groups. Degradation of sphingolipids occurs in the lysosomes of the reticuloendothelial system; the figure on the following page illustrates this process. In the case of Gaucher disease, the sugars in the cerebroside head groups are successively hydrolyzed from the outer end of the head group, but the last sugar attached to the sphingosine backbone cannot be removed. The carrier rate for β-glucoceramidase mutations among Ashkenazi Jews is close to 10%, and Gaucher disease is inherited in an autosomal recessive manner.

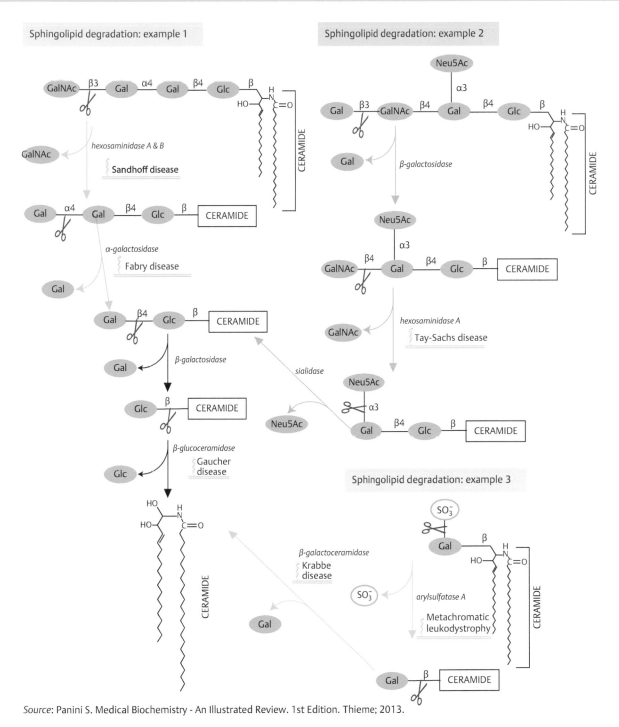

Sphingolipid degradation: example 1

Sphingolipid degradation: example 2

Sphingolipid degradation: example 3

Source: Panini S. Medical Biochemistry - An Illustrated Review. 1st Edition. Thieme; 2013.

A is incorrect. Accumulation of glycosaminoglycans occurs in the mucopolysaccharidoses, a group of lysosomal storage diseases generally associated with skeletal and facial deformities, cardiovascular problems, and frequently with impaired mental and neurological function. These features are not exhibited by the patient described here.

C is incorrect. Proteoglycans are composed of a protein core linked to hundreds of glycosaminoglycan polymers. The protein core, in turn, is covalently linked to a hyaluronic acid chain. Degradation of these extracellular components primarily involves endocytosis followed by hydrolysis of the protein core by lysosomal proteases, and hydrolysis of the carbohydrate polymers by lysosomal glycosidases. Genetic deficiencies in this process involve mutations in the lysosomal glycosidases and result in accumulation of glycosaminoglycans. These disorders are commonly referred to as mucopolysaccharidoses, and most frequently result in skeletal and facial deformities, cardiovascular problems, and sometimes impaired mental and neurological function.

D is incorrect. Glycerophospholipid degradation and remodeling is carried out by phospholipases A_1, A_2, C, and D. Isoforms of phospholipases A_2 and C are additionally involved in signal transduction pathways and eicosanoid biosynthesis. Only a few genetic deficiencies in phospholipase activity have been identified, and those deficiencies are associated with disease resulting from impaired signal transduction or eicosanoid synthesis, not from accumulation of undegraded glycerophospholipids.

E is incorrect. Accumulation of glycogen in hepatic cells can occur with various glycogen storage diseases. These disorders are not associated with bone pain or the unique wrinkled paper appearance of hepatic macrophages seen in this patient.

8. Correct: C. It inhibits a lipoxygenase.

The new drug most likely inhibits a lipoxygenase. The bronchoconstriction that is characteristic of asthma is stimulated by leukotrienes (and inhibited by β2 agonists). shown in the figure in Answer 4, leukotrienes are synthesized from arachidonate in a pathway that begins with the activity of lipoxygenases. Inhibition of lipoxygenases (5-lipoxygenase, specifically) by drugs such as zileuton, thus, will decrease the levels of leukotrienes and relieve asthmatic symptoms.

A is incorrect. Cyclooxygenase activity is associated with PGH synthase and the synthesis of prostaglandins and thromboxanes from arachidonic acid. Inhibition of cyclooxygenase would not decrease leukotrienes levels, and thus would not relieve symptoms of asthma. In fact, in some asthmatic patients, inhibition of cyclooxygenase exacerbates bronchoconstriction by increasing diversion of arachidonic acid to leukotriene synthesis.

B is incorrect. Linoleic acid is an essential fatty acid; it cannot be synthesized in the human body.

D is incorrect. Isoprostanes are generated by free radical reactions with arachidonic acid and their presence in physiological systems is an indication of oxidative stress. They have no known effect on bronchoconstriction.

E is incorrect. The release of arachidonic acid from phospholipids is inhibited by corticosteroids, which interfere with the action of phospholipase A_2 (PLA_2). Inhibition of PLA_2 does, indeed, decrease leukotriene synthesis, and thus bronchoconstriction. However, this girl is known to have an adverse reaction to corticosteroids, so the new drug she is given should not be a corticosteroid.

9. Correct: B. Lipase = Capillary lipoprotein; Lipoprotein = VLDL.

This patient's insulin insensitivity decreases the activity of capillary lipoprotein lipase, which catalyzes the hydrolysis of triglycerides carried by VLDL and chylomicrons in the serum. The free fatty acids that are released then enter nearby tissues, primarily adipocyte and myocyte, where they may be oxidized to generate energy or be re-esterified with glycerol to make triglycerides for storage. Capillary lipoprotein lipase is activated by insulin, so in diabetic individuals conversion of VLDL and chylomicrons to their respective remnants is impaired. Because this patient has not eaten in 12 hours, the major carrier of triglycerides in her serum will be VLDL. Recall that chylomicrons carry dietary lipids, and are generally cleared from circulation within a few hours of a meal (a few hours longer in diabetics). VLDL carries endogenous lipids and are release from the liver, which generates triglycerides from fatty acids that it synthesizes from excess carbohydrate. VLDL also carries triglycerides that are taken up by hepatocytes from chylomicron remnants and IDL. See the figure on the following page for a summary of chylomicron and VLDL synthesis and uptake of fatty acids into adipocytes and myocytes.

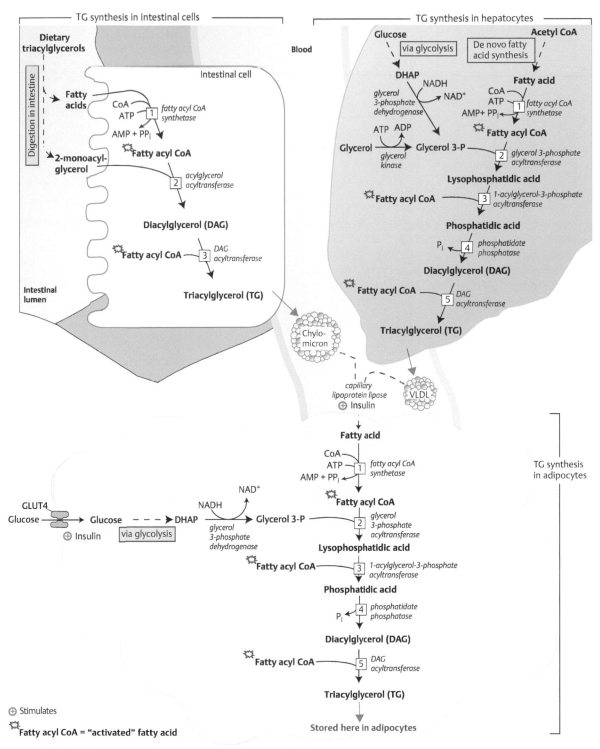

Source: Panini S. Medical Biochemistry - An Illustrated Review. 1st Edition. Thieme; 2013.

A is incorrect. Although the primary triglyceride-carrying lipoprotein particle in this patient is, indeed, VLDL, the cause of hypertriglyceridemia is not associated with inhibited hormone-sensitive lipase activity. Hormone-sensitive lipase is found in adipocytes and is responsible for initiating the lipolysis of triglycerides resulting in release of free fatty acids and glycerol to the serum. It is inhibited by insulin and activated by glucagon. In diabetic individuals, the enzyme will more active than normal;

this contributes to hypertriglyceridemia by increasing the transport of fatty acids to the liver, which uses them to generate VLDL.

C is incorrect. Although the primary triglyceride-carrying lipoprotein particle in this patient is, indeed, VLDL, the cause of hypertriglyceridemia is not associated with alterations in pancreatic lipase activity. Pancreatic lipase is a digestive enzyme and its activity is not regulated by insulin.

D, E, and F are incorrect. Chylomicrons carry dietary triglycerides; their concentration will be quite low 12 hours into a fast.

10.   Correct: E. Phytanic acid.

This patient's symptoms and treatment are consistent with adult Refsum disease, a progressive neurological disease associated with accumulation of phytanic acid in the serum. Phytanic acid, a derivative of chlorophyll, is found in the milk and fat of ruminant animals. Individuals with *adult* Refsum disease have a deficiency in the first enzyme involved in phytanic acid metabolism, phytanoyl CoA hydroxylase. Symptoms of the disease can often be reversed by elimination of phytanic acid from the diet. Phytanic acid metabolism occurs in peroxisomes; *infantile* Refsum disease is caused by mutations that impair normal peroxisome biogenesis, and produces more severe symptoms. See the figure below for a summary of peroxisomal fatty acid metabolism.

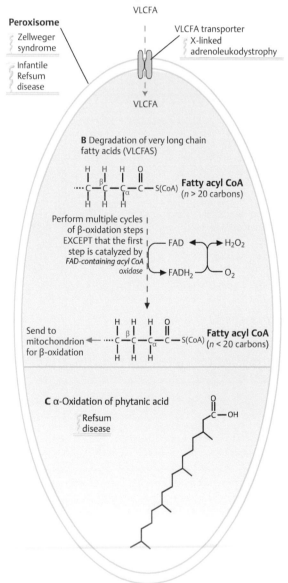

B is incorrect. Oleic acid (18:1) is a common unsaturated fatty acid; elevated levels are not associated with any particular disease.

C is incorrect. Accumulation of dicarboxylic acids in the serum and urine is associated with increased ω-oxidation of medium-chain fatty acids and is usually due to a defect in β-oxidation of fatty acids, such as medium-chain acyl-CoA dehydrogenase deficiency. Symptoms are not neurological in nature, and these diseases cannot be treated by dietary elimination of milk and fat of ruminant animals.

D is incorrect. Cerotic acid (26:0) accumulates in X-linked adrenoleukodystrophy (see the figure on the left), another neurological disease. It cannot be treated by dietary modification.

E is incorrect. Pristanic acid is the product of the reaction catalyzed by phytanoyl CoA dehydrogenase, the enzyme that is deficient in this patient.

11.   Correct: C. Ethylene glycol antifreeze.

This boy has most likely consumed ethylene glycol antifreeze. Ethylene glycol is metabolized to oxalic acid by the ethanol-metabolizing enzymes alcohol dehydrogenase and acetaldehyde dehydrogenase, producing glycolic acid. Additional enzymes convert glycolic acid to oxalic acid, glycine, and α-hydroxy β-ketoadipate. See the figure on the following page for a summary of ethylene glycol and methanol metabolism. Generation of large quantities of glycolic acid results in metabolic acidosis, as indicated by this boy's low serum pH, low bicarbonate level, and compensatory hyperventilation. In addition, oxalate, the conjugate base of oxalic acid, binds tightly to calcium ions, causing hypocalcemia and formation of calcium oxalate crystals in tissues and urine. Accumulation of oxalate crystals in the kidneys can result in acute renal failure. This boy's elevated creatinine and BUN levels are indicative of renal complications.

Source: Panini S. Medical Biochemistry - An Illustrated Review. 1st Edition. Thieme; 2013.

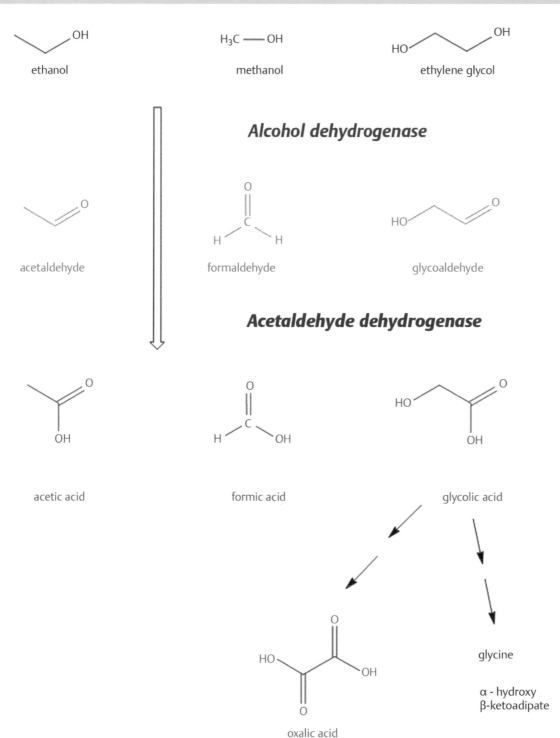

ethanol

methanol

ethylene glycol

Alcohol dehydrogenase

acetaldehyde

formaldehyde

glycoaldehyde

Acetaldehyde dehydrogenase

acetic acid

formic acid

glycolic acid

glycine

α - hydroxy
β-ketoadipate

oxalic acid

A is incorrect. Denatured alcohol is a solvent containing ~ 90% ethanol and additives such as methanol, acetone, pyridine, and isopropanol to make it undrinkable. Its toxicity is due largely to the presence of methanol, which causes metabolic acidosis, but not renal failure.

B is incorrect. Consumption of dish soap results primarily in severe gastrointestinal complications, not metabolic acidosis or renal complications.

D is incorrect. A few household plants, including philodendron and diffenbachia, contain very high levels of oxalate in their leaves. Consumption results in a painful burning sensation and erythema of the oral cavity, and is not associated with metabolic complications.

E is incorrect. Metabolism of methanol, also known as wood alcohol, via alcohol dehydrogenase and acetaldehyde dehydrogenase produces formic acid. Formic acid accumulation leads to metabolic acidosis, which this boy has, but does not result in renal failure or appearance of crystals in the urine.

12.   Correct: C. Octanoylcarnitine.

Octanoylcarnitine would most likely have been detected in his blood sample. Deficient activity of medium-chain acyl-CoA dehydrogenase (MCAD), an enzyme involved in β-oxidation of fatty acids, results in accumulation of medium-chain fatty acids such as octanoic acid. See the figure below for a review of the reactions involved in β-oxidation of fatty acids. These accumulated fatty acids form acylcarnitines, which leak into the serum and appear in both the serum and urine. Newborn screening in most states involves analysis for elevated levels of medium-chain acylcarnities. Note that testing for MCAD deficiency also frequently involves urinary analysis for dicarboxylic acids, as accumulation of medium-chain fatty acids results in increased ω-oxidation, producing medium-chain dicarboxylic acids. Medium-chain acylglycines are also detected in the serum and urine.

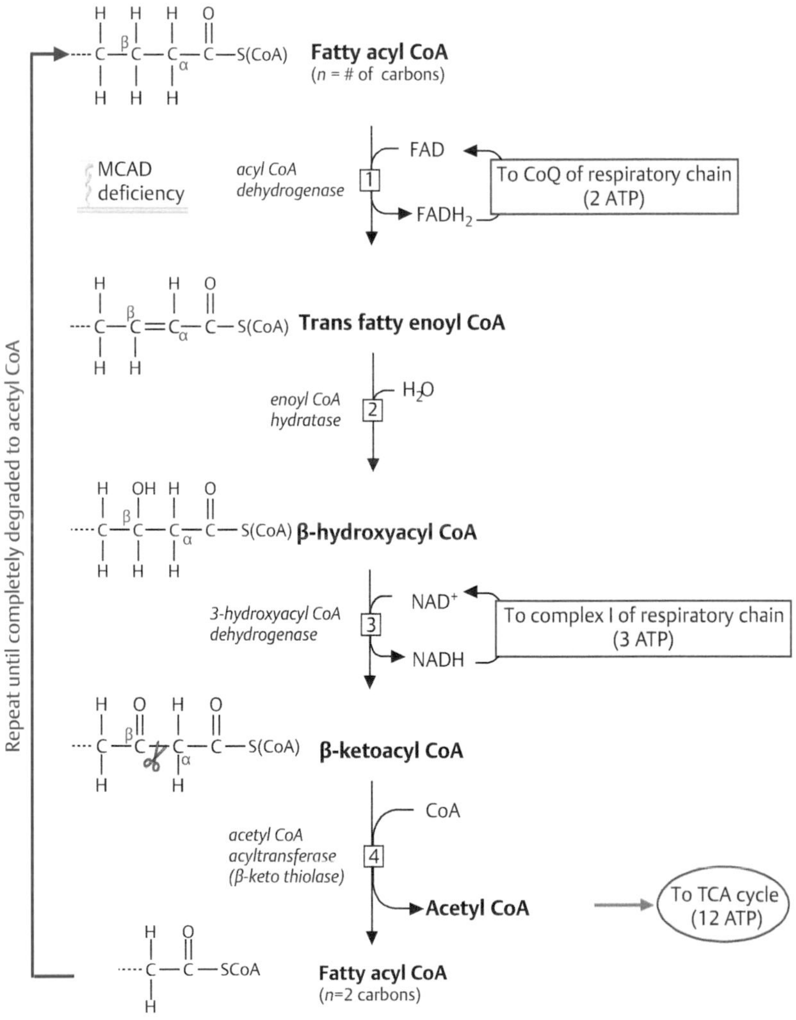

Source: Panini S. Medical Biochemistry - An Illustrated Review. 1st Edition. Thieme; 2013.

A is incorrect. β-hydroxybutyrate is a ketone body. A deficiency in β-oxidation of fatty acids will result in decreased synthesis of ketone bodies.

B is incorrect. MCAD deficiency often produces a secondary carnitine *deficiency* due to increased secretion of medium-chain acylcarnitines.

D is incorrect. Phenyllactate accumulates in the serum of individuals afflicted with phenylketonuria.

E is incorrect. Increased serum phytanic acid levels are associated with individuals with deficiencies in either peroxisomal biogenesis or phytanoyl CoA hydroxylase.

13. Correct: E. Fatty infiltration of the liver.

MCAD deficiency frequently causes hepatomegaly and hepatic steatosis. During fasting or illness, fatty acids are mobilized from adipocytes and used to generate energy in various tissues. The liver has a particularly large demand for fatty acids in order to generate ATP for gluconeogenesis. In individuals with disorders of fatty acid oxidation, then, hepatic complications including steatosis are likely to arise. This is partly due simply to accumulation of medium-chain fatty acids, but also to development of secondary carnitine deficiency due to loss of carnitine as it is bound to the excess medium-chain fatty acids and excreted. The secondary carnitine deficiency results in inability to transport fatty acids into hepatic mitochondria for oxidation and thus contributes to steatosis.

A is incorrect. MCAD deficiency is not a peroxisomal disorder.

B is incorrect. MCAD deficiency has little, if any effect on cholesterol metabolism and plaque formation.

C is incorrect. Cytoplasmic lysosomal vacuoles are indicative of some lysosomal storage diseases. MCAD deficiency is not a lysosomal storage disease.

D is incorrect. Impaired fatty acid oxidation will have no effect on myelin sheath formation or decay.

14. Correct: B. Avoidance of fasting.

This child would most likely have benefited from frequent feedings and avoidance of fasting. Fasting or any other condition, such as infection, that triggers fasting metabolism will result in development of severe hypoglycemia with hypoketosis in individuals with MCAD deficiency. The hepatic inability to oxidize fatty acids completely to acetyl CoA results in insufficient allosteric activation of pyruvate carboxylase to support gluconeogenesis. Furthermore,

hepatic ATP production is not adequate to support gluconeogenesis, and the deficiency in acetyl CoA severely impairs ketone synthesis. Finally, accumulation of octanoic acid is toxic to mitochondria and further impairs hepatic function, leading to additional complications such as hyperammonemia.

A is incorrect. A high fat, low carbohydrate diet would be detrimental to an individual who has MCAD deficiency. Treatment goals should be to reduce reliance on fatty acid oxidation for energy production.

C is incorrect. Dairy products do not contain substances that would aggravate metabolic complications in an individual with MCAD deficiency.

D is incorrect. MCAD deficiency impairs the ability to oxidize all fatty acids other than short chain fatty acids. The longer chain fatty acids are oxidized down to medium-chain length, at which point the β-oxidation process gets stalled and medium-chain fatty acids and their abnormal metabolites begin to accumulate. Thus, eliminating only medium-chain fatty acids from the diet will not be beneficial. Furthermore, elimination of dietary fat of very long, long, or medium-chain length will not be helpful because those very types of fatty acids are made endogenously and will be released to the serum from adipocytes, and thus used for β-oxidation in various tissues, during the metabolic fasting states.

E is incorrect. Supplementation with cobalamin would not correct MCAD deficiency, as cobalamin is not a cofactor for acyl-CoA dehydrogenases.

15. Correct: A. Hormone sensitive lipase.

This boy's ketosis is linked to increased activity of hormone sensitive lipase. Ketosis, which has been shown to be beneficial for some epileptic patients, is stimulated when the serum insulin/glucagon ratio is very low, as will be the case in this patient who is most likely eating a very high fat, low carbohydrate diet. The low insulin/glucagon ratio activates hormone sensitive lipase in adipocytes, as reviewed in the figure on the following page. This lipase is activated by glucagon and epinephrine, and inactivated by insulin. Activation of hormone sensitive lipase stimulates adipocyte lipolysis, thus providing free fatty acids for use in β-oxidation. Individuals who consume a ketogenic diet have such a low insulin/glucagon ratio that they rely heavily on gluconeogenesis to maintain adequate serum glucose; the combination of increased fatty acid β-oxidation occurring simultaneously with gluconeogenesis results in hepatic ketone production.

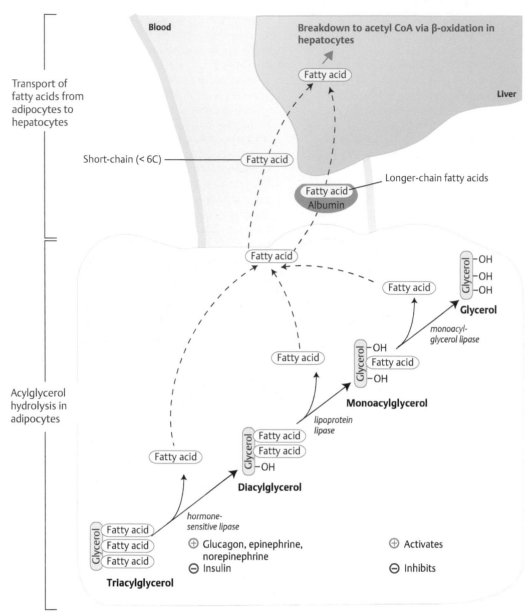

Source: Panini S. Medical Biochemistry - An Illustrated Review. 1st Edition. Thieme; 2013.

B is incorrect. Capillary lipoprotein lipase catalyzes the hydrolysis of triglycerides found in chylomicrons and VLDL. It is activated by insulin and stimulates the storage of fat as fuel and will be inactive under conditions that favor ketogenesis.

C is incorrect. HMG CoA reductase, the rate-limiting step in cholesterol biosynthesis, is activated by insulin and inhibited by glucagon; it will be inactive under conditions that favor ketogenesis.

D is incorrect. Acetyl CoA carboxylase, the rate-limiting step in fatty acid synthesis, is activated by insulin and inhibited by glucagon; it will be inactive under conditions that favor ketogenesis.

E is incorrect. Pyruvate dehydrogenase catalyzes the oxidation of pyruvate to acetyl CoA. It is inactivated by acetyl CoA, will be thus inactive under conditions that favor β-oxidation of fatty acids and ketogenesis.

16.   Correct: B. Increased production of resolvins and protectins.

The pain-relieving effects of increased consumption of fatty fish is most likely due to increased production of resolvins and protectins. Salmon and halibut are fatty fish, and contain significant amounts of ω-3 fatty acids. The ω-3 fatty acids have been linked with several beneficial health effects including reduction of inflammation, which would be helpful in relieving this patient's pain. The anti-inflammatory effects of ω-3 fatty acids are due to their use as precursors for the synthesis of resolvins, protectins, and maresins; eicosanoids that prevent or resolve inflammation. Furthermore, the ω-3 fatty acids act as competitive inhibitors of some of the enzymes involved in synthesis of inflammatory prostaglandins.

A is incorrect. Although inhibition of COX-2 would decrease prostaglandin synthesis and thus provide some relieve to this patient, ω-3 fatty acids found in salmon and halibut do not exhibit their greatest effect by directly inhibiting this enzyme.

C is incorrect. Increased production of prostaglandins would only increase the inflammatory response, and thus potentially increase pain.

D is incorrect. The ω-3 fatty acids associated with fatty fish such as salmon and halibut are not antioxidants.

E is incorrect. Although inhibition of phospholipase A_2 would decrease prostaglandin synthesis and thus provide some relieve to this patient, ω-3 fatty acids found in salmon and halibut do not inhibit this enzyme.

---

17. Correct: E. Oxaloacetate.

Depletion of heptatic oxaloacetate contributes to the accumulation of acetone, which has a fruity odor. Acetone, along with acetoacetate and β-hydroxybutyrate, is a ketone body. Ketone body synthesis, which occurs only when hepatic acetyl CoA concentrations are high, occurs under conditions such as fasting where hepatocytes are simultaneously running the β-oxidation and gluconeogenic pathways. β-oxidation of fatty acids, which is stimulated by a low insulin/glucagon ratio, generates large quantities of acetyl CoA, NADH, and $FADH_2$ in hepatic mitochondria. Gluconeogenesis, which is also stimulated by a low insulin/glucagon ratio, converts oxaloacetate (generated either from TCA cycle intermediates or from pyruvate by pyruvate carboxylase) to glucose. Depletion of oxaloacetate for gluconeogenesis results in accumulation of acetyl CoA because the citrate synthase reaction in the TCA cycle cannot consume all of the acetyl CoA generated by β-oxidation. The accumulated acetyl CoA is then used for ketone body synthesis.

A is incorrect. Acetyl CoA concentrations are elevated, not depleted, under conditions that stimulate ketogenesis.

B is incorrect. Depletion of carnitine would impair β-oxidation of fatty acids, and would thus impair ketogenesis.

C is incorrect. Hepatic glycerol concentrations may influence the rates of gluconeogenesis or triglyceride synthesis, but should have very little effect on ketogenesis.

D is incorrect. Under fasting conditions, when ketogenesis is stimulated, hepatic mitochondrial NADH levels *increase* as β-oxidation is activated. This increase in mitochondrial NADH inhibits the TCA cycle, and thus contributes to the accumulation of acetyl CoA that is necessary for ketogenesis.

---

18. Correct: C. Carnitine palmitoyltransferase II.

This patient's physical symptoms and laboratory results are consistent with a carnitine palmitoyltransferase II (CPT II) deficiency. As shown in the figure in

Answer 3, CPT II catalyzes the last step in the transport of activated fatty acids across the inner mitochondrial matrix. In this step, fatty acylcarnitines are converted to fatty acyl CoA, and carnitine is released. Deficiency in this enzyme results in accumulation of long chain acylcarnitines in the serum and depletion of free serum carnitine; this patient's serum free carnitine is low, and his total carnitines and palmitoylcarnitine (C16:0) are high. The net effect is that long and very long chain fatty acids cannot enter the mitochondria to undergo β-oxidation. In the adult-onset form of this disorder, the deficiency is limited to muscle tissue, and the symptoms of muscle weakness and rhabdomyolysis occur only under conditions that require muscle reliance on fatty acids for fuel, such as vigorous or prolonged exercise, illness, and fasting. The patient's leukocyte and creatine kinase levels indicate the likely presence of an infection and rhabdomyolyis, respectively.

A is incorrect. A deficiency in the Na^+-dependent carnitine transporter, which carries carnitine from the serum across cell membranes, results in decreases in both free and total carnitine levels. Free carnitine levels decrease due to insufficient renal resorption of carnitine, and acylcarnitine levels decrease due to the inability to provide carnitine for the reaction catalyzed by CPT I. Furthermore, this disorder generally presents in early childhood, with both muscular and hepatic symptoms.

B is incorrect. Deficiency in carnitine palmitoyltransferase I, which converts fatty acyl CoAs to fatty acylcarnitines, results in an increase in free serum carnitine, and decreases in acylcarnitines of all lengths. Furthermore, this disorder generally presents in early childhood with fasting hypoglycemia and hypoketonemia.

D is incorrect. Deficiency in medium-chain acyl-CoA dehydrogenase results in an increase in octanoylcarnitine, due to accumulation of medium-chain fatty acids in the mitochondria. It also generates secondary carnitine deficiency. Furthermore, this disorder generally presents with fasting hypoglycemia and hypoketonemia.

E is incorrect. Propionyl CoA carboxylase is a biotin-dependent enzyme that is required for complete oxidation of odd-chain fatty acids. A deficiency in this enzyme would have no expected direct effect on serum carnitine or acylcarnitine levels.

---

19. Correct: A. Pancreatic lipase.

This girl's symptoms are most likely due to decreased activity of pancreatic lipase. Cystic fibrosis can cause pancreatic insufficiency; dried mucus blocks the pancreatic duct, resulting in decreased secretion of digestive enzymes and bicarbonate into the intestinal lumen. Pancreatic lipase is responsible for the digestion of ~90% of dietary triglycerides. Gastric and lingual lipases digest the remainder, as summarized in the figure below. Inadequate digestion of lipids due to

123

insufficient pancreatic lipase activity is the cause of this patient's steatorrhea, and probably contributes to her fatigue and weight loss. Recall also that bicarbonate secretion into the intestinal lumen is crucial for adequate suspension of dietary lipids into micelles; bile salts are protonated, and thus not amphipathic, at the lower intestinal pH that results from impaired pancreatic bicarbonate secretion. Poorly suspended lipids may lead to small bowel obstruction.

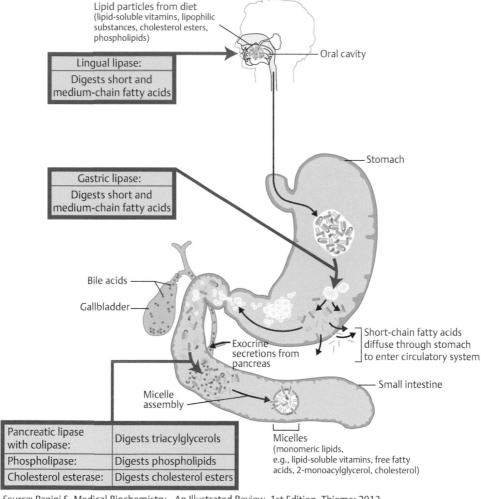

Source: Panini S. Medical Biochemistry - An Illustrated Review. 1st Edition. Thieme; 2013.

B is incorrect. Although α-amylase is secreted by the pancreas and its activity will be decreased in this patient, the resulting decrease in digestion of starch will not cause steatorrhea.

C is incorrect. Microsomal transfer protein plays a key role in the synthesis of chylomicrons and VLDL. Deficiency is the cause of abetalipoproteinemia and does result in steatorrhea, but is not associated with cystic fibrosis.

D is incorrect. Pepsin is a gastric protease. Decreased pepsin activity is not associated with cystic fibrosis, and would not cause steatorrhea.

E is incorrect. 7 α-hydroxylase catalyzes the committed and regulated step in bile salt synthesis. Deficiency is not associated with cystic fibrosis, although it would result in decreased bile production, and possibly steatorrhea.

20. Correct: B. They indirectly inhibit β-oxidation.

Inhibition of fatty acid synthase will result in accumulation of malonyl CoA, its substrate. Malonyl CoA, in turn, inhibits carnitine palmitoyltransferase I and import of fatty acids to the mitochondria for β-oxidation. Thus, ATP production via β-oxidation is inhibited. (For a review of fatty acid synthesis and transport of fatty acids across the mitochondrial membrane, see the figures in Answers 2 and 3, respectively.)

A is incorrect. Inhibition of fatty acid synthesis will not result in production or accumulation of a substance that would inhibit glycolysis.

C is incorrect. Inhibition of fatty acid synthesis will not result in production or accumulation of a substance that would inhibit the TCA cycle.

D is incorrect. Inhibition of fatty acid synthesis will not result in production or accumulation of a substance that would inhibit the electron transport chain.

E is incorrect. Inhibition of fatty acid synthesis will not result in production or accumulation of a substance that would inhibit ATP synthase.

Chapter 8

Cholesterol and Steroid Metabolism

Cholesterol   Estradiol   Cholic acid

LEARNING OBJECTIVES

► Describe the four phases of cholesterol synthesis and the regulation of 3-hydroxy-3-methylglutaryl coenzyme-A (HMG-CoA) reductase by energy availability, hormones, and pharmacological manipulation.

► Describe the effects of up-regulating or down-regulating plasma cholesterol levels on the transcriptional regulation of genes involved in cholesterol homeostasis.

► Summarize the process by which cholesterol is eliminated from the body, recognizing the roles of 7-α-hydroxylase, conjugation reactions, and bacterial deconjugation.

► Describe the pathways for synthesis of aldosterone, cortisol, and the sex hormones, knowing the roles of key enzymes that are associated with known metabolic disorders or important pharmaceutical treatments.

► Compare and contrast the life cycle of the various lipoprotein particles with respect to their composition, metabolism, and transport, and explain the mechanisms of the effects of statins, ezetimibe, and bile acid resins on serum levels of the different lipoprotein particles.

► Describe the functions of important apolipoproteins and lipoprotein receptors.

► Categorize and describe the various hyperlipidemias.

► Describe the synthesis of vitamin D.

► Describe the process of atherosclerotic plaque formation.

8.1 Questions

Easy	Medium	Hard

1. A 44-year-old female visits her physician after noticing a small lump in her breast. Subsequent imaging and a biopsy indicate that the woman has an estrogen receptor positive breast cancer. As part of her therapy, she is prescribed Rivizor. Which of the following enzymes does Rivizor most likely inhibit?

A. Aromatase

B. 21-α-hydroxylase

C. 5-α-reductase

D. 17-α-hydroxylase

E. Desmolase

2. An 8-year-old boy with abnormally small genitalia and a history of hypotonic dehydration and ketotic hypoglycemia is referred to an endocrinologist for evaluation. After a careful physical examination and acquisition of history, the endocrinologist orders laboratory determination of baseline serum hormones, followed by an adrenocorticotropic hormone (ACTH) stimulation test. The results are shown in the table below. This patient most likely has a deficiency in which of the following enzymes?

Basal serum hormones	Patient	Normal range
Aldosterone	<30 ng/dL	40–150 ng/dL
Dehydroepiandrosterone	15 µg/dL	20–130 µg/dL
Androstenedione	25 ng/dL	50–100 ng/dL
Cortisol	9 µg/dL	5–25 µg/dL
Post-ACTH stimulation serum cortisol	10 µg/dL	

ACTH, adrenocorticotropic hormone.

A. Aromatase

B. 21-α-hydroxylase

C. 11-β-hydroxylase

D. 17-α-hydroxylase

E. Desmolase

3. Evolocumab, a monoclonal antibody, is used to treat some patients whose hypercholesterolemia is not controlled by standard therapies. Evolocuamb is directed against proprotein convertase subtilisin kexin 9 (PCSK9), a protein that associates tightly with low-density lipoprotein (LDL) receptors. PSCK9 gain-of-function mutations are associated with the familial hypercholesterolemia phenotype, while loss-of-function mutations are associated with lifetime LDL levels and decreased risk of cardiovascular disease. Which of the following is the most likely function of PCSK9 in LDL metabolism?

A. It decreases the equilibrium dissociation constant (K_d) for binding of LDL to LDL receptors

B. It facilitates recycling of LDL receptors

C. It stimulates LDL receptor-driven formation of oxidized low-density lipoprotein (oxLDL)

D. It stimulates proteolysis of endocytosed LDL receptors

4. A 25-year-old male who was hospitalized following a myocardial infarction 3 months ago visits his physician for a follow-up appointment. At the time of his hospitalization, his serum LDL cholesterol level was 480 mg/dL (normal, <200 mg/dL), and he had large xanthomas on his legs and hands. Family history and genetic testing were indicative of homozygous familial hypercholesterolemia, and the patient was placed on the highest tolerable dose of statins, as well as ezetimibe. At this visit, his serum LDL cholesterol was 450 mg/dL. He reported that since his release from the hospital, he has faithfully adhered to his prescribed statin and ezetimibe therapy. The man's physician prescribes mipomersen, an inhibitor of apo-B100 synthesis. Which of the following might the physician expect to observe during the patient's mipomersen treatment?

A. Steatorrhea

B. Hepatic steatosis

C. Muscle pain and increased muscle fatigability

D. Increased number and size of xanthomas

E. Elevated serum triglycerides

5. A 65-year-old male who was recently diagnosed with benign prostatic hyperplasia was prescribed finasteride, an inhibitor of 5-α-reductase. Production of which of the following hormones will decrease while this patient is taking finasteride?

A. Testosterone

B. Estradiol

C. Dihydrotestosterone

D. Androstenedione

E. Pregnenolone

6. Due to recurrent vomiting, poor feeding, and failure to thrive, a 6-week-old boy was admitted to the pediatric hospital for observation and testing. The following laboratory values were obtained:

	Patient	Normal range
Plasma Na⁺ (mEq/L)	129	135-145
Plasma K⁺ (mEq/L)	6.26	3.5-5
Plasma renin (ng/dL)	5214	6.3-149

Plasma and urine analyses of several steroids were performed in order to determine if the infant's symptoms were due to a deficiency in steroid metabolism. ACTH challenge resulted in a significant increase in cortisol production. Which of the following plasma/urine steroid profiles would be most consistent with this patient's presentation at the time of his admission?

	Aldosterone	Corticosterone	Cortisol
A	Low	Elevated	Normal
B	Low	Low	Low
C	Normal	Elevated	Elevated
D	Elevated	Normal	Normal
E	Elevated	Elevated	Elevated

7. Abiraterone, an irreversible mechanism-based inhibitor of CYP17 (17-α-hydroxylase/17, 20-lyase), is in clinical trials for treatment of aggressive prostate cancer. Patients in these clinical trials are carefully monitored and treated for side effects associated with inhibition of CYP17. These adverse side effects are most likely due to production of which of the following hormones?

A. Testosterone

B. Aldosterone

C. Cortisol

D. Estradiol

E. Androstenedione

8. A 24-year-old male presents to his primary care physician, concerned about bumps that have been developing on his elbow over the past few months. His family history reveals that the patient's father recently died of a heart attack at age 45. Which of the following proteins is most likely expressed at an abnormally *high* levels in this patient?

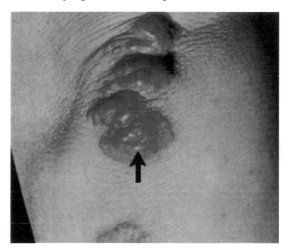

Source: Riede U, Werner M. Color Atlas of Pathology: Pathologic Principles · Associated Diseases · Sequela. 1st Edition. 2004.

A. Phosphofructokinase-1

B. Apo B-48

C. HMG-CoA reductase

D. Cholesterol 7-α-hydroxylase

E. Lipoprotein lipase

9. A 15-year-old male was referred to a gastroenterologist by his optometrist who was concerned that the boy exhibited signs of hypovitaminosis A. The boy reported a long history of recurrent diarrhea, producing foul-smelling, non-watery stools that were difficult to flush. He also reported mild peripheral neuropathy. Physical examination revealed slight hepatomegaly. The gastroenterologist ordered a fasting lipid profile, as well as serum vitamin analysis. The relevant laboratory results are shown below, where the image on the right was obtained. Subsequently, a biopsy of the duodenal mucosa was obtained. An image from that biopsy is shown in the right hand panel below. The image in the left panel is of normal mucosa, for comparison and the image on the left is shown for comparison (i.e., a normal tissue sample). A mutation in the gene for which of the following proteins most likely has contributed to this patient's symptoms?

	Patient	Reference range
Vitamin A	< 12 mg/dL	30–80 mg/dL
Vitamin E	< 0.3 mg/dL	0.5–1.8 mg/dL
Total cholesterol	30 mg/dL	125–230 mg/dL
Triglycerides	4 mg/dL	55–110 mg/dL
LDL cholesterol	10 mg/dL	80–120 mg/dL
HDL cholesterol	30 mg/dL	35–80 mg/dL

HDL, high-density lipoprotein; LDL, low-density lipoprotein.

A. Lipoprotein lipase
B. Pancreatic lipase
C. Cystic fibrosis transmembrane conductance regulator
D. LDL receptor
E. Apolipoprotein B (APOB)

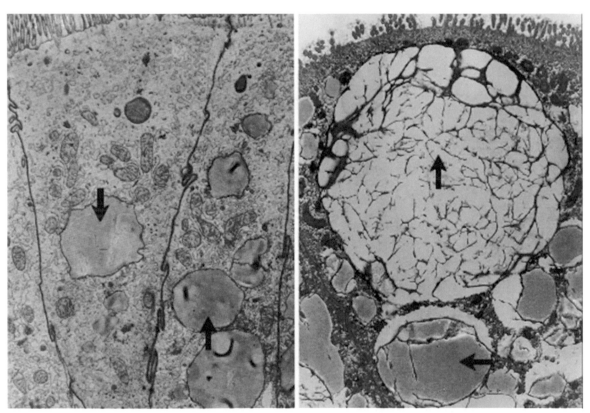

Source: Riede U, Werner M. Color Atlas of Pathology: Pathologic Principles · Associated Diseases · Sequela. 1st Edition. 2004.

10. Lipoprotein particles were isolated from a patient with hyperlipidemia and then separated by centrifugation. Images of the particles, all at the same level of magnification, are shown in the figure below. Which of the following most accurately indicates the identities of the various lipoprotein particles?

	Panel A	Panel B	Panel C	Panel D
A	HDL	LDL	Chylomicron	VLDL
B	Chylomicron	HDL	LDL	VLDL
C	VLDL	Chylomicron	LDL	HDL
D	LDL	HDL	VLDL	Chylomicron
E	Chylomicron	VLDL	LDL	HDL

HDL, high-density lipoprotein; LDL, low-density lipoprotein; VLDL, very low-density lipoprotein.

11. A 15-year-old female with a history of chronic kidney disease fractures her hip after tripping and falling on a sidewalk curb. Her fracture can be attributed, at least in part, to decreased serum levels of which of the following substances?

A. Cholecalciferol

B. 7-dehydrocholesterol

C. 1,25-dihydroxycholecalciferol

D. Ergocalciferol

E. 25-hydroxycholecalciferol

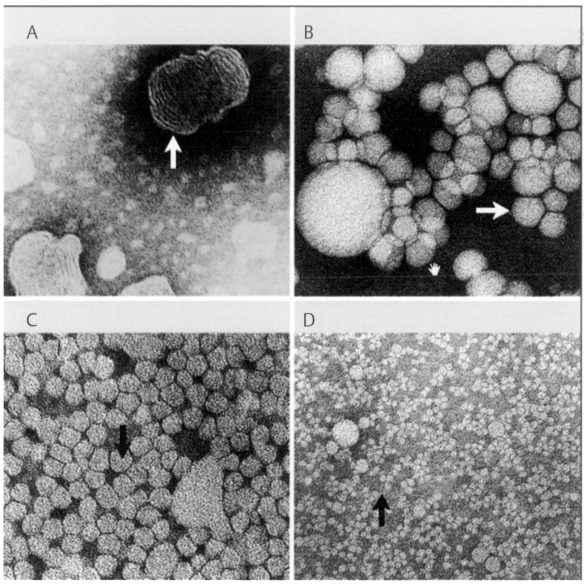

Source: Riede U, Werner M. Color Atlas of Pathology: Pathologic Principles · Associated Diseases · Sequela. 1st Edition. 2004.

12. An 18-year-old male was subjected to thorough evaluation following a myocardial infarction. A lipid panel revealed that his serum LDL levels were markedly elevated, and ultrasonography revealed several mobile echogenic foci with posterior acoustic shadowing in his gall bladder. Subsequent genetic testing was indicative of a rare deficiency. A deficiency in which of the following enzymes or proteins is most consistent with this patient's presentation?

A. 7-α-hydroxylase

B. Cholecystokinin

C. HMG-CoA reductase

D. Hypotaurine dehydrogenase

E. LDL receptor

13. A 32-year-old male with no history of medical concerns died while sleeping. His family requested an autopsy, during which the pathologist obtained the aortic segments shown in panels B and C of the figure below (panel A is an aortic segment from another individual, for comparison). The pathological sequence of events that most likely caused this individual's death can be linked directly to increased activity of which of the following proteins?

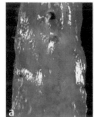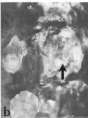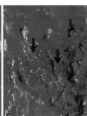

Source: Riede U, Werner M. Color Atlas of Pathology: Pathologic Principles · Associated Diseases · Sequela. 1st Edition. 2004.

A. Capillary lipoprotein lipase

B. Desmolase

C. Lecithin:cholesterol acyltransferase (LCAT)

D. LDL receptor

E. Scavenger receptor A

14. Anacetrapib, an inhibitor of the cholesteryl ester transfer protein (CETP), is in Phase III clinical trials for treatment of hypercholesterolemia. Which of the following processes does this drug inhibit?

A. Transfer of cholesterol from peripheral tissues to HDL

B. Transfer of cholesterol from HDL to peripheral tissues

C. Transfer of cholesterol from VLDL, IDL, and LDL to HDL

D. Transfer of cholesterol from HDL to VLDL, IDL, and LDL

15. A 54-year-old woman with a body mass index (BMI) of 28.5 and a family history of cardiovascular disease presents to her primary care physician with complaints of painful cramping in the calf of her right leg. The cramps occur when she walks and disappear after a few minutes of rest. Physical examination reveals that the right calf is cooler to the touch than the left calf. Her physician orders a fasting lipid panel, the results of which are shown here:

	Patient	Ideal
Total triglycerides	350 mg/dL	<150 mg/dL
Total cholesterol	450 mg/dL	<200 mg/dL
LDL cholesterol	110 mg/dL	<100 mg/dL
HDL cholesterol	52 mg/dL	>40 mg/dL

HDL, high-density lipoprotein; LDL, low-density lipoprotein.

A genetic deficiency in which of the following proteins is most consistent with this patient's presentation?

A. Apolipoprotein A-1

B. Apo-B48

C. Apolipoprotein E

D. LDL receptor

E. LCAT

16. A 47-year-old male with moderate hypercholesterolemia is prescribed cholestyramine (a bile acid sequestrant). While he is taking this drug, hepatic utilization of which of the following substances will increase most significantly?

A. Betaine

B. NADPH (nicotinamide adenine dinucleotide phosphate, reduced)

C. Pyridoxal phosphate

D. Taurine

E. Tetrahydrofolate

17. A 47-year-old male with moderate hypercholesterolemia is prescribed lovastatin (a statin) and ezetimibe. While he is taking these drugs, which of the following protein modification processes will increase most significantly?

A. Allosteric activation of capillary lipoprotein lipase by Apo CII

B. Phosphorylation of HMG-CoA reductase

C. Phosphorylation of LDL receptors

D. Polyubiquitination of HMG-CoA reductase

E. Proteolytic cleavage of sterol regulatory element binding protein

8.2 Answers and Explanations

Easy	Medium	Hard

1. Correct: A. Aromatase.

Rivizor inhibits aromatase, which catalyzes the conversion of the androgens androstenedione and testosterone to the estrogens estrone and estradiol. (For a review of sex steroid hormone biosynthesis, see the figure below.) Inhibition of aromatase reduces the level of circulating estrogens and inhibits the growth of estrogen receptor positive tumors.

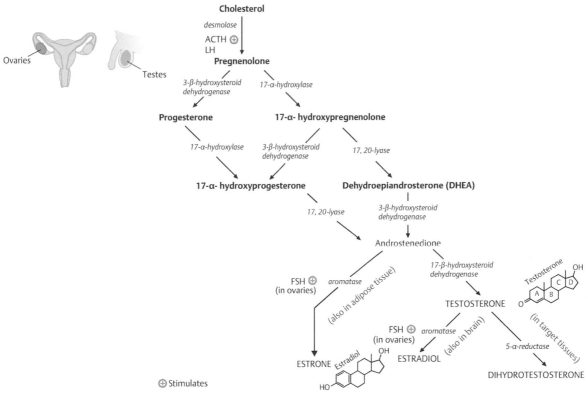

Source: Panini S. Medical Biochemistry - An Illustrated Review. 1st Edition. Thieme; 2013.

B is incorrect. Inhibition of 21-α-hydroxylase would decrease synthesis of aldosterone and would not decrease estrogen levels. This enzyme does not participate in sex hormone synthesis.

C is incorrect. Inhibition of 5-α-reductase would decrease synthesis of dihydrotestosterone and would not decrease estrogen levels.

D is incorrect. Inhibition of 17-α-hydroxylase would decrease synthesis of all sex hormones and cortisol. There would be too many adverse side effects if this enzyme were inhibited; specific inhibition of aromatase is less problematic.

E is incorrect. Inhibition of desmolase would decrease synthesis of all steroid hormones and cause adverse side effects.

2. Correct: E. Desmolase.

This patient most likely has a deficiency in desmolase. The child has low levels of the sex hormones, androstenedione and dehydroepiandrosterone, and very low levels of aldosterone; these laboratory results are consistent with his physical presentation and history and indicate deficiencies in the synthesis of both mineralocorticoids and sex hormones.[1] Furthermore, his relatively low baseline cortisol level did not increase upon stimulation with ACTH, indicating a deficiency in glucocorticoid synthesis. Because the boy is unable to synthesize normal amounts of all three types of steroid hormones, we can conclude that he has a deficiency in the first steps of the steroid synthesis pathway, before pregnenolone enters the three branches of

---

[1]Case based on Parajes S, Kamrath C, Rose IT, et al. A novel entity of clinically isolated adrenal insufficiency caused by a partially inactivating mutation of the gene encoding for P450 side chain cleavage enzyme (CYP11A1). J Clin Endocrinol Metab. 2011;96(11). doi:10.1210/jc.2011-1277.

steroid hormone synthesis. (See the figure below for a summary of steroid hormone synthesis.) The deficiency is most likely in desmolase, the enzyme that catalyzes the conversion of cholesterol to pregnenolone. (Note that this enzyme is also known as CYP450$_{scc}$ and cholesterol side chain cleavage enzyme.) Other possibilities that would explain these observations, but are not listed here, are deficiencies in the Steroid Acute Regulatory (StAR) protein, which controls entry of cholesterol to the mitochondria for the first steps of steroid hormone synthesis, or in 3-β-hydroxysteroid dehydrogenase.

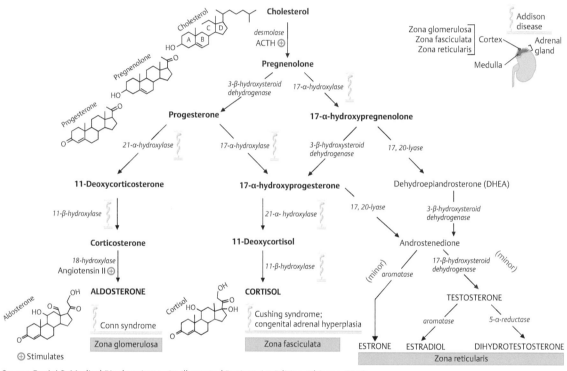

Source: Panini S. Medical Biochemistry - An Illustrated Review. 1st Edition. Thieme; 2013.

A is incorrect. Aromatase converts androgens (androstenedione and testosterone) to estrogens (estrone and estradiol). A deficiency would not result in decreased levels of the hormones listed in this patient's laboratory results.

B is incorrect. While a deficiency in 21-α-hydroxylase, the most common deficiency found in patients with congenital adrenal hyperplasias, will result in deficiencies in synthesis of both cortisol and aldosterone; it does not impair sex hormone synthesis. Indeed, in some patients with 21-α-hydroxylase deficiency, excess androgens are produced due to accumulation of pregnenolone, resulting in excess virilization in males and prenatal masculinization in females.

C is incorrect. 11-β-hydroxylase is involved in the synthesis of both aldosterone and cortisol, but is not involved with androgen synthesis. A deficiency would not result in decreased levels of dehydroepiandrosterone or androstenedione.

D is incorrect. A deficiency in 17-α-hydroxylase will impair androgen synthesis, but not mineralocorticoid or glucocorticoid synthesis. In fact, some patients with

17-α-hydroxylase deficiency generate excess aldosterone due to shunting of pregnenolone to that pathway.

3. Correct: D. It stimulates proteolysis of endocytosed LDL receptors.

PCSK9 stimulates proteolysis of endocytosed LDL receptors. Upon binding of LDL receptor to serum LDL particles, a process mediated by LDL-associated apolipoprotein B-100 (apo-B100), the ligand–receptor complex is endocytosed. Prior to fusion of the endosome with a lysosome, LDL is released from the LDL receptor, and the receptor is recycled to the cell surface. PCSK9 binds tightly to the LDL receptor and inhibits recycling of the receptor. This results in proteolysis of the receptor upon fusion of the endosome with a lysosome; the net effect is that fewer LDL receptors are exposed on the plasma membrane. Exposure of fewer LDL receptors leads to increased serum LDL levels.

A is incorrect. A decrease in the K_d for binding of LDL to LDL receptors would result in tighter binding of LDL and ultimately a decrease in serum LDL levels.

However, PCSK9 gain-of-function mutations are associated with increased serum LDL levels.

B is incorrect. Stimulation of LDL receptor recycling would result in higher numbers of LDL receptors on the plasma membrane. This would decrease serum LDL levels. However, PCSK9 gain-of-function mutations are associated with increased serum LDL levels.

C is incorrect. The LDL receptor does not mediate oxidation of LDL to oxLDL. The oxidation process is not enzyme-mediated and occurs spontaneously as circulating LDL is exposed to oxidants in the serum.

4. Correct: B. Hepatic steatosis.

The physician should monitor this patient closely for signs of hepatic steatosis. Mipomersen is an antisense therapeutic that binds to the messenger ribonucleic acid (mRNA) for apo-B100. The resulting decreased expression of apo-B100 impairs the liver's ability to form and excrete very low-density lipoprotein (VLDL), which carries triglycerides, cholesterol, and other lipids from the liver to extrahepatic tissues. As VLDL deliver triglycerides to extrahepatic tissues, they are processed and converted to intermediate density lipoproteins (IDL) and then LDL. (For a review of VLDL processing, see the figure below.) Thus, mipomersen treatment results in decreased serum LDL levels. However, because hepatic VLDL formation is inhibited by mipomersen, lipids accumulate in the liver and may cause significant steatosis.

A is incorrect. Steatorrhea, or fatty stools, results from malabsorption of dietary fat. Mipomersen will not affect intestinal absorption of dietary fats or incorporation of those fats into chylomicrons. Recall that the apolipoprotein associated with chylomicrons is apolipoprotein B-48 (apo-B48); apo-100, the target of mipomersen, is only associated with VLDL and its subsequent metabolites (IDL and LDL). Mipomersen activity is specific to apo-B100 and does not inhibit apo-B48 synthesis.

C is incorrect. Muscle pain and increased muscle fatigability are associated with statin treatment. The statins inhibit HMG-CoA reductase, which catalyzes the synthesis of mevalonic acid in the cholesterol biosynthetic pathway. Mevalonic acid is the precursor of the activated isoprenes which, in addition to cholesterol synthesis, are also used for biosynthesis of coenzyme Q. Some individuals who take statins experience muscle pain/fatigue due to decreased mitochondrial function resulting from low coenzyme Q levels.

D is incorrect. Xanthomas are subcutaneous cholesterol-rich deposits. Xanthomas associated with the tendons on the hands, feet, and heel often accompany familial hypercholesterolemia. If mipomersen is effective in lowering the patient's serum LDL levels, the xanthomas may decrease in size. The treatment should not cause the xanthomas to increase in size.

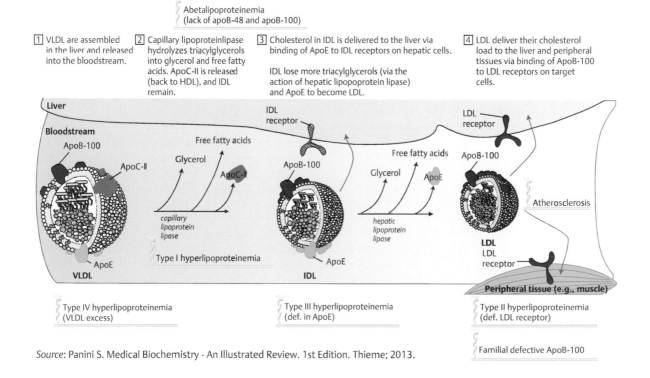

Abetalipoproteinemia
(lack of apoB-48 and apoB-100)

1. VLDL are assembled in the liver and released into the bloodstream.

2. Capillary lipoproteinlipase hydrolyzes triacylglycerols into glycerol and free fatty acids. ApoC-II is released (back to HDL), and IDL remain.

3. Cholesterol in IDL is delivered to the liver via binding of ApoE to IDL receptors on hepatic cells.

   IDL lose more triacylglycerols (via the action of hepatic lipopoprotein lipase) and ApoE to become LDL.

4. LDL deliver their cholesterol load to the liver and peripheral tissues via binding of ApoB-100 to LDL receptors on target cells.

Type IV hyperlipoproteinemia
(VLDL excess)

Type III hyperlipoproteinemia
(def. in ApoE)

Type II hyperlipoproteinemia
(def. LDL receptor)

Familial defective ApoB-100

Source: Panini S. Medical Biochemistry - An Illustrated Review. 1st Edition. Thieme; 2013.

E is incorrect. Decreased expression of apo-B100, with the resulting decrease in hepatic output of VLDL, would result in *decreased* lipid triglycerides.

5. Correct: C. Dihydrotestosterone.

Dihydrotestosterone levels will decrease in this patient. 5-α-reductase catalyzes the conversion of testosterone to dihydrotestosterone, the most potent androgen. (For a review of the enzymes and intermediates involved in steroid hormone synthesis, see the figure in Answer 1.)

A is incorrect. Testosterone is the substrate for 5-α-reductase; if anything, its concentration may increase.

B is incorrect. 5-α-reductase is not a part of the pathway for estradiol synthesis; inhibition of 5-α-reductase will not reduce estradiol levels.

D is incorrect. Androstenedione is the precursor of testosterone, which is the substrate for 5-α-reductase. Its concentration may increase during treatment with finasteride.

E is incorrect. Pregnenolone is the precursor of all steroid hormones; its concentration will not be affected by inhibiting 5-α-reductase.

6. Correct: A. Aldosterone = Low; Corticosterone = Elevated; Cortisol = Normal.

This infant's extremely high plasma renin level, along with his impaired renal resorption of sodium and increased elimination of potassium, is indicative of a problem with production of aldosterone. Because treatment with ACTH results in a significant increase in cortisol levels, we can deduce that the most likely defect is in 18-hydroxylase, also known as aldosterone synthase, which is the only enzyme unique to the aldosterone synthetic pathway (see the figure in Answer 2). An 18-hydroxylase deficiency would result in lower than normal aldosterone levels and elevated corticosterone. The effect on serum cortisol levels would be minimal.

B is incorrect. Although this answer choice correctly identifies that aldosterone levels will be low, it is incorrect because it states that corticosterone and cortisol levels would also be low. This might be correct if the ACTH challenge had not resulted in significantly increased cortisol levels. The ACTH challenge result tells us that the cortisol pathway is working correctly; hence, cortisol and corticosterone are both being made at normal levels. Corticosterone will be high, though it is the precursor of aldosterone.

C is incorrect. The infant's sodium, potassium, and renin values are indicative of a deficiency in synthesis of aldosterone; aldosterone levels will be low.

D is incorrect. The infant's sodium, potassium, and renin values are indicative of a deficiency in synthesis of aldosterone; aldosterone levels will be low.

E is incorrect. The infant's sodium, potassium, and renin values are indicative of a deficiency in synthesis of aldosterone; aldosterone levels will be low.

7. Correct: B. Aldosterone.

These patients should be monitored, and if needed, be treated for increased synthesis of aldosterone. (For a review of the enzymes and intermediates involved in steroid hormone synthesis, see the figure in Answer 2.) CYP 17 is involved in the synthesis of the sex hormones and cortisol. The enzyme has two activities, a 17-α-hydroxylase activity and a 17, 20-lyase activity. Both activities are required for androgen and estrogen synthesis, while only the 17-α-hydroxylase activity is necessary for synthesis of cortisol. Inhibition of the 17-α-hydroxylase activity will result in accumulation of pregnenolone and progesterone. These intermediates will be diverted toward the pathway for aldosterone synthesis.

A is incorrect. Inhibition of CYP17 will result in decreased synthesis of testosterone.

C is incorrect. Inhibition of CYP17 will result in decreased synthesis of cortisol.

D is incorrect. Inhibition of CYP17 will result in decreased synthesis of estradiol.

E is incorrect. Inhibition of CYP17 will result in decreased synthesis of androstenedione.

8. Correct: C. HMG-CoA reductase.

HMG-CoA reductase will most likely be expressed at abnormally high levels in this patient. The xanthomas observed on this patient's elbow and his family history of early cardiovascular disease are consistent with a diagnosis of familial hypercholesterolemia or familial combined hyperlipidemia. In either case, serum LDL levels will be elevated. In most cases of familial hypercholesterolemia, there is a deficiency in LDL receptor function, although some patients may have defective apo B-100 or overly active PCSK9 enzyme. The molecular cause of familial combined hyperlipidemia is not well understood. In individuals with either hypercholesterolemia or combined hyperlipidemia, cholesterol transport from plasma into cells is inefficient, and the cell's demands for cholesterol will be met primarily by *de novo* cholesterol synthesis. Transcription of HMG-CoA reductase, the committed and rate-limiting enzyme in cholesterol biosynthesis, is stimulated under these conditions.

A is incorrect. The patient's xanthomas and his family history are consistent with familial hypercholesterolemia or familial combined hyperlipidemia. Neither of these disorders would be expected to affect the activity of phosphofructokinase-1.

B is incorrect. The patient's xanthomas and his family history are consistent with familial hypercholesterolemia or familial combined hyperlipidemia. Neither of these disorders would be expected to affect the expression of apo-B48.

D is incorrect. This patient most likely has markedly elevated serum LDL cholesterol levels, due to ineffective transport of LDL from plasma into hepatocytes and other cells. This would result in decreased hepatocyte cholesterol concentrations, and subsequently *decreased* expression of 7-α-hydroxylase.

E is incorrect. The patient's xanthomas and his family history are consistent with familial hypercholesterolemia or familial combined hyperlipidemia. Neither of these disorders would be expected to increase expression of lipoprotein lipase, which is regulated primarily by insulin.

9. Correct: E. Apolipoprotein B (APOB).

This patient most likely has hypobetalipoproteinemia caused by a deficiency in APOB. The patient exhibits signs of fat malabsorption, fatty stools and deficiencies in fat-soluble vitamins. Furthermore, his very low fasting serum lipid levels and hepatomegaly indicate that hepatic secretion of lipids is also impaired. Finally, the accumulation of lipids in his enterocytes indicates that lipids do enter the enterocytes, but are not able to leave. A mutation in the gene for APOB would explain all of these observations. In enterocytes, the APOB gene product is Apo-B48, which plays an essential role in the assembly of chylomicrons that transport dietary lipids, including fat-soluble vitamins, out of enterocytes to body tissues. In the liver, the APOB gene product is Apo-B100, which plays an essential role in the assembly of VLDL particles that transport endogenous lipids from hepatocytes to extra-hepatic tissues. Impaired VLDL synthesis will result in low-fasting triglycerides, as well as low LDL cholesterol, as VLDL is the precursor of LDL.

A is incorrect. Lipoprotein lipase is located on the capillary lumen and catalyzes the hydrolysis of triglycerides carried by chylomicrons and VLDL. A deficiency in this enzyme would cause an elevation of serum triglyceride levels. Furthermore, this deficiency would not result in impaired absorption of fat-soluble vitamins or decreased serum cholesterol levels.

B is incorrect. While a deficiency in pancreatic lipase would result in fat malabsorption, it would neither affect hepatic release of lipids nor cause lipid accumulation in enterocytes.

C is incorrect. While a deficiency in cystic fibrosis transmembrane conductance regulator would result in decreased pancreatic secretion of digestive enzymes, resulting in fat malabsorption, it would neither affect hepatic release of lipids nor cause lipid accumulation in enterocytes.

D is incorrect. A deficiency in the LDL receptor would not affect absorption of dietary lipids and would result in an increase, rather than a decrease, in fasting LDL levels.

10. Correct: E. Panel A = Chylomicron; Panel B = VLDL; Panel C = LDL; Panel D = HDL.

During centrifugation, the lipoprotein particles separate according to density. The larger and least dense particles are chylomicrons, followed by VLDL, LDL, and high-density lipoprotein (HDL). (For a review of lipoprotein particle features, see the figure below.)

A is incorrect. This set of responses does not place the lipoprotein particles in the correct order of size from the largest, least dense, and particle (panel A) to the smallest, most dense, and particle (panel D).

B is incorrect. This set of responses does not place the lipoprotein particles in the correct order of size from the largest, least dense, and particle (panel A) to the smallest, most dense, and particle (panel D).

Mature chylomicron

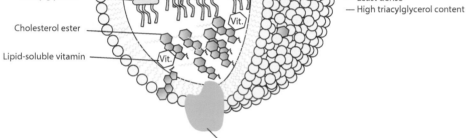

Chylomicron properties:
— Largest
— Least dense
— High triacylglycerol content

VLDL, IDL, LDL

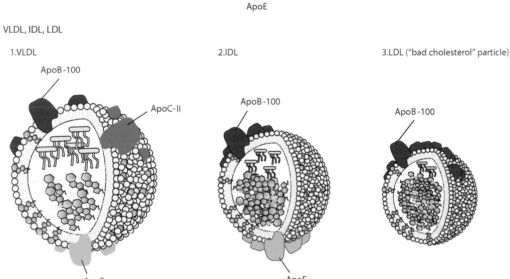

HDL ("good cholesterol" particle)

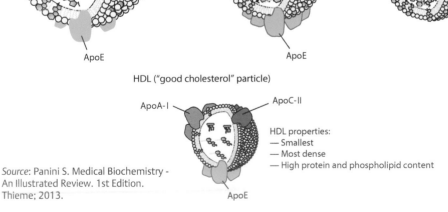

HDL properties:
— Smallest
— Most dense
— High protein and phospholipid content

Source: Panini S. Medical Biochemistry - An Illustrated Review. 1st Edition. Thieme; 2013.

C is incorrect. This set of responses does not place the lipoprotein particles in the correct order of size from the largest, least dense, and particle (panel A) to the smallest, most dense, and particle (panel D).

D is incorrect. This set of responses does not place the lipoprotein particles in the correct order of size from the largest, least dense, and particle (panel A) to the smallest, most dense, and particle (panel D).

11. Correct: C. 1,25-dihydroxycholecalciferol.

This patient most likely has decreased serum levels of 1,25-dihydroxycholecalciferol. Given the very young age of this patient, and the fact that her severe injury was caused by a minor fall, it is quite likely that her bone fracture is due to increased bone fragility resulting from chronic kidney disease. While the kidney contributes to the regulation of bone metabolism by several mechanisms, the mechanism of interest in this question is vitamin D synthesis, which is summarized in the figure below. Conversion of 25-hydroxycholecalciferol to 1,25-dihydroxycholecalciferol (calcitriol), the biologically active form of vitamin D, is catalyzed by 1-α-hydroxylase in the kidney. Individuals with chronic kidney disease often have low serum levels of 1,25-hydroxycholecalciferol, causing impaired intestinal absorption of calcium and phosphate ions and decreased renal reabsorption of calcium. The consequence of low serum 1,25-hydroxycholecalcifrol levels is hypocalcemia and hypophosphatemia, resulting in poor bone mineralization.

A is incorrect. Cholecalciferol (vitamin D_3) is synthesized from cholesterol in the skin and is obtained in the diet from some meat products and fortified foods. It can also be generated from ergocalciferol (vitamin D_2) found in some plant foods. Dietary deficiency of vitamin D or lack of exposure to sunlight can cause osteomalacia in adults or rickets in children. This individual's bone fragility, however, is more likely associated with kidney disease, which will not cause cholecalciferol deficiency.

B is incorrect. 7-dehydrocholesterol is a precursor for cholecalciferol synthesis in the skin; it does not appear in the serum, and its concentration is not sensitive to kidney function.

D is incorrect. Ergocalciferol (vitamin D_2) is a dietary source of vitamin D found in some plant foods, such as mushrooms. It is converted to cholecalciferol in intestinal cells and does not appear in the serum.

E is incorrect. 25-hydroxycholecalciferol is generated by hydroxylation of cholecalciferol in the liver and then released to the serum where it binds vitamin D-binding protein. This is the body's storage form of vitamin D. It will decrease when the diet is deficient in vitamin D and/or in persons who have low exposure to the sun. Its concentration is not sensitive to kidney function.

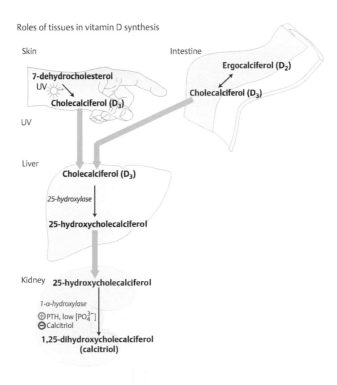

Roles of tissues in vitamin D synthesis

Source: Panini S. Medical Biochemistry - An Illustrated Review. 1st Edition. Thieme; 2013.

12. Correct: A. 7-α-hydroxylase.

This patient most likely has a deficiency in 7-α-hydroxylase. 7-α-hydroxylase catalyzes the first step in the synthesis of bile acids from cholesterol; it is stimulated by intracellular cholesterol and is inhibited by bile acids. (See the figure below for a review of bile salt metabolism.) A deficiency in this enzyme results in decreased bile acid synthesis and increased hepatocellular cholesterol levels. The increased hepatocellular cholesterol concentrations repress activation of the sterol regulatory element binding protein (SREBP) and thus decreases the expression of LDL receptors. This results in significantly elevated serum LDL levels and premature cardiovascular disease. The increased hepatocellular cholesterol concentration, coupled with the decreased synthesis of bile salts, significantly increases the probability of the formation of cholesterol stones in the gall bladder, as evidenced by this individual's ultrasonograph. Recall that bile salts help to keep cholesterol solubilized in the bile.

B is incorrect. Cholecystokinin is a peptide hormone released by the gut during digestion of lipids and protein; it stimulates contraction of the gall bladder and subsequent release of bile to the duodenum. It also stimulates secretion of enzymes from the pancreas. Deficiencies in cholecystokinin generation are very rare and are associated with autoimmune polyglandular syndrome. The clinical signs include malabsorption due to decreased solubility (and thus absorption) of dietary lipids and to decreased release of digestive enzymes from the pancreas.

C is incorrect. A deficiency in HMG-CoA reductase, the rate-limiting and controlled step in cholesterol biosynthesis, would result in decreased levels of intracellular cholesterol, and thus increased expression of LDL receptors. This would decrease serum LDL levels.

D is incorrect. Hypotaurine dehydrogenase catalyzes the last step the synthesis of taurine from

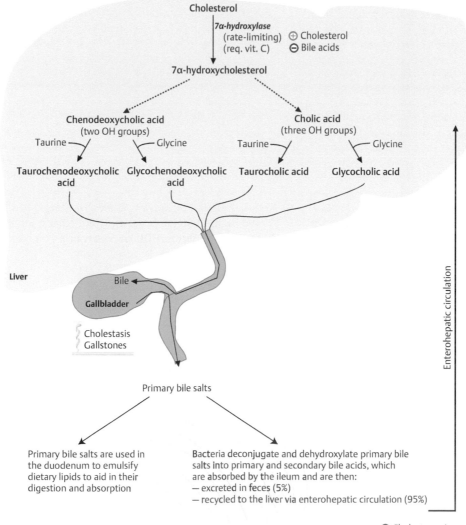

⊕ Stimulates
⊖ Inhibits

Source: Panini S. Medical Biochemistry - An Illustrated Review. 1st Edition. Thieme; 2013.

cysteine. A deficiency in taurine synthesis might impair generation of bile salts that are conjugated with taurine if this individual consumed a vegan diet deficient in taurine. (The great majority of taurine in the human body is obtained from the diet.) A taurine deficiency severe enough to cause cholelithiasis, however, would most likely present with other physiological problems resulting from insufficient function of taurine in regulating osmolality.

E is incorrect. A deficiency in LDL receptor function would certainly elevate serum LDL levels. However, it would not be expected to increase susceptibility to formation of gallstones, as seen in this patient.

---

13. Correct: E. Scavenger receptor A.

Increased function of scavenger receptor A most likely contributed to this patient's death. This individual most likely died due to premature atherosclerotic cardiovascular disease (ACVD), as suggested by the large atherosclerotic plaques in panel B and the atherosclerotic ulcer (resulting from plaque rupture) in panel C. Premature ACVD is linked to abnormally high levels of serum cholesterol, most often of the LDL form. Plaque formation begins with minor damage to the vascular endothelial lining. Monocytes are attracted to the injury, are converted to macrophages, and enter the subintimal space where they exhibit increased expression of scavenger receptor A. Scavenger receptor A binds to oxidized LDL particles in the serum and stimulates endocytosis of the oxidized LDL. The macrophages thus become foam cells, which stimulate the process of plaque formation.

A is incorrect. Capillary lipoprotein lipase catalyzes the hydrolysis of triglycerides found in chylomicrons and VLDL. Increased activity of this enzyme does not contribute directly to atherosclerotic plaque formation or to the elevated serum LDL levels associated with plaque formation.

B is incorrect. Desmolase catalyzes the first step in steroid hormone synthesis. Its activity is not associated with the development of premature atherosclerotic cardiovascular disease.

C is incorrect. LCAT facilitates the transport of cholesterol from extrahepatic tissues to HDL. Increased activity of this enzyme would, if anything, have a beneficial effect on this individual's pathology, as it would facilitate the removal of cholesterol from his plaques and increase his serum HDL levels. High serum HDL levels are associated with lower risk of ACVD.

D is incorrect. Most likely, this individual has *decreased* LDL receptor activity, resulting in high serum LDL levels and increased risk of ACVD.

---

14. Correct: D. Transfer of cholesterol from HDL to VLDL, IDL, and LDL.

CETP facilitates the transfer of cholesterol esters (CE) from HDL to VLDL, IDL, and LDL and plays a key role in the maturation of HDL particles. The figure below summarizes the interactions between HDL and other lipoprotein particles. Initially, lecithin:cholesterol acyltransferase (LCAT) facilitates the transfer of cholesterol from peripheral tissues to nascent HDL. The cholesterol-ester-rich HDL then transfers cholesterol esters to LDL, IDL, and VLDL particles in exchange for triglycerides (TG) in a process catalyzed by CETP. Hepatic lipoprotein lipase removes triglycerides from HDL (not shown in the figure), leaving poorly lipidated HDL, which are degraded. Inhibition of CETP prevents the delipidation and subsequent degradation of HDL, thus increasing serum HDL levels; it also helps to decrease serum LDL cholesterol levels by inhibiting transport of cholesterol into LDL, IDL, and VLDL. Note that hypertriglyceridemia is thought to decrease serum HDL levels because it increases CETP action.

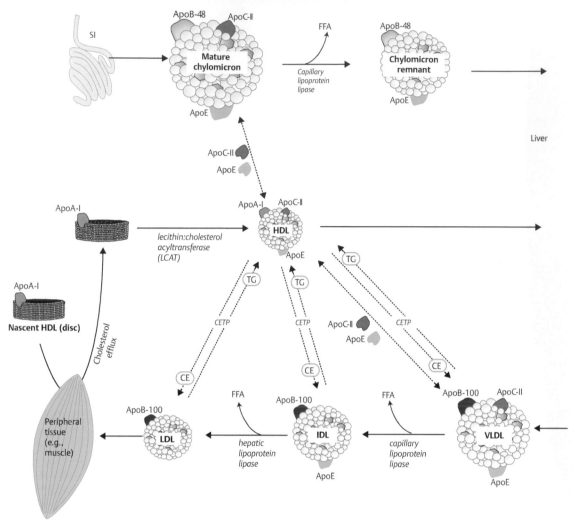

Source: Panini S. Medical Biochemistry - An Illustrated Review. 1st Edition. Thieme; 2013.

A is incorrect. This is the reaction catalyzed by LCAT.

B is incorrect. This is the reverse of the reaction catalyzed by LCAT.

C is incorrect. This is the reverse of the reaction catalyzed by CETP.

15. Correct: C. Apolipoprotein E.

This patient's elevated serum triglyceride and cholesterol levels with (relatively) low LDL and normal HDL are consistent with a deficiency in apolipoprotein E. Because of impaired apolipoprotein E activity, chylomicron remnants and IDL are not efficiently removed from circulation. (See the figure in Answer 4, which illustrates IDL processing; chylomicron remnants are not shown in this figure, but are also taken up via apolipoprotein E-binding IDL receptors in hepatocytes.) This results in high serum triglyceride and cholesterol levels. Furthermore, LDL cholesterol levels tend to be normal or only slightly elevated because of impaired conversion of IDL to LDL. Apolipoprotein E deficiency or Type III hyperlipoproteinemia is referred to as dysbetalipoproteinemia because of the elevated levels of serum APOB species associated with

chylomicrons and IDL. This disorder usually presents with peripheral atherosclerotic cardiovascular disease, as exhibited by this patient.

A is incorrect. A deficiency in apolipoprotein A-1 would impair the generation of HDL cholesterol, and thus abnormally result in low serum HDL levels. This patient's HDL is normal.

B is incorrect. A deficiency in apo-B100, known as abetalipoproteinemia, generally also accompanies deficiency in apo-B48, as the two proteins are derived from the same gene by alternative splicing. [Alternatively, a deficiency in the microsomal transfer protein (MTP) will also result in low serum apolipoprotein B levels.] These deficiencies result in accumulation of triglycerides in enterocytes and hepatocytes and in low serum triglyceride and cholesterol levels.

D is incorrect. A deficiency in LDL receptor results in very high serum LDL levels. This patient's LDL level is normal.

E is incorrect. Deficiency in LCAT impairs the transport of cholesterol from peripheral tissues to HDL. With this deficiency, HDL cholesterol levels are quite low (this patient's HDL is close to normal), and accumulated cholesterol in peripheral tissues often results in reduced vision due to corneal opacities.

16. Correct: B. NADPH.

Hepatic utilization of NADPH will increase. Cholestyramine inhibits the absorption and enterohepatic circulation of bile acids and salts (see the figure in Answer 12). Normally, about 95% of bile acids and salts are returned to the liver, thus keeping hepatic need for de novo bile acid synthesis low. When enterohepatic recycling of bile salts is impaired, the liver produces new bile salts from cholesterol. The process of synthesizing bile acids utilizes several cytochrome P450 enzymes, including cholesterol 7-α-hydroxylase, that utilize NADPH. Furthermore, increased demand for cholesterol for bile acid synthesis will also increase the rate of cholesterol synthesis, another process that utilizes large quantities of NADPH.

A is incorrect. Betaine (trimethylglycine) is used as a methylating agent for the synthesis of methionine in the liver. There is no reason to expect that its use would increase under conditions requiring increased hepatic synthesis of bile acids and salts.

C is incorrect. None of the enzymes involved in either cholesterol or bile salt synthesis require pyridoxal phosphate.

D is incorrect. Hepatic consumption of taurine will most likely not change significantly and will certainly not change as significantly as NADPH. Recall that in addition to dehydroxylating them, intestinal bacteria deconjugate most of the primary bile salts. Thus, the liver consumes taurine even while

recycling the bile acids that return to it via enterohepatic circulation.

E is incorrect. None of the enzymes involved in either cholesterol or bile salt synthesis require tetrahydrofolate.

17. Correct: E. Proteolytic cleavage of sterol regulatory element binding protein.

The sterol regulatory element binding protein will be subject to increased proteolysis. The statin drugs are competitive inhibitors of HMG-CoA reductase, and ezetimibe inhibits intestinal absorption of dietary and biliary cholesterol. The net effect of these two drugs is to decrease intracellular cholesterol levels. As shown in the figure below, a decreased intracellular cholesterol level promotes the release of the sterol regulatory element binding protein (SREBP)-SREBP cleavage-activating protein (SCAP) complex from the endoplasmic reticulum. The complex moves to the Golgi apparatus, where SREBP undergoes sequential proteolysis to release the active form. Active SREBP dimerizes and migrates to the nucleus, where it binds the sterol regulatory element and stimulates transcription of several proteins, including HMG-CoA reductase and LDL receptors, that will increase intercellular cholesterol levels. Importantly, the statins inhibit newly transcribed HMG-CoA reductase, and the newly transcribed LDL receptors increase cellular uptake of LDL cholesterol from the serum, thus decreasing serum LDL levels.

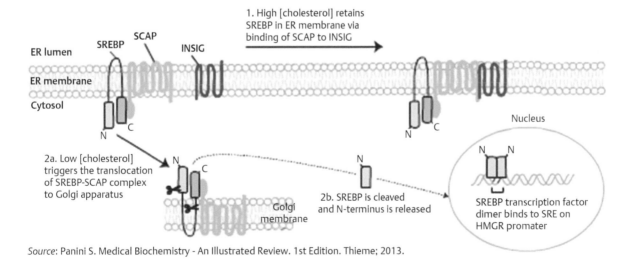

Source: Panini S. Medical Biochemistry - An Illustrated Review. 1st Edition. Thieme; 2013.

A is incorrect. Allosteric activation of capillary lipoprotein lipase by Apo CII will increase if chylomicron or VLDL triglyceride levels increase. Statins and ezetimibe, however, generally have the effect of decreasing serum triglycerides.

B is incorrect. Inactivation of HMG-CoA reductase by phosphorylation is facilitated by 5' adenosine monophosphate (AMP)-dependent protein kinase, which is activated by low cellular energy levels (low [AMP]), glucagon, and sterols (which will decrease during treatment with statins and ezetimibe).

C is incorrect. LDL receptors are not regulated by covalent phosphorylation.

D is incorrect. Polyubiquitination of HMG-CoA reductase stimulates is proteolysis and is stimulated by high intercellular sterol concentrations. These drugs decrease intercellular cholesterol.

Chapter 9

Protein, Amino Acid, and One Carbon Metabolism

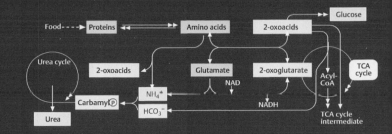

LEARNING OBJECTIVES

▶ Describe the digestion of protein, knowing the names, functions, and locations of the relevant digestive enzymes and describing the activation of pancreatic zymogens.

▶ Describe the uptake of peptides, amino acids, and cobalamin in the gastrointestinal tract and identify defects in uptake that lead to clinical symptoms.

▶ Compare and contrast degradation of body protein via ubiquitin-mediated proteolysis and lysozomes.

▶ List specific examples of ketoacid/amino acid transamination reactions and explain the relevance of transamination reactions in nitrogen metabolism.

▶ Describe the importance of the reactions catalyzed by glutamine synthetase, glutaminase, and glutamate dehydrogenase.

▶ Explain the role of the urea cycle in ammonia excretion and identify urea cycle defects based on laboratory test results.

▶ Describe inborn errors of metabolism related to amino acid degradation and/or transport.

▶ Describe the pathways for catecholamine, serotonin, and melanin biosyntheses, knowing required cofactors.

▶ Explain the functions of the cofactors tetrahydrofolate, *S*-adenosylmethionine (SAM), and cobalamin, their roles in the activated methyl cycle, and the "methyl trap" hypothesis regarding cobalamin deficiency and secondary folate deficiency.

▶ Identify which amino acids are ketogenic and which are glucogenic, and describe the end products of amino acid catabolism.

9.1 Questions

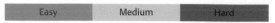

Easy   Medium   Hard

1. A research report was recently published in which the level of cobalamin in postmortem human frontal cortex was measured in several subjects. As shown in the figure below, the study revealed a significant difference in total cobalamin levels between subjects known to have autism or schizophrenia and age-matched control subjects. Which of the following would be a likely consequence of the altered cobalamin levels in the frontal cortex?

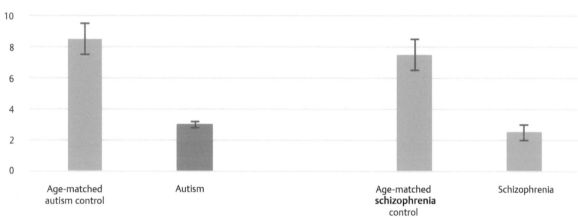

Source: Zhang Y, Hodgson NW, Trivedi MS, et al. Decreased Brain Levels of Vitamin B12 in Aging, Autism and Schizophrenia. PLOS ONE. 2016.

A. Decreased recycling of pyrimidines

B. Decreased levels of homocysteine

C. Increased levels of phenylalanine

D. Increased *de novo* purine synthesis

E. Decreased methylation of deoxyribonucleic acid (DNA)

2. A 53-year-old female underwent surgery to remove a mass from her pancreas. Pathological analysis of the resected tissue resulted in a diagnosis of pancreatic ductal adenocarcinoma; a neoplasm that cannot survive in the absence of exogenous glutamine. In these cells, glutamine provides nitrogen for the synthesis of which of the following molecules?

A. Tyrosine

B. Lysine

C. Urea

D. Serine

E. Nicotinamide

3. A 40-year-old male unexpectedly and suddenly died. His family requested an autopsy. During her review of the medical history, the pathologist noted that the man had an 8-year history of severe arthritic pain and stiffness in his knees, hips, and back. She also noticed a comment that a laboratory technician had made on a recent urinalysis report; the technician remarked that he thought that the urine sample had darkened significantly between the time it arrived in the laboratory and the time at which he ran the analysis. During the autopsy, the pathologist obtained the sample of the patient's aorta that is photographed in the figure below. Which of the following substances most likely contributed to the change in urine color that the laboratory technician observed?

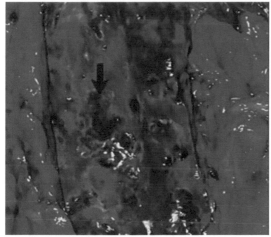

Source: Riede U, Werner M. Color Atlas of Pathology: Pathologic Principles · Associated Diseases · Sequela. 1st Edition. 2004.

A. Porphobilinogen

B. Myoglobin

C. Cystine

D. Homogentisate

E. Tyrosine

4. A 12-year-old boy who had always been in the lower 10th percentile on growth charts presented to his pediatrician with complaints of intermittent lack of coordination and tremors. His mother reports that these episodes usually occur following illness, such as a severe cold, diarrhea, or the flu, and frequently are accompanied by emotional instability. She also mentions that the boy has been extremely sensitive to sun exposure since birth. Subsequent testing leads the pediatrician to prescribe nicotinamide, to be taken when the episodes occur. Urinalysis will most likely reveal elevated levels of which of the following amino acids?

A. All amino acids will be elevated

B. Cysteine

C. Cystine

D. Glutamine

E. Tryptophan

5. A 45-year-old woman with a body mass index (BMI) of 35 and a history of cystinuria that was controlled well by dietary protein restriction and urinary alkalinization underwent bariatric surgery in order to facilitate weight loss. However, a few months after the procedure, her urinary cystine levels began to rise in spite of careful adherence to the treatment plan that had worked well prior to the surgery. Her physician suspected that the elevated urine cystine levels could be due to malabsorption of a particular nutrient, resulting from the gastric bypass. A deficiency in which of the following vitamins or minerals would most likely explain the aggravation of this patient's condition?

A. Iron

B. Pyridoxine

C. Niacin

D. Cobalamin

E. Thiamine

6. The 6-year-old boy pictured with his parents in the figure below recently completed kindergarten. At the end of the school year, his teacher reported that he was socially well-adjusted, had a reading vocabulary of approximately 100 words, and could neatly write his first and last names. His parents report that he has no history of significant illness, is physically active, and learned to ride a bicycle at age 4. This boy most likely has a deficiency in the metabolism of which of the following amino acids?

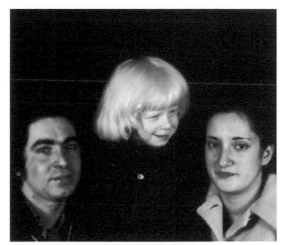

Source: Riede U, Werner M. Color Atlas of Pathology: Pathologic Principles · Associated Diseases · Sequela. 1st Edition. 2004.

A. Phenylalanine

B. Tryptophan

C. Valine

D. Histidine

E. Tyrosine

7. A 19-year-old woman who received no prenatal care gave birth to the full-term infant whose back is pictured in the figure below. Assuming that the infant's birth defect is not genetically linked, but can be attributed to a significant maternal dietary deficiency, which of the following metabolites would most likely be elevated in the mother's serum?

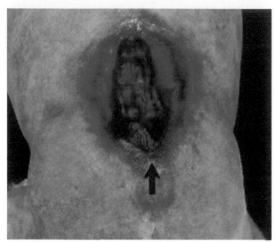

Source: Riede U, Werner M. Color Atlas of Pathology: Pathologic Principles · Associated Diseases · Sequela. 1st Edition. 2004.

A. Isoleucine

B. Uric acid

C. Homocysteine

D. Glutamine

E. Phenylalanine

8. The figure below shows urinary pH values observed in healthy individuals who consumed isocaloric diets with varying amounts of protein: a low protein (LP), moderate protein (MP), or high protein (HP) diet. Each of these diets contained similar compositions of all 20 amino acids. A fourth group of individuals was placed on the MP diet supplemented daily with 3 g of one of the 20 individual dietary amino acids (MP+). Eighteen of the 20 dietary amino acids had no effect on urinary pH when supplemented at 3 g to the MP diet. However, two amino acids, when supplemented at 3 g to the MP diet, generated the effect on urinary pH shown for the MP+ group in the figure. Which of the following are most likely the amino acids that elicit the observed change in urinary pH when added to the diets of the MP+ group?

A. Glutamic acid and aspartic acid

B. Histidine and lysine

C. Methionine and cysteine

D. Glutamine and asparagine

E. Phenylalanine and tyrosine

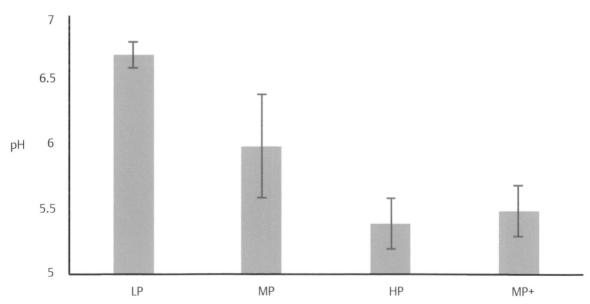

Source: Remer T. Acid-Base in Renal Failure: Influence of Diet on Acid-Base Balance. Seminars in Dialysis. 2001.

9. An 8-year-old boy has a known genetic deficiency in argininosuccinate synthase that is well-controlled by dietary restriction of protein. He is admitted to the hospital following a recent febrile illness and has been experiencing lethargy, vomiting, and seizures. Administration of which of the following amino acids or amino acid derivatives will most likely relieve his symptoms?

A. N-acetylglutamate

B. Arginine

C. Aspartate

D. Glutamine

E. Lysine

10. A woman in the fourth month of her first pregnancy is concerned regarding the recent gradual development of a discolored patches of skin on her face. See the figure below. The discoloration is due, most likely, to increased activity of which of the following enzymes?

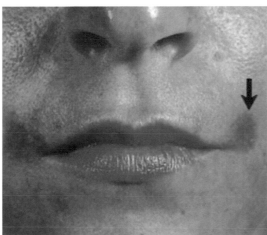

Source: Riede U, Werner M. Color Atlas of Pathology: Pathologic Principles · Associated Diseases · Sequela. 1st Edition. 2004.

A. Homogentisate oxidase

B. Uroporphyrinogen decarboxylase

C. Tyrosinase

D. Biliverdin reductase

E. Tryptophan monooxygenase

11. A 24-year-old male was admitted to the emergency department complaining of shortness of breath, nausea, and abdominal pain of about 18 hours in duration. Arterial blood gas and serum metabolic panels were obtained. Laboratory results are shown below.

Glucose	300 mg/dL
β-hydroxybutyrate	3.5 mmol/L (normal <0.5 mmol/L)
pH	7.15
Bicarbonate	12 mEq/L

As this patient's illness progresses, which of the following substances will be used by his kidneys at higher-than-normal levels?

A. Aspartate

B. Cobalamin

C. Glucose

D. Glutamine

E. Tetrahydrofolate

Consider this narrative for questions 12 to 14.

A young Mennonite couple sought genetic testing and counseling prior to trying to conceive a child. Testing indicated that they were both carriers of a mutation in the gene for branched chain ketoacid dehydrogenase.

12. If the couple were to give birth to a child that was homozygous for mutations in this gene, which of the following dietary therapies would most likely be necessary?

A. A low-carbohydrate diet and avoidance of fasting

B. A very low protein diet and a complete amino acid supplement with carefully determined levels of valine, leucine, and isoleucine

C. A very low protein diet and a complete amino acid supplement with carefully determined levels of phenylalanine and tyrosine

D. A very low protein diet and avoidance of fasting

E. A high-carbohydrate, low-fat diet and avoidance of fasting

13. If the couple were to give birth to a child that was homozygous for mutations in this gene, which of the following physical features would most likely be present in the child?

A. Albinism

B. Fragile bones

C. Musty-smelling urine

D. Spina bifida

E. Sweet-smelling earwax

14. If the couple were to give birth to a child that was homozygous for mutations in this gene, supplementation with which of the following vitamins might be part of the child's treatment plan?

A. Biotin

B. Cobalamin

C. Folate

D. Niacin

E. Thiamine

15. Hereditary Parkinson's disease is most commonly associated with inactivating mutations in parkin, a ubiquitin E3 ligase. In individuals that carry this mutation and develop Parkinson's disease, the disease etiology most likely involves alterations in which of the following intracellular processes?

A. Amino acid uptake

B. DNA replication

C. Lysosomal protein degradation

D. Proteasomal protein degradation

E. Protein synthesis

16. A 64-year-old male with a history of chronic alcohol abuse was admitted to the emergency department following several days of mental confusion and seizures. His serum pH was 7.5, and his serum ammonia concentration was 390 µM (normal: 20–50 µM). After admission, he received an intravenous (IV) treatment that facilitated elimination of which of the following substances in his urine?

A. Bicarbonate

B. Free ammonia

C. Glutamine and glycine

D. Urea

E. Urea and free ammonia

17. A one-month-old infant is diagnosed with dihydrobiopterin reductase deficiency following genetic testing that was prompted by the results of newborn screening. This child should be treated for deficiencies in the synthesis of which of the following biomolecules?

A. SAM

B. Catecholamines and serotonin

C. Catecholamines and tetrahydrofolate

D. Nicotinamide and serotonin

E. Tetrahydrofolate and SAM

18. A 20-year-old female presents to her primary care physician with complaints of significant weight loss, fatigue, and diarrhea over the last 3 months. Laboratory tests indicate iron-deficiency anemia. The right panel in the figure below is an image of tissue obtained during a biopsy of her small intestine. (For comparison, the left panel is an image of tissue obtained from a healthy individual.) The diarrhea and weight loss this patient has experienced is most directly linked to decreased activity of which of the following proteases?

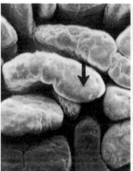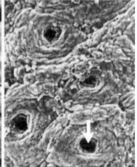

Source: Riede U, Werner M. Color Atlas of Pathology: Pathologic Principles · Associated Diseases · Sequela. 1st Edition. 2004.

A. Cathepsin

B. Elastase

C. Enteropeptidase

D. Pepsin

E. Trypsin

19. A 25-year-old college student has been on a hunger strike for 3 days, protesting the use of animals in medical research. As the fast progresses and muscle tissue is degraded, which of the following amino acids will be used by the liver primarily to generate serum glucose, and which will be used to generate serum ketone bodies?

	Precursor of glucose	**Precursor of ketone bodies**
A	Alanine	Arginine
B	Alanine	Leucine
C	Glutamine	Proline
D	Leucine	Lysine
E	Proline	Cysteine

20. A 2-day-old boy is in the neonatal intensive care unit. He is hyperventilating and lethargic, refuses oral nutrition, and has had several seizures. Serum analysis reveals the following:

	Patient	Normal
Ammonia	4,000 µM	<50 µM
Citrulline	3 µM	9–38 µM
Ornithine	900 µM	20–130 µM

Measurement of which of the following metabolites in the serum or urine would be most helpful for determining the biochemical deficiency that is causing this patient's illness?

A. Ammonia in the urine

B. Glutamine in the serum

C. Orotic acid in the urine

D. Urea in the serum

E. Uric acid in the serum

21. A 45-year-old woman who underwent a partial gastrectomy as part of her treatment for stomach cancer 5 years ago presents to her physician with complaints of fatigue and shortness of breath. Blood work indicates that her folate levels are normal, and her mean corpuscular volume is larger than normal. Which of the following treatment options would most likely benefit this patient?

A. Injections of cobalamin

B. Injections of intrinsic factor

C. Injections of ferrous sulfate

D. Oral cobalamin

E. Oral intrinsic factor

F. Oral ferrous sulfate

9.2 Answers and Explanations

Easy	Medium	Hard

1. Correct: E. Decreased methylation of deoxyribonucleic acid (DNA).

Decreased cobalamin levels would result in decreased methylation of DNA. Cobalamin (vitamin B_{12}) is the cofactor for methionine synthase, which catalyzes the methylation of homocysteine to generate methionine. Methionine is the precursor for *S*-adenosylmethionine (SAM) an important methylating agent that is involved in the synthesis of several neurotransmitters, as well as in the epigenetic methylation of DNA. (See the figure below for a review of methylation reactions facilitated by SAM.) The decreased levels of cobalamin found in the brain tissue of individuals afflicted with autism or schizophrenia, then, could lead to decreased activity of methionine synthase and lower levels of SAM. This would decrease synthesis of some neurotransmitters, as well as decrease methylation of DNA.

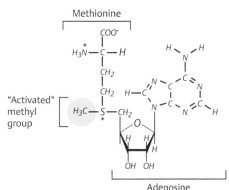

SAM functions as a methyl donor for various reactions, such as:
– Norepinephrine → Epinephrine (Catecholamine synthesis)
– Cytidine → 5-methylcytidine (DNA methylation)
– Adenosine → N^6-methyladenosine (DNA methylation)
– THF → N^5-methyl THF (Methyl transfers)
– Arg + Gly → Creatine (Energy storage in muscle)
– Lys → ε-*N*-timethyllysine → Carnitine (Fatty acid transport into mitochondria)
– Ornithine → Putrescine → Spermidine → Spermine (Growth factor synthesis)

Source: Panini S. Medical Biochemistry - An Illustrated Review. 1st Edition. Thieme; 2013.

A is incorrect. Cobalamin is not a cofactor for enzymes involved in pyrimidine recycling. Furthermore, none of the reactions involved in pyrimidine recycling involves methylation by SAM, which requires cobalamin for its synthesis.

B is incorrect. Homocysteine is the substrate for the cobalamin-dependent reaction catalyzed by methionine synthase. Thus, low cobalamin levels would possibly *increase* concentrations of homocysteine.

C is incorrect. Cobalamin is not a cofactor for enzymes involved in phenylalanine metabolism. Furthermore, phenylalanine metabolism does not involve methylation reactions for which SAM is a co-substrate.

D is incorrect. *De novo* purine synthesis could be *impaired* by a deficiency in cobalamin that results in significant methionine synthase deficiency. The methyl group that is transferred to homocysteine by methionine synthase is derived from N^5-methyl-tetrahydrofolate. If methionine synthase activity is greatly impaired, N^5-methyl-tetrahydrofolate will accumulate, as the methionine synthase reaction is the only reaction for which N^5-methyl-tetrahydrofolate is a substrate. Eventually the majority of the pool of tetrahydrofolate will be stuck in the methyl form, thus decreasing the levels of more reduced tetrahydrofolate species that are needed for purine *de novo* biosynthesis.

2. Correct: D. Serine.

Glutamine will provide nitrogen for the synthesis of serine. Glutamine is deamidated to produce glutamate, the nitrogen donor (via transamination) for synthesis of all non-essential amino acids except tyrosine, which is synthesized directly by hydroxylation of phenylalanine. Rapidly proliferating cells have high demand for glutamine, as they must produce proteins and nucleotides, which also obtain nitrogen from glutamine, for cell growth and division. Serine is generated from the glycolytic intermediate, 3-phosphoglycerate, in a three-step process involving oxidation, transamination, and hydrolysis of phosphate. During the transamination step, the amino nitrogen for serine is provided by glutamate. That glutamate, in turn, is produced by deamidation of glutamine, either by hydrolysis via the activity of glutaminase or by direct donation of the glutamine side-chain nitrogen in the synthesis of purine nucleotides, pyrimidine nucleotides, or asparagine.

A is incorrect. Tyrosine is the only non-essential amino acid for which glutamate (derived from glutamine) does not provide the α-amino group via transamination. Tyrosine is derived by hydroxylation of phenylalanine, an essential amino acid.

B is incorrect. Lysine is an essential amino acid and cannot be synthesized by human cells.

C is incorrect. Although glutamine does (indirectly) provide nitrogen for the synthesis of urea in the urea cycle, the urea cycle is only active in hepatocytes and is not active in tumor cells.

E is incorrect. Nicotinamide, a precursor in the synthesis of nicotinamide adenine dinucleotide (NAD) and nicotinamide adenine dinucleotide phosphate (NADP), is synthesized from either vitamin B_3 (niacin) or the essential amino acid tryptophan.

3. Correct: D. Homogentisate.

The change in urine color was most likely due to the product of homogentisate oxidation. The patient's history of arthritic pain and stiffness in the large joints, as well as the brown discoloration of connective tissue observed on the patient's aorta are consistent with alkaptonuria, a deficiency in homogentisate oxidase activity. Homogentisate oxidase participates in the pathway for catabolism of phenylalanine and tyrosine and catalyzes the oxidation of homogentisate to maleylacetoacetate. (For a review of phenylalanine metabolism, see the figure on the following page) The deficiency results in accumulation of homogentisate, which is rapidly cleared by the kidney and excreted. Upon exposure to air, homogentisate in the urine is gradually oxidized to form a black-pigmented polymer. Over time, homogentisate accumulates in collagenous tissues and polymerizes there, resulting in damage to the tissue and black discoloration (ochronosis). Deposition in the large joints causes degenerative arthritis, and deposition on heart valves can result in valvular heart disease. Some patients develop visible black pigmentation on cartilaginous tissues, such as the ears, and on the sclera.

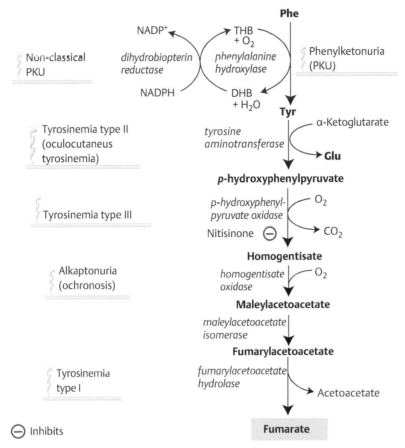

Source: Panini S. Medical Biochemistry - An Illustrated Review. 1st Edition. Thieme; 2013.

A is incorrect. Porphobilinogen accumulates in the urine of individuals with acute intermittent porphyria (AIP), due to a deficiency in the second enzyme in the heme biosynthetic pathway (porphobilinogen deaminase). Urinary porphobilinogen undergoes oxidation resulting in a color change to dark red. However, the other symptoms of AIP, including abdominal pain and neuropsychological issues, were not observed in this patient. In addition, ochronosis, as observed in this patient's aorta, is not associated with AIP.

B is incorrect. Rhabdomyolysis results in tea-colored urine due to an overload of myoglobin released by damaged skeletal muscle tissue. The urine is discolored upon voiding and does not undergo significant color change over time due to oxidation.

C is incorrect. Cystine in the urine is the result of a deficiency in an amino transporter that facilitates resorption of cystine. In some patients, the urine will have a "rotten-egg" smell, but it will not be discolored.

E is incorrect. Accumulation of tyrosine does not result in readily observed changes in urine color.

4. Correct: E. Tryptophan.

The boy's urine will most likely contain elevated levels of tryptophan, as his symptoms and the prescription for nicotinamide are consistent with a diagnosis of Hartnup disease. This disorder results from a defect in the neutral amino acid transporter. Individuals with this disorder can develop deficiencies in tryptophan, an essential amino acid whose dietary uptake and renal resorption are mediated by this transporter (see the figure on the following page). The tryptophan deficiency is generally not severe enough to impair protein synthesis, but does sometimes result in impaired niacin synthesis that can be alleviated by treatment with nicotinic acid or nicotinamide. (Recall that synthesis of niacin from tryptophan can account for approximately 50% of the body's needs for NAD and NADP synthesis.) Conditions such as poor protein nutrition, exposure to sun, or febrile illness trigger pellagra-like symptoms, including dermatitis on sun-exposed skin and altered neurological and/or mental function.

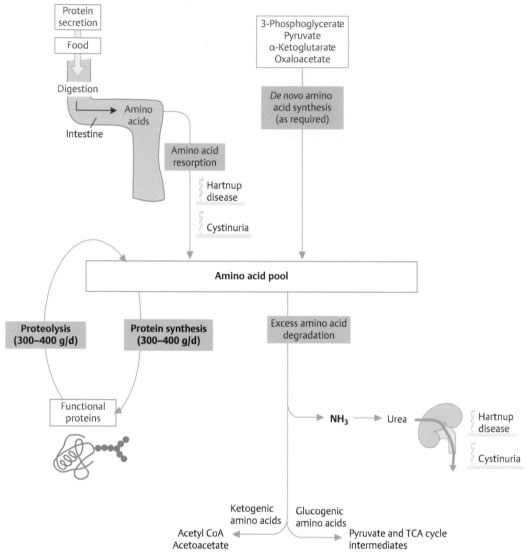

Source: Panini S. Medical Biochemistry - An Illustrated Review. 1st Edition. Thieme; 2013.

A is incorrect. Elevation of all amino acids in the urine would be indicative of a severe catabolic state, or significant renal or liver malfunction. The boy's symptoms are intermittent and not consistent with this type of condition.

B is incorrect. Because most serum cysteine is spontaneously oxidized to cystine, the probability of urinary accumulation of cysteine due to defects in renal resorption or to extremely high serum cysteine levels is quite low. There is no known disease associated with hypercysteinuria.

C is incorrect. Cystinuria is caused by a deficiency in the transport of cystine (cysteine disulfide) by the dibasic amino acid transporter. The symptoms are associated with formation of renal cystine crystals and subsequent formation of stones.

D is incorrect. Elevated levels of glutamine in the urine would be expected in diseases associated with hyperammonemia. Symptoms are much more severe and would not be corrected by treatment with nicotinamide.

5. Correct: D. Cobalamin.

The aggravation of this patient's cystinuria is most likely due to impaired intestinal absorption of cobalamin. Cystinuria results from a genetic deficiency in the amino acid transporter that facilitates renal resorption of cystine (cysteine disulfide). It can sometimes be managed effectively by dietary protein restriction, which reduces the body's load of methionine and cysteine, the precursors of cystine, and urinary alkalinization, which increases cystine solubility in the urine. Assuming that this patient was still adhering closely to this treatment plan after her surgery, it is likely that her urinary cystine levels started to rise because of an alteration in metabolism that resulted in increased cystine production. Cystine is produced by oxidation of cysteine, which is generated from methionine in the pathway shown in the figure in Answer 21 [note that cysteine (Cys) appears as a product in the reaction shown at the bottom of the figure]. Cysteine is the product of hydrolysis of cystathionine, which in turn is produced from homocysteine. Synthesis of cystathionine, and thus also cysteine and cystine, is only one possible fate of homocysteine; homocysteine can also be methylated to form methionine in a cobalamin-dependent reaction catalyzed by homocysteine methyltransferase (aka methionine synthase). A deficiency in cobalamin will decrease the rate of conversion of homocysteine to methionine, resulting in accumulation of homocysteine and in more synthesis of cysteine and cystine. Normally, the human liver stores enough cobalamin to meet the body's needs for a few years. However, this patient may have a lower than normal store of cobalamin due to her long-term low-protein diet, as dietary cobalamin is provided only from animal products. If her gastric bypass procedure significantly impaired intestinal uptake of cobalamin, the effects of the cobalamin deficiency could be observed within a few months.

A is incorrect. Iron does not play a role in the metabolism of sulfur-containing amino acids.

B is incorrect. A deficiency in pyridoxine could affect metabolism of sulfur-containing amino acids, but would result in a *decrease* in cysteine/cystine levels. Pyridoxine is a cofactor for cystathionine β-synthase, which catalyzes the synthesis of cystathionine (the precursor of cysteine) from homocysteine. A deficiency in pyridoxine would result in increased homocysteine levels and decreased cystathionine.

C is incorrect. Niacin is the precursor of nicotinamide, a component of NAD and NADP. A deficiency in niacin would not affect the metabolism of sulfur-containing amino acids.

E is incorrect. Thiamine provides the cofactor for α-ketoacid dehydrogenases and transketolases, neither of which play a role in sulfur-containing amino acid metabolism.

6. Correct: E. Tyrosine.

This child most likely has a deficiency in tyrosine metabolism. Compared to his parents, this child has very light skin and hair. Although his eyes are not visible in the photograph with Question 6, they are most likely blue. The boy has albinism, which results from an inability to generate melanin from tyrosine. (See the figure below for a review of tyrosine metabolism.) In many cases, albinism results from a genetic defect in tyrosinase, which catalyzes the first step in synthesis of melanin from tyrosine. In other cases, the defect may be in copper or tyrosine transport or in stabilization of tyrosinase by an accessory protein. Finally, some patients that exhibit albinism have a genetic defect in either phenylalanine hydroxylase or dihydrobiopterin reductase, two enzymes that participate in the conversion of phenylalanine to tyrosine. The latter patients, however, also exhibit

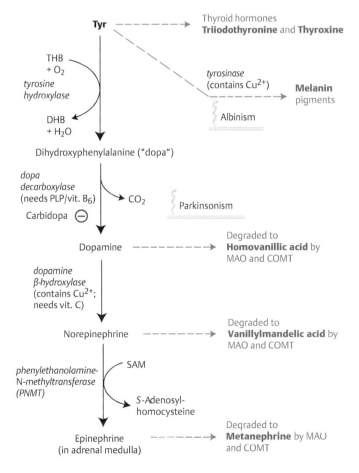

⊖ Inhibits

Source: Panini S. Medical Biochemistry - An Illustrated Review. 1st Edition. Thieme; 2013.

signs of severe impairment of neurological function, which is not observed in this child.

A is incorrect. A deficiency in phenylalanine metabolism would cause albinism, due to impaired biosynthesis of tyrosine. However, defects in phenylalanine metabolism (due to deficiencies in either phenylalanine hydroxylase or dihydrobiopterin reductase) also cause severe impairment of neurological function, which is not observed in this child.

B is incorrect. A deficiency in tryptophan metabolism may result in inadequate synthesis of serotonin and melatonin but will not cause albinism.

C is incorrect. A deficiency in valine metabolism would not affect melanin synthesis, and thus would not result in albinism. Defects in valine metabolism are associated with maple syrup urine disease. The hallmarks of maple syrup urine disease include mental retardation and production of urine with an odor of burnt maple syrup.

D is incorrect. Defects in histidine metabolism are generally asymptomatic and do not result in albinism.

7. Correct: C. Homocysteine.

The mother's folate deficiency could result in accumulation of homocysteine in her serum. This infant has spina bifida, a neural tube defect that can be linked to genetic and/or environmental factors including inadequate intake of folic acid during pregnancy. Inadequate levels of folate early in pregnancy are thought to impair nucleotide biosynthesis and epigenetic modifications that are required for correct fetal neural tube development. If the mother did, indeed, have a folate deficiency, the activity of methionine synthase, which requires both N^5-methyl tetrahydrofolate (derived from folate) and cobalamin, could be diminished. The substrate for methionine synthase is homocysteine. Thus, folate deficiency is sometimes observed to cause homocysteinemia.

A is incorrect. This infant's spina bifida is potentially caused by a deficiency in folic acid. Folic acid is the precursor for the cofactor tetrahydrofolate, which is not involved in isoleucine metabolism.

B is incorrect. Elevated uric acid levels are generally due to either renal malfunction or increased uric acid production due to elevated purine nucleotide catabolism. A folate deficiency, which could cause this infant's spina bifida, would not contribute to either of these causes of hyperuricemia.

D is incorrect. Elevated serum glutamine levels are a sign of hyperammonemia, which is generally a result of impaired urea cycle function. The urea cycle does not require tetrahydrofolate and, thus, would not be affected by a folate deficiency.

E is incorrect. This infant's spina bifida is potentially caused by a deficiency in folic acid. Folic acid is the precursor for the cofactor tetrahydrofolate, which is not involved in phenylalanine metabolism.

8. Correct: C. Methionine and cysteine.

Catabolism of methionine and cysteine results in decreased urinary pH. The data show that as dietary protein content increases, urinary pH decreases. The results of the experiments in which two particular amino acids are added to the MP diet suggest that the effect of amino acid consumption on urinary pH is caused primarily by those two specific amino acids and not just due to increased metabolism of amino acids in general. Urinary pH decreases in response to increased elimination of acidic metabolic intermediates (such as lactic acid or ketone bodies) or non-volatile acids (sulfuric acid and phosphoric acid). Of the 20 common dietary amino acids, only cysteine and methionine generate acid (sulfuric acid) during normal metabolism.

A is incorrect. Increased consumption of glutamic acid and aspartic will not result in changes in urinary pH in healthy individuals. Complete metabolism of these amino acids generates only carbon dioxide (CO_2) and urea and will not produce non-volatile acids that could alter urinary pH.

B is incorrect. Increased consumption of histidine and lysine will not result in changes in urinary pH in healthy individuals. Complete metabolism of these amino acids generates only CO_2 and urea and will not produce non-volatile acids that could alter urinary pH.

D is incorrect. Increased consumption of glutamine and asparagine will not result in changes in urinary pH in healthy individuals. Complete metabolism of these amino acids generates only CO_2 and urea and will not produce non-volatile acids that could alter urinary pH.

E is incorrect. Increased consumption of phenylalanine and tyrosine will not result in changes in urinary pH in healthy individuals. Complete metabolism of these amino acids generates only CO_2 and urea and will not produce non-volatile acids that could alter urinary pH.

9. Correct: B. Arginine.

The boy will most likely benefit from administration of arginine. Argininosuccinate synthase catalyzes the condensation of citrulline with aspartate in the urea cycle, which is shown in the figure on the following page. In some patients, the hyperammonemia that results from this urea cycle defect can be controlled by limiting dietary protein consumption. However, catabolic states, such a febrile illness, can lead to hyperammonemia due to increased demand on the urea cycle. Ammonia accumulates in this patient because the low argininosuccinate synthase activity impairs synthesis of arginine, which is the precursor of ornithine and an allosteric activator of N-acetylglutamate (NAG) synthase. The urea cycle cannot function unless ornithine levels are adequate, and NAG is a potent allosteric activator of carbamoyl phosphate synthase I, which catalyzes the condensation of ammonium and bicarbonate ions. Administration of arginine to this patient will stimulate the synthesis of NAG, and thus the activity of carbamoyl phosphate synthase I. It will also provide arginine for synthesis of ornithine via the enzyme arginase. (Note that although ornithine synthesis via the urea cycle is impaired in this patient, some ornithine will be produced from glutamate by its oxidation to glutamate semialdehyde, followed by transamination. However, under conditions that require increased flux through the urea cycle, the cellular concentration of ornithine will most likely be inadequate.)

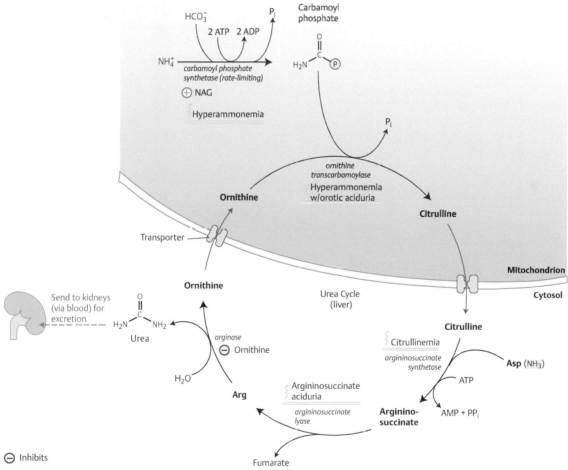

Source: Panini S. Medical Biochemistry - An Illustrated Review. 1st Edition. Thieme; 2013.

A is incorrect. Administration of *N*-acetylglutamate would stimulate the activity of carbamoyl phosphate, but would not facilitate the generation of ornithine, which is depleted in this patient.

C is incorrect. Administration of aspartate might be somewhat beneficial if this patient's genetic defect decreases the affinity of argininosuccinate synthase for aspartate. However, one of the other answer choices has a much greater probability of being beneficial.

D is incorrect. If anything, administration of glutamine may exacerbate this patient's condition. Recall that when ammonia levels are high, as in cases of urea cycle defects, the body "soaks up" some of the ammonia by condensing it with glutamate to form glutamine.

E is incorrect. Administration of lysine will have no beneficial effect on urea cycle function in this patient.

10. Correct: C. Tyrosinase.

Increased pigmentation is most likely due to increased activity of tyrosinase. Pigmentation in human tissues is due to the presence of melanin, which is derived from tyrosine. Melanin production in melanocytes begins with the hydroxylation of tyrosine to dopamine, followed by oxidation of dopamine to dopaquinone. Both of these reactions are catalyzed by tyrosinase. Regulation of melanogenesis is complex and involves many factors including UV light, melanin-stimulating hormone, estrogen, and progesterone. Melanin synthesis is stimulated in response to estrogen and is inhibited in response to progesterone. Changing estrogen and progesterone levels during pregnancy can result in increased pigmentation on areas of the face, arms, and other areas of the body frequently exposed to sunlight. Hyperpigmentation can also occur along the linea alba.

A is incorrect. Homogentisate oxidase is an enzyme involved in the catabolism of phenylalanine and tyrosine. Deficiency in homogentisate oxidase activity results in accumulation of black pigment in connective tissues and urine, a disorder called alkaptonuria.

B is incorrect. Uroporphyrinogen decarboxylase catalyzes a step in the synthesis of heme. Deficiencies in this enzyme result in porphyria cutanea tarda, with symptoms including photosensitivity resulting in blistering of the skin.

D is incorrect. Biliverdin reductase catalyzes the conversion of biliverdin to bilirubin in the degradation of heme. Accumulation of heme (purple), biliverdin (green-yellow), and bilirubin (red-orange) in macrophages near the site of a wound cause coloration observed in bruises. The spot on this woman's face is not a bruise.

E is incorrect. Tryptophan hydroxylase (aka tryptophan monooxygenase) catalyzes the first step in the synthesis of serotonin and melatonin from tryptophan. Neither of these hormones, nor the intermediate 5-hydroxytryptophan, are associated with production of pigment.

11. Correct: D. Glutamine.

This patient's kidneys will increase their catabolism of glutamine in order to generate more serum bicarbonate in an effort to compensate for metabolic acidosis. This patient's laboratory results are consistent with ketoacidosis. During any type of acidosis, the kidney works to neutralize the serum by producing more serum bicarbonate and eliminating protons in the urine. It utilizes large quantities of glutamine to do this (acidosis stimulates protein degradation in the muscle, providing glutamine to the kidney). Glutamine metabolism in the kidney generates ammonium ions via the actions of glutaminase and glutamate dehydrogenase. Ammonia molecules diffuse into the tubules, where they associate with protons (also passed into the tubules) to generate ammonium ions. In this way, some serum protons are eliminated in the urine. The α-ketoglutarate that is generated in the glutamate dehydrogenase reaction runs through reactions of the tricarboxylic acid (TCA) cycle to generate oxaloacetate, which is converted to phosphoenolpyruvate (PEP) by PEP carboxykinase. PEP is converted to pyruvate and then acetyl CoA and oxidized in the TCA cycle, generating CO_2 for

formation of carbonic acid. Carbonic acid dissociates to form bicarbonate, which is transported to the serum to facilitate buffering of protons.

A is incorrect. Aspartate is utilized at greater than normal levels by the liver when the urea cycle is activated and by any tissue that has a greater than normal demand for *de novo* nucleotide synthesis. This is not the case with this patient.

B is incorrect. In order to compensate for this patient's acidosis, the kidney will generate more bicarbonate and ammonium ions. The reactions used for this process do not require cobalamin as a cofactor.

C is incorrect. Although the renal tubule cells may be transporting more glucose from the filtrate back to the serum, the cells will not be using (i.e., consuming) more glucose than normal. Rather, they will be relying largely on glutamine as an energy source.

E is incorrect. In order to compensate for this patient's acidosis, the kidney will generate more bicarbonate and ammonium ions. The reactions used for this process do not require tetrahydrofolate as a cofactor.

12. Correct: B. A very low protein diet and a complete amino acid supplement with carefully determined levels of valine, leucine, and isoleucine.

This child will require a diet containing only the necessary amounts of the branched chain amino acids: valine, leucine, and isoleucine. As illustrated in the figure below, branched chain α-ketoacid dehydrogenase catalyzes the second step in the metabolism of the branched chain amino acids. In individuals who are homozygous for mutations in this protein, the branched chain amino acids and their α-keto derivatives accumulate. If untreated, these individuals develop severe neurological damage. Although the pathology is not well understood, it is believed that high levels of leucine competitively inhibit transport of other amino acids into cells. In order to keep the concentrations of the branched chain amino acids and their α-keto derivatives low, these individuals must consume a diet that is very low in protein (branched chain amino acids are ubiquitous in food proteins). In order to prevent negative nitrogen balance, they must also consume a complete amino acid cocktail that contains normal dietary levels of most amino acids, but only the minimal amount of branched chain amino acids needed to meet the body's demand for protein synthesis. Note that although not mentioned in this answer choice, these individuals should also avoid fasting, as that will trigger muscle proteolysis and increase the levels of branched chain amino and ketoacids in the serum.

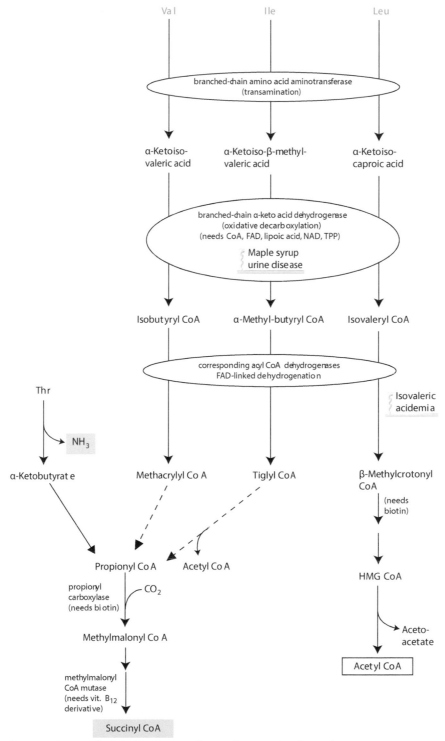

Source: Panini S. Medical Biochemistry - An Illustrated Review. 1st Edition. Thieme; 2013.

A is incorrect. Branched chain α-ketoacid dehydrogenase does not participate in carbohydrate metabolism, so there would be no need to avoid carbohydrates.

C is incorrect. Branched chain α-ketoacid dehydrogenase does not participate in phenylalanine metabolism, so there would be no need to avoid phenylalanine. Phenylalanine should be avoided by individuals who are homozygous for mutations in either phenylalanine hydroxylase or dihydrobiopterin reductase.

D is incorrect. Although these individuals need to carefully control dietary intake of branched chain amino acids, a very low protein diet without amino acid supplementation would be unsustainable. It will still be necessary to consume at least the minimal amounts of the nine essential amino acids, which include the branched chain amino acids.

E is incorrect. Branched chain α-ketoacid dehydrogenase does not participate in the metabolism of fatty acids, so there would be no need to limit fatty acid intake.

13. Correct: E. Sweet-smelling earwax.

Deficiency in branched chain α-ketoacid dehydrogenase is associated with the smell of burnt sugar or maple syrup in the urine and earwax. The enzyme deficiency results in accumulation of branched chain amino acids and their α-ketoacid derivatives (see the figure in Answer 12). The ketoacid derivative of isoleucine smells of maple syrup; hence, this disorder is known as maple syrup disease or maple syrup urine disease.

A is incorrect. Albinism results from deficiencies in the synthesis of melanin or in the regulation of melanin synthesis. Melanin is generated from tyrosine; its synthesis and regulation are not influenced by branched chain α ketoacid dehydrogenase.

B is incorrect. Genetically linked fragile bones are generally associated with osteogenesis imperfecta, a deficiency in collagen synthesis.

C is incorrect. Musty-smelling urine is associated with phenylketonuria, a deficiency in phenylalanine metabolism caused by mutations in either phenylalanine hydroxylase or dihydrobiopterin reductase.

D is incorrect. Spina bifida is associated with inadequate folate consumption around the time of conception and early pregnancy.

14. Correct: E. Thiamine.

The child may benefit from supplementation with thiamine. Branched chain α-ketoacid dehydrogenase is a member of a family of large multisubunit enzyme complexes that utilize five cofactors: thiamine pyrophosphate (derived from thiamine), lipoic acid, coenzyme A, flavin adenine dinucleotide (FAD) and NAD$^+$. (A good mnemonic for remembering this list is **T**ender **L**oving **C**are **F**or **N**ancy.) Other members of this enzyme family are the pyruvate dehydrogenase complex, and the α-ketoglutarate complex. Some individuals with deficiencies in these enzymes have mutations that can be partially compensated for by increasing thiamine levels.

A is incorrect. Biotin is a required cofactor for carboxylases, including pyruvate carboxylase and acetyl CoA carboxylase.

B is incorrect. Cobalamin is the required cofactor for methylmalonyl CoA mutase and methionine synthase.

C is incorrect. Folate is required for generation of tetrahydrofolate, a one-carbon carrier that participates in the synthesis of several biomolecules but has no role in the degradation of branched chain amino acids.

D is incorrect. Niacin is utilized to synthesize NAD+ and NADP+. Although NAD+ is a required

cofactor for the branched chain α-ketoacid dehydrogenase, supplementation with niacin is not known to be beneficial, most likely due to the fact that cellular NAD+ concentrations are regulated by cellular energy levels.

15. Correct: D. Proteasomal protein degradation.

Deficiency in Parkin results in impaired proteosomal protein degradation. Ubiquitin E3 ligases bind to target proteins and facilitate their ubiquitination, which is catalyzed by E2 ubiquitin-conjugating enzymes. There are more than 600 known different E3 ligases, providing selectivity for the ubiquitination process. Ubiquitination targets proteins for hydrolysis by proteasomes. Individuals with deficient Parkin activity fail to degrade proteins that are normally targeted by Parkin for ubiquitination.

A is incorrect. E3 ligases do not participate in amino acid uptake.

B is incorrect. DNA replication does not require the participation of E3 ligases, which facilitate protein degradation.

C is incorrect. Lysosomal protein degradation is catalyzed by cathepsins, which are acid-activated proteases. Proteins enter lysosomes and are degraded following endocytosis, pinocytosis or phagocytosis (extracellular proteins), or autophagy (intracellular proteins). Ubiquitination of proteins, facilitated by E3 ligases, is not part of this process.

E is incorrect. E3 ligases participate in protein degradation, not synthesis.

16. Correct: C. Glutamine and glycine.

This patient most likely received treatment with sodium phenyl acetate and/or sodium benzoate in order to facilitate removal of glutamine and glycine from his serum. The laboratory results indicate that this patient is likely is suffering from hepatic encephalopathy, caused by alcohol-induced hepatic cirrhosis; his liver is damaged to such an extent that the urea cycle is not functioning at full capacity, resulting in hyperammonemia. Frequently, an IV mixture of sodium phenyl acetate and sodium benzoate is administered to in-patients with hyperammonemia. Phenylbutyrate forms conjugates with glutamine, and benzoate forms conjugates with glycine. These conjugates are eliminated in the urine, thus removing glutamine (which contains two amino groups) and glycine (one amino group) from the body and decreasing the amount of amino acid nitrogen available for ammonia formation.

A is incorrect. The treatment goal is to reduce serum ammonia concentrations, which in turn will correct the patient's alkalosis. The drug that is typically administered in cases of hyperammonemia will not directly influence renal bicarbonate elimination.

B is incorrect. While the goal of treatment is to reduce serum ammonia levels, the drug that is typically administered in cases of hyperammonemia does not increase the rate of renal ammonium ion elimination.

D is incorrect. This patient's hyperammonemia is most likely due to poor liver function. Administration of a drug that would restore liver function would correct the hyperammonemia and increase urea production, and thus urinary urea excretion. However, the only drug available to efficiently reduce serum ammonia levels in these cases does not function by this mechanism.

E is incorrect. As described in the explanations for choices B and C, the drug that is administered to relieve hyperammonia does not result in increased urinary elimination of free ammonia or urea.

17. Correct: B. Catecholamines and serotonin.

This child will have impaired synthesis of catecholamines and serotonin. Tetrahydrobiopterin is the reducing agent utilized by phenylalanine hydroxylase, tyrosine hydroxylase, and tryptophan monooxygenase. Tetrahydrobiopterin is oxidized to dihydrobiopterin during the reactions catalyzed by these enzymes; dihydrobiopterin reductase utilizes NADPH to reduce dihydrobiopterin back to tetrahydrobiopterin. A deficiency in this reductase will impair the activity of all enzymes that utilize tetrahydrobiopterin. Phenylalanine hydroxylase and tyrosine hydroxylase are in the pathway for synthesis of catecholamines, and tryptophan monooxygenase catalyzes the first step in the synthesis of serotonin (which is a precursor of melatonin). Thus, individuals deficient in dihydrobiopterin reductase will need to be treated for deficiencies in catecholamine and serotonin production.

A is incorrect. Biosynthesis of SAM is not dependent on adequate levels of tetrahydrobiopterin, the product of dihydrobiopterin reductase.

C is incorrect. This child would have impaired catecholamine synthesis, but tetrahydrofolate concentrations will not be affected by a dihydrobiopterin reductase deficiency.

D is incorrect. Nicotinamide and serotonin are both derived from tryptophan. However, only serotonin synthesis requires a tetrahydrobiopterin reductase-dependent enzyme, tryptophan monooxygenase. Nicotinamide synthesis will not be affected in this patient.

E is incorrect. Synthesis of SAM and tetrahydrofolate are not dependent on tetrahydrobiopterin. Thus, a deficiency in dihydrobiopterin reductase will not affect levels of SAM or tetrahydrofolate.

18. Correct: C. Enteropeptidase.

This patient's diarrhea and weight loss is most likely due to impaired digestion of dietary protein due to insufficient activity of enteropeptidase. The patient's biopsy indicates significant damage to her intestinal epithelial cells, with marked atrophy or total loss of villi consistent with celiac disease. Enterocyte damage may be caused by an allergic reaction to gliadin proteins in gluten, which is found in barley, wheat, and rye, resulting in atrophy of the villi in the small intestine and subsequent development problems with malabsorption of macronutrients, minerals, and vitamins. Malabsorption of macronutrients results in diarrhea and weight loss. Protein malabsorption specifically is due in large part to decreased levels of enteropeptidase, a membrane-associated protein located in the microvilli of enterocytes. Enteropeptidase catalyzes the proteolytic activation of trypsinogen, a zymogen released from the pancreas. Active trypsin then proteolytically activates other pancreatic zymogens. Without activation of trypsinogen by enteropeptidase, the concentration of active digestive proteases is low, and dietary protein is not digested. This results in malabsorption of amino acids, contributing to weight loss and diarrhea.

A is incorrect. Cathepsins are lysosomal proteases and are not involved in intestinal protein digestion.

B is incorrect. Although elastase activity will be low in this individual, the decreased elastase activity is caused by low trypsin activity, which in turn is caused by decreased enteropeptidase activity.

D is incorrect. Pepsin is a gastric peptidase; its activity will not be affected by the intestinal disease exhibited by this patient.

E is incorrect. Although trypsin activity will be low in this individual, the decreased trypsin activity is caused by low enteropeptidase activity.

19. Correct: B. Precursor of glucose = Alanine; Precursor of ketone bodies = Leucine.

Alanine will be used for gluconeogenesis, and leucine will be used to generate ketone bodies. Glucogenic amino acids are those that can be converted to TCA cycle intermediates. Malate generated in the TCA cycle can be transported to the cytosol, where it is oxidized to oxaloacetate and then converted to PEP by PEP carboxykinase; PEP then feeds into the gluconeogenic pathway. The only exception is serine, which can be converted directly to dihydroxyacetone phosphate, a glycolytic/gluconeogenic intermediate. The ketogenic amino acids are degraded to acetoacetate or acetyl CoA. Only two amino acids, leucine and lysine, are exclusively ketogenic; other ketogenic amino acids generate TCA cycle intermediates in addition to either acetyl CoA or acetoacetate. The figure on the following page illustrates the catabolic fates and common derivatives of the 20 common amino acids.

Ketogenic and glucogenic amino acids

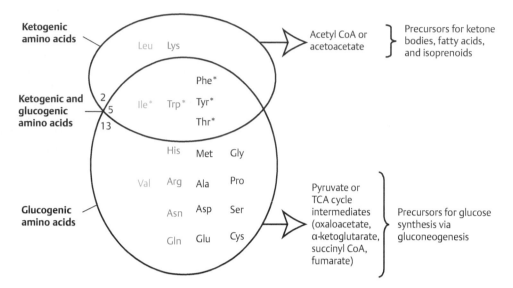

Amino acid degradation: overview

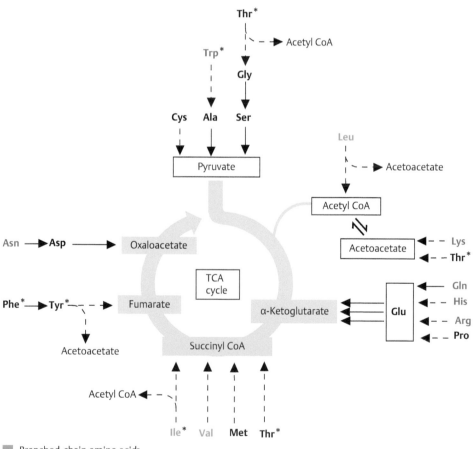

■ Branched-chain amino acids

■ Contains amino group in side chain

* Amino acid with ketogenic and glucogenic degradation products

Source: Panini S. Medical Biochemistry - An Illustrated Review. 1st Edition. Thieme; 2013.

A is incorrect. Both alanine and arginine are glucogenic.

C is incorrect. Both glutamine and proline are glucogenic.

D is incorrect. Both leucine and lysine are ketogenic.

E is incorrect. Both proline and cysteine are glucogenic.

20. Correct: C. Orotic acid in the urine.

Measurement of the orotic acid level in urine would be most beneficial in the diagnosis of this patient. This infant has hyperammonemia along with significant hyperornithinemia, which is suggestive of an inherited urea cycle defect. Elevated ornithine accompanied by low citrulline levels could be attributed to deficiencies in carbamoyl phosphate synthetase I, ornithine transcarbamoylase, or N-acetylglutamate (NAG) synthase (recall that NAG is a potent activator of carbamoyl phosphate synthetase I). [For a review of the urea cycle, see the figure in Answer 9.] The most common of these is ornithine transcarbamoylase (OTC) deficiency, an X-linked trait. In patients with OTC deficiency, carbamoyl phosphate that accumulates in the mitochondria leaks into the cytosol where it becomes a substrate for aspartate transcarbamoylase and subsequent synthesis of orotate in the pyrimidine synthesis pathway, shown in the figure on the following page. Because 5-phosphoribosyl-1-pyrophosphate (PRPP, the activated form of ribose 5-phosphate) levels are not elevated, as is the case when pyrimidine synthesis is normally activated, orotate accumulates in the cytosol, is eventually released from hepatocytes, and is excreted in the urine. Elevated urine orotate levels are diagnostic of OTC deficiency caused hyperammonemia. If this patient's urinary orotate level is normal, further testing will need to be done in order to distinguish between carbamoyl phosphate synthetase I deficiency and NAG synthase deficiency.

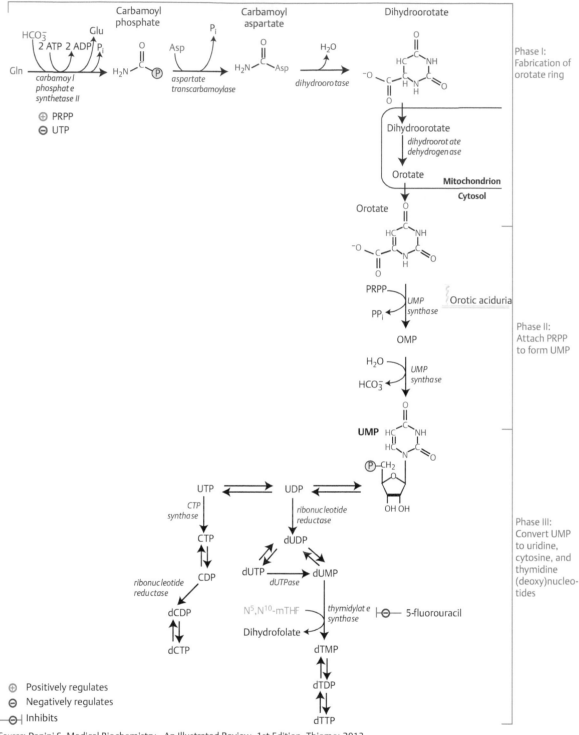

Source: Panini S. Medical Biochemistry - An Illustrated Review. 1st Edition. Thieme; 2013.

A is incorrect. In cases of hyperammonemia, urinary ammonia levels may also be elevated; this does not provide information that would be useful in determining the root cause of the hyperammonemia.

B is incorrect. Serum glutamine levels are always elevated in cases of hyperammonemia, regardless of the root cause. Recall that when ammonia levels are elevated, the glutamate dehydrogenase reaction runs in the direction of synthesis of glutamate from α-ketoglutarate and ammonia. Glutamate then combines with ammonia to form glutamine in the reaction catalyzed by glutamine synthetase.

D is incorrect. Because this child has a urea cycle defect, serum urea levels will be low regardless of which enzyme is deficient.

E is incorrect. Hyperuricemia in newborns could be caused by a defect in purine metabolism, such as Lesch–Nyhan syndrome, or by deficiency in glucose 6-phosphatase (von Gierke disease). It is not linked to hyperammonemia and urea cycle defects.

21. Correct: A. Injections of cobalamin.

This patient will most likely benefit from injections of cobalamin. She has macrocytic anemia, which is generally associated with deficiencies in either folate (vitamin B_9) or cobalamin (vitamin B_{12}). Recall that the methylene and formyl forms of tetrahydrofolate are required for nucleotide biosynthesis, and impaired nucleotide synthesis in turn inhibits DNA replication in erythroid cells, resulting in release of immature megaloblastic erythrocytes. As illustrated in the figure below, a deficiency in cobalamin will result in inadequate methionine synthase (aka homocysteine methyltransferase) activity. This will cause accumulation of N_5-methyl-tetrahydrofolate

(N_5-mTHF), which has no other possible metabolic fate. The result is that the body's available tetrahydrofolate is trapped in the methyl form, causing a secondary folate deficiency. In this patient's case, the normal serum folate level indicates that her megaloblastic anemia is due to a deficiency in cobalamin. Her partial gastrectomy most likely has resulted in decreased parietal cell production of intrinsic factor, which is required for adequate uptake of dietary cobalamin. Oral supplementation with cobalamin is not the best choice of treatment, as the orally supplemented cobalamin will not be well-absorbed due to the intrinsic factor deficiency. Hence, injections of cobalamin are preferred.

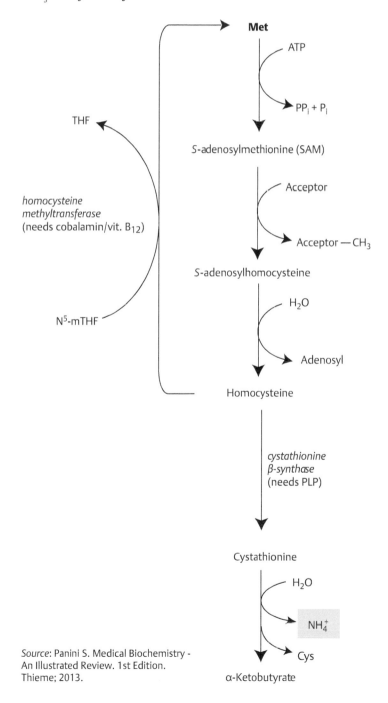

Source: Panini S. Medical Biochemistry - An Illustrated Review. 1st Edition. Thieme; 2013.

165

B in incorrect. Although this patient's partial gastrectomy has apparently resulted in decreased parietal cell production of intrinsic factor, injection of intrinsic factor will not facilitate increased absorption of dietary cobalamin.

C is incorrect. Macrocytic anemia is symptomatic of folate or cobalamin deficiency. Supplementation with iron will not be beneficial.

D is incorrect. Oral cobalamin treatment will not be as beneficial as parenteral cobalamin treatment, as the deficiency is most likely due to decreased production of intrinsic factor and subsequently poor absorption. In patients who refuse or cannot tolerate regular cobalamin injections, a mega-dose of oral cobalamin is sometimes therapeutic.

E is incorrect. Although this patient's partial gastrectomy has apparently resulted in decreased parietal cell production of intrinsic factor, oral administration of intrinsic factor is not known to be beneficial.

F is incorrect. Macrocytic anemia is symptomatic of folate or cobalamin deficiency. Supplementation with iron will not be beneficial.

Chapter 10

Nucleotide, Heme, and Iron Metabolism

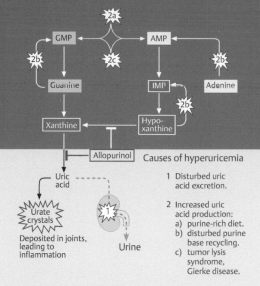

LEARNING OBJECTIVES

▶ Describe the *de novo* biosynthesis of the purine and pyrimidine nucleotides, knowing key intermediates, key regulated steps, and the amino acids and one-carbon metabolites that are involved.

▶ Describe inborn errors of metabolism in the purine and pyrimidine *de novo* and salvage pathways.

▶ Describe the ribonucleotide reductase reaction and its role in chemotherapy.

▶ Summarize purine nucleotide catabolism, knowing key enzymes and intermediates and their role in the development of hyperuricemia and gout.

▶ Explain the thymidylate synthase reaction and its role in the mechanisms of action of 5-fluorouracil and the antifolates.

▶ Describe the pathway for heme biosynthesis, with particular attention to the rate-limiting step, cofactor requirements, the role of iron, the effects of lead poisoning, and deficiencies resulting in porphyria cutanea tarda and acute intermittent porphyria.

▶ Describe heme catabolism, knowing key intermediates, the differences between direct and indirect bilirubin, and the causes of Gilbert's syndrome and the following types of jaundice: neonatal, hemolytic, hepatocellular, and obstructive.

▶ Describe the processes and key proteins involved in iron hemostasis, and interpret results of laboratory iron panels.

▶ Compare and contrast different causes of anemia using biochemical mechanisms to explain how laboratory results can differentiate between them.

10.1 Questions

Easy	Medium	Hard

1. A 55-year-old woman who was recently diagnosed with stage IV breast cancer and has not yet begun therapy complains of extreme fatigue. A peripheral blood smear indicates microcytic, hypochromic anemia, and iron tests indicate that her serum ferritin levels are high. Tumor-induced increased expression of which of the following proteins would best explain this patient's anemia?

Causes of hyperuricemia

A. Apoferritin

B. Divalent metal transporter-1 (DMT1)

C. Ferrochetolase

D. Heme oxidase

E. Hepcidin

2. An 8-day-old Caucasian infant who was mildly jaundiced 1 day after birth presents at her pediatrician's office. The child's mother reports that although she's been following instructions for BiliBlanket phototherapy at home, the baby's skin seems to be developing a deeper yellow color. Which of the following combination of laboratory results and physical observations would indicate that this infant suffers from biliary atresia, rather than the physiologic jaundice of newborns that was initially diagnosed?

	Direct bilirubin	Indirect bilirubin	Stool color
A	Normal	Normal	Pale/gray
B	Increased	Normal	Normal
C	Normal	Increased	Pale/gray
D	Increased	Normal	Pale/gray
E	Normal	Increased	Normal

3. During a routine well-child examination, the mother of a 6-year-old girl reports to the pediatrician that over the last few months the girl has become lethargic and irritable. Furthermore, the girls' school teacher reports that the child is not performing well academically. Physical examination indicates pallor and pale conjunctiva. The pediatrician orders a complete blood count and iron panel (relevant results shown in the table below), and subsequently a bone marrow aspiration and biopsy.

	Patient	Normal range
Hemoglobin	4.6 g/dL	11–13 g/dL
Mean corpuscular volume	45.7 fL	78–102 fL
Serum iron	212 µg/dL	50–175 µg/dL
Ferritin	595 ng/mL	18–300 ng/mL
Total iron binding capacity	240 µg/dL	250–460 µg/dL

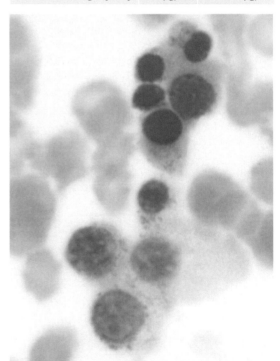

Source: Siegenthaler W. Siegenthaler's Differential Diagnosis in Internal Medicine: From Symptom to Diagnosis. 1st Edition. Thieme; 2007.

Which of the following proteins is most likely defective or inhibited in this patient?

A. Divalent metal transporter-1

B. Ferrochetolase

C. Hemoglobin β-chain

D. Hepcidin

E. Thymidylate synthase

F. Glucose-6-phosphate dehydrogenase

4. A 74-year-old man, recently diagnosed with an aggressive form of non-Hodgkin's lymphoma, underwent his first round of chemotherapy. Two days later, he went to the emergency room complaining of weakness, nausea, and intense bilateral flank pain. Physical examination indicated edema, and urinalysis indicated hematuria. A computed tomography (CT) scan was indicative of nephrolithiasis. An increase in the activity of which of the following enzymes contributed to this patient's emergent condition?

A. Renal amino acid transporter SLC3A1

B. Thymidylate synthase

C. Glutaminase

D. Xanthine oxidase

E. Caspases

5. X-linked sideroblastic anemia is a rare disorder resulting from mutations in the *ALAS2* gene, which codes for δ-aminolevulinic acid (ALA) synthase in erythroid cells. In many patients with this disorder, hemoglobin levels can be improved significantly by administration of a vitamin. Which of the following vitamins would most likely correct anemia associated with ALAS2 deficiency?

A. Pyridoxine

B. Folic acid

C. Cobalamin

D. Ascorbic acid

E. Cholecalciferol

6. A 55-year-old man complained to his primary care physician that in the last few months he'd been experiencing episodes of severe pain in the metatarsophalangeal joint of his right foot. The pain, which lasts for a several hours and then dissipates, is limited to that joint and is accompanied by redness and swelling. The physician obtained a sample of synovial fluid from the joint. A micrograph of the fluid, viewed through a polarizing filter is shown in the figure below. Which of the following most likely contributes to the development of this patient's symptoms?

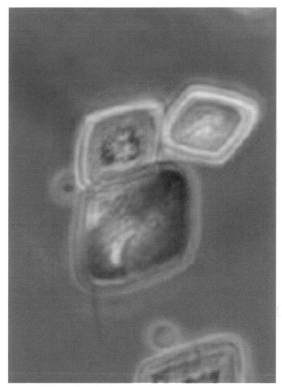

Source: Theml H, Diem H, Haferlach T. Color Atlas of Hematology. Practical Microscopic and Clinical Diagnosis. 2nd Edition. Thieme; 2004.

A. Consumption of a diet high in red meat and butter

B. Consumption of a diet high in seafood and alcohol

C. A genetic defect resulting in increased release of pyrophosphate from chondrocytes

D. A bacterial infection

E. A genetic deficiency in tyrosine catabolism

7. A 40-year-old man with a 10-year history of worsening fatigue, joint pain, and low libido recently underwent genetic testing that revealed that he is homozygous for a missense mutation in the *HFE* gene. Initially, his treatment protocol includes weekly phlebotomy of about 500 mL. Which of the following blood tests is most appropriate for monitoring the progress of his treatment?

A. Hemoglobin concentration

B. Mean corpuscular volume

C. Serum ferritin

D. Total iron binding capacity

E. Total serum iron

8. On his 21st birthday, a male college student who had previously never consumed alcohol went on a drinking binge with his friends. He was admitted to the emergency department after complaining of severe abdominal pain and exhibiting psychotic behavior. There, it was noted that he was hypertensive and tachycardic. Following urinalysis, the attending physician ordered intravenous (IV) treatment with glucose and hematin. Which of the following substances was most likely elevated in this patient's urine?

A. β-hydroxybutyrate

B. Lactate

C. Porphobilinogen

D. Uric acid

E. Uroporphyrin

9. A 40-year-old woman who has been experiencing gradually worsening joint pain and swelling in her hands and wrists is prescribed leflunomide, which gives rise to a metabolite that inhibits dihydroorotate reductase. As a result of this treatment, which of the following substances will be produced at lower concentrations in this patient?

A. Uric acid

B. Carbamoyl phosphate

C. Guanosine monophosphate

D. Cytidine monophosphate

E. Glutathione

10. A 25-year-old man had blood drawn for a comprehensive metabolic panel and a complete blood count (CBC) during his annual physical examination. He had fasted for 24 hours prior to the examination. The results of the CBC were all within normal range, and the results of part of the metabolic panel are shown here:

	Patient	Normal
Total bilirubin	2.7 mg/dL (90% indirect)	0–1 mg/dL
AST	16 U/L	8–20 U/L
ALT	13 U/L	8–20 U/L
Alk Phos	74 U/L	46–108 U/L

Abbreviations: Alk Phos, alkaline phosphatase; ALT, alanine aminotransferase; AST, aspartate aminotransferase.

The patient returned 2 months later for a follow-up blood draw to be used for a repeat of the CBC and a liver function test. He did not fast prior to this appointment, and all results were in the normal range. A similar scenario occurred at his annual physical examination the following year. Which of the following genetic alterations most likely is the cause of this man's abnormal test results?

A. A mutation in the active site of cholesterol 7α-hydroxylase

B. A mutation in the promotor region of bilirubin UDP-glucuronyltransferase

C. A mutation in the active site of heme oxidase

D. A mutation in the β-subunit of hemoglobin

E. A mutation in the binding site of multidrug resistance–associated protein 2

11. A 55-year-old woman who was diagnosed with plaque psoriasis 3 months ago presented to her dermatologists with complaints that the topical treatment she'd been initially prescribed was not effective. The dermatologist prescribed oral methotrexate, one 10 mg dose per week. However, the pharmacist who filled the order erroneously indicated that the dose was 10 mg per day. Two weeks later, the woman became quite ill. She experienced labored breathing, fever, and chills. Blood tests were indicative of low red and white blood cell counts, as well as a low platelet count. This woman's illness is most directly attributable to *increased* concentrations of which of the following biomolecules in her bone marrow?

A. Adenosine monophosphate (AMP)

B. δ-Aminolevulinic acid

C. N^5-Methyltetrahydrofolate

D. Protoporphyrin

E. Deoxyuridine triphosphate (dUTP)

12. A 60-year-old vegetarian man who had been donating whole blood every 2 months for the last 20 years started taking over-the-counter omeprazole (a H⁺-pump inhibitor) to treat his worsening heartburn. A few months after beginning the omeprazole therapy, and continuing with his habit of donating blood, he presented to his physician with complaints of fatigue and shortness of breath. A CBC was ordered, along with a peripheral blood smear, which revealed microcytic, hypochromic erythrocytes. This patient's presenting illness is most likely due to decreased activity of which of the following proteins?

A. δ-Aminolevulinic acid synthase
B. Divalent metal transporter-1
C. Frataxin
D. Heme oxidase
E. Hepcidin

13. A 65-year-old man diagnosed with stage III squamous cell carcinoma underwent resection of a tumor from his temporal region. He subsequently received radiation therapy, along with a drug that directly decreased cellular concentrations of deoxynucleoside diphosphates. Which of the following is most likely the chemotherapy this patient received?

A. 5-Fluorouracil
B. Folinic acid (N^5-formyltetrahydrofolate)
C. Hydroxyurea
D. Methotrexate
E. Zidovudine (AZT)

Consider this scenario when answering questions 14 and 15.

A 9-month-old male infant was brought to his pediatrician for a well-child examination. His mother expressed concern that the boy had not yet been able to sit and had not started crawling. Physical examination revealed a child in the lower tenth percentile for weight and height, poor muscle tone, and random involuntary movements. One year later the child, who had only recently begun to crawl, was admitted to the emergency department following 2 days of vomiting and anuria. Physical examination indicated bilateral flank tenderness, and his mother reported that during the last few months she had regularly noticed a substance that looked like orange sand in the child's diapers. Ultrasonography of the kidneys was performed and revealed bilateral hyperechoic particles.

14. Which of the following metabolic pathways is most likely functioning at a significantly *higher* level in this patient than in other children of comparable age?

A. Activated methyl cycle
B. *De novo* purine synthesis
C. *De novo* pyrimidine synthesis
D. Purine salvage
E. Pyrimidine salvage
F. Urea cycle

15. The metabolic change alluded to in Question 14 is due most directly to increased cellular concentrations of which of the following substances?

A. Adenosine monophosphate
B. Carbamoyl phosphate
C. Hypoxanthine
D. 5-Phosphoribosyl-1-pyrophosphate
E. Ribose-5-phosphate

16. A 50-year-old homeless man with a history of chronic hepatitis B and alcohol abuse presents at the free clinic with complaints of blisters on his hands and forearms. Physical examination reveals extensive scaring, hyperpigmentation on his face, and excessive hair growth on his temples and cheeks. Upon questioning, he indicates that recently his urine has appeared wine-colored. What is the most likely cause of this patient's blistering?

A. Binding of antibodies to type VII collagen
B. Impaired adenosine triphosphate (ATP) synthesis in cutaneous tissue
C. Niacin deficiency
D. Sunlight-triggered formation of reactive oxygen species
E. Viral infection

10.2 Answers and Explanations

Easy	Medium	Hard

1. Correct: E. Hepcidin.

This patient's anemia is most likely due to increased hepcidin expression. Hepcidin, a peptide hormone synthesized primarily by the liver, stimulates the degradation of ferroportin, the protein responsible for transporting ferrous iron out of enterocytes and other cells, such as hepatocytes and macrophages. Increased serum levels of hepcidin thus decrease the amount of iron available for transport to erythroid cells where it is needed for heme synthesis. This results in the production of microcytic, hypochromic erythrocytes. (For a review of iron metabolism, see the figure below.) In cases of elevated hepcidin expression, serum ferritin levels will usually be normal or elevated, because there is not a true iron deficiency; ample (or even excess) iron is stored in hepatocytes and macrophages. Many patients with advanced cancer, like the one described here, develop anemia of chronic disease. The chronic inflammation that accompanies malignancy results in a significant increase in serum interleukin-6 levels, which stimulates hepatic production of hepcidin.

A is incorrect. Apoferritin is ferritin without iron bound. Increased expression of apoferritin in cells should not have a significant influence on iron bioavailability, as the associated increased storage capacity will not influence mobilization of iron to serum.

B is incorrect. DMT1 facilitates the transport of dietary iron into enterocytes. Increased expression of this protein would increase enterocyte iron levels and would not create a deficiency of iron for heme synthesis.

C is incorrect. Ferrochetolase catalyzes the last step in heme biosynthesis, the incorporation of Fe^{+2} into the protoporphyrin ring. Increased expression of this enzyme would not result in low erythroid heme levels, with subsequent production of microcytic, hypochromic erythrocytes.

D is incorrect. Heme oxidase catalyzes the first step in the degradation of heme. It does not play a role in iron or heme metabolism or regulation.

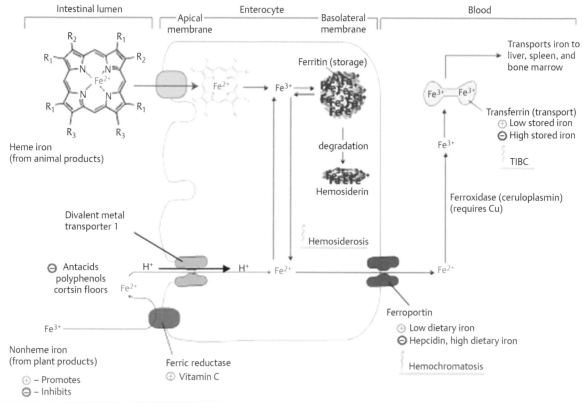

Source: Panini S. Medical Biochemistry - An Illustrated Review. 1st Edition. Thieme; 2013.

2. **Correct: D. Direct bilirubin = Increased; Indirect bilirubin = Normal; Stool color = Pale/gray.**

Biliary atresia results in little or no flow of bile from the liver to the gallbladder. Thus, bilirubin that is conjugated with glucuronic acid in hepatocytes and then secreted in the bile remains trapped in the liver. (See the figure below for a review of heme catabolism.) Eventually, it begins to leak into the serum. This conjugated bilirubin causes the jaundice observed in this patient, and is also known as direct bilirubin. [Recall that conjugated bilirubin is relatively soluble in serum and will react directly with diazo dyes to produce a reddish-purple product that can be easily quantitated. Unconjugated bilirubin is much less soluble in serum and does not react with diazo dyes unless it is made soluble by the addition of methanol to the serum. In the laboratory, two bilirubin measurements are taken; conjugated, or

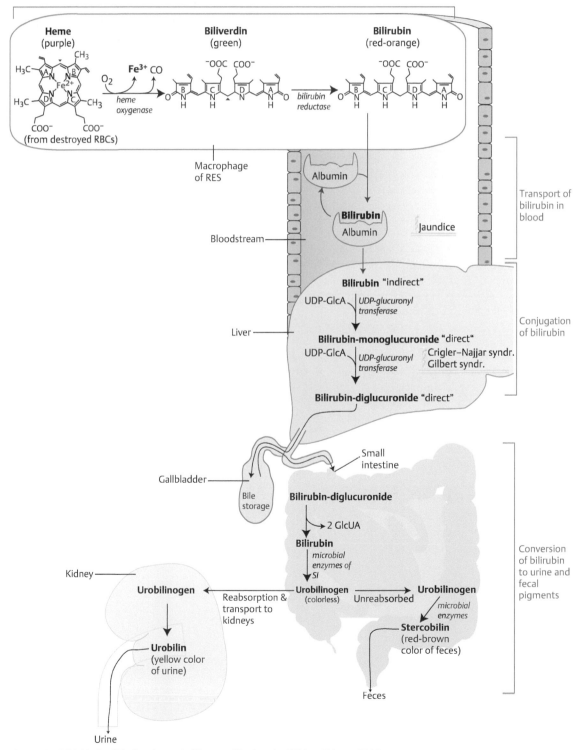

Source: Panini S. Medical Biochemistry - An Illustrated Review. 1st Edition. Thieme; 2013.

direct, bilirubin is determined in serum without the addition of methanol, and total bilirubin, the sum of the conjugated and unconjugated bilirubin species, is determined in a mixture of serum and methanol. The amount of unconjugated bilirubin can be determined by taking the difference between the total and direct bilirubin, and is thus known as indirect bilirubin. A good mnemonic for differentiating between direct and indirect bilirubin is that consonants go together (direct = conjugated), as do vowels (indirect = unconjugated).] Because conjugated bilirubin is not being secreted in the bile to the small intestine, intestinal conversion of bilirubin to stercobilin is not occurring. Stercobilin gives the feces its red-brown color, and the lack of it results in pale or gray-colored stools.

Choice A is incorrect. Having normal levels of direct and indirect bilirubin would not lead to jaundice, as seen in this patient.

Choice B is incorrect. This response correctly indicates an increase in direct bilirubin, resulting from leakage of conjugated bilirubin from the gallbladder to the serum due to the biliary atresia. However, it incorrectly predicts normal stool color; the lack of secretion of bilirubin to the intestine will result in a lack of stercobilin, which gives the stool its normal brown color.

Choice C is incorrect. An increase in indirect, unconjugated bilirubin is more consistent with hemolytic anemia, internal hemorrhage, or low glucuronyltransferase activity. In any of these cases, hepatocyte capacity to conjugate bilirubin is exceeded, resulting in leakage of unconjugated bilirubin to the serum. The bilirubin that does get conjugated, however, is still secreted to the intestine via the bile, so stool color would be normal.

Choice E is incorrect. An increase in indirect, unconjugated bilirubin is more consistent with hemolytic anemia, internal hemorrhage, or low glucuronyltransferase activity. In any of these cases, hepatocyte capacity to conjugate bilirubin is exceeded, resulting in leakage of unconjugated bilirubin to the serum.

3. Correct: B. Ferrochetolase.

This patient most likely has impaired ferrochetolase activity. The patient's low hemoglobin level and mean corpuscular volume are indicative of microcytic anemia, which is generally due to a deficiency in hemoglobin production resulting from an iron deficiency or other problem with heme or hemoglobin synthesis. The elevated serum iron and ferritin levels, together with the appearance of iron granules (sideroblasts) in the erythroid cells, indicate that the problem is not due to iron deficiency. The most likely problem is a congenital or acquired deficiency in heme synthesis. Ferrochetolase is the only enzyme listed here that plays a role in heme synthesis. Although there could be a genetic deficiency, the most likely cause of this patient's anemia is lead poisoning; lead is a known inhibitor of ferrochetolase, and elevated serum lead levels are associated with sideroblastic anemia.

A is incorrect. DMT1 is involved in the transport of Fe^{+2} across the enterocyte apical membrane. A deficiency or inhibition of DMT1 would result in decreased intestinal uptake, and thus storage, of iron. The result would be low ferritin levels; this patient's ferritin level is high. Furthermore, iron deficiency would not produce the sideroblasts observed in this patient's biopsy.

C is incorrect. A deficiency in hemoglobin β-chain synthesis results in β-thalassemia. Although β-thalassemia is a microcytic anemia, it is not associated with iron accumulation unless the patient has had repeated transfusions and is experiencing iron overload. Sideroblasts are not observed in β-thalassemia.

D is incorrect. Hepcidin, a key regulatory protein hormone in iron hemostasis, is produced in the liver and inhibits ferroportin, the transporter that moves iron out of enterocytes and other cells. A deficiency or inhibition of hepcidin would result in increased serum levels of iron and ferritin, as seen in this patient. However, hemoglobin synthesis would not be inhibited, and there would be no anemia.

E is incorrect. A deficiency or inhibition of thymidylate synthase would impair nucleotide synthesis. If the inhibition were severe enough, erythroid maturation would be impaired, resulting in macrocytic anemia rather than microcytic.

F is incorrect. Glucose-6-phosphate dehydrogenase deficiency is associated with hemolytic anemia and does not produce microcytic erythrocytes.

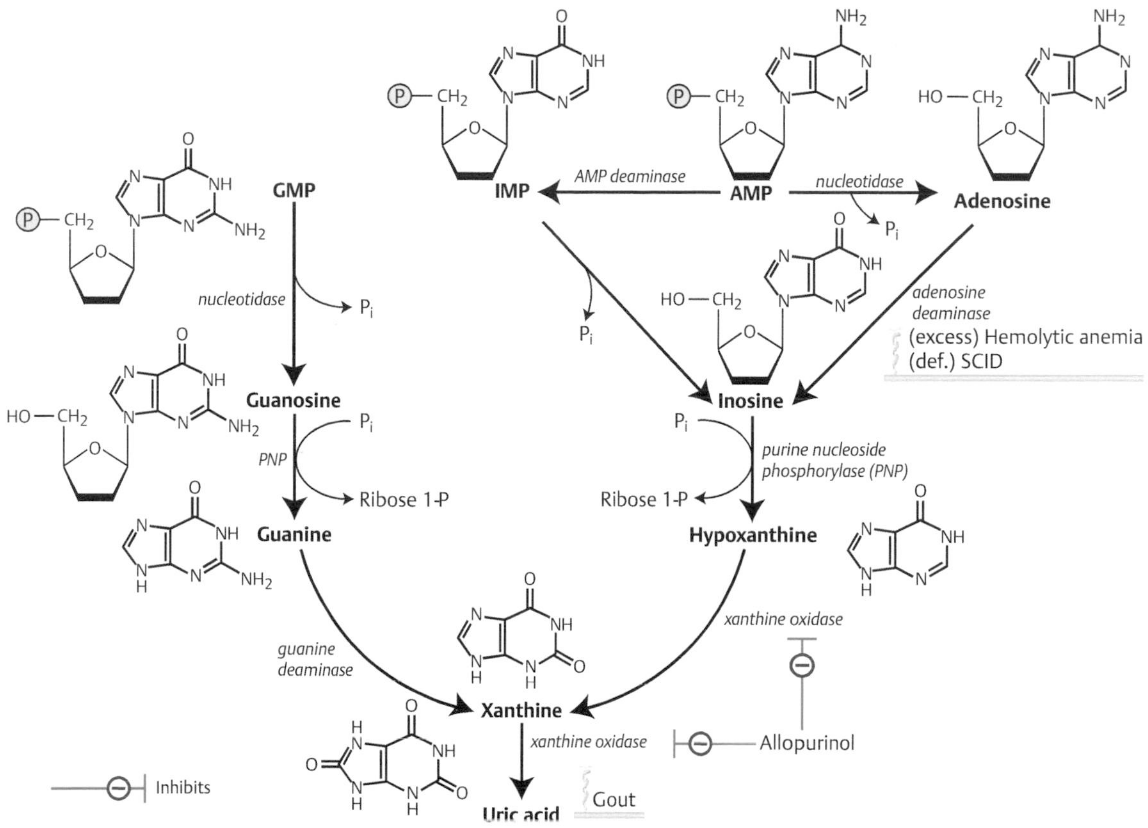

Source: Panini S. Medical Biochemistry - An Illustrated Review. 1st Edition. Thieme; 2013.

4. Correct: D. Xanthine oxidase.

This patient's nephrolithiasis is most likely attributable to uric acid stones resulting from increased xanthine oxidase activity. This patient has tumor lysis syndrome; the chemotherapeutic drugs that he's been administered are rapidly killing his tumor(s), thus releasing large quantities of purine nucleotides and other cellular components. Catabolism of the excess purines results in hyperuricemia, which can lead to accumulation of renal uric acid crystals. Xanthine oxidase catalyzes a key step in purine catabolism; its activity will increase as a result of the excess purine levels. See the figure above for a review of purine catabolism.

A is incorrect. Renal amino acid transporter SLC3A1 facilitates the transport of basic amino acids and cystine. A deficiency in this transporter results in the accumulation of cystine in the urine and may result in the formation of renal cystine crystals. Cystinuria results from a genetic defect; this patient's nephrolithiasis was triggered by his chemotherapy treatment.

B is incorrect. Depending on the chemotherapeutic agent that this patient has been administered, thymidylate synthase activity might be *inhibited* in this patient; it won't be stimulated.

C is incorrect. Glutaminase catalyzes the hydrolysis of glutamine to glutamate. Its activity is not implicated in the formation of renal stones.

E is incorrect. Caspases are proteases that mediate programmed cell death. Upon chemotherapeutic treatment, tumor cell caspases will be activated. However, the increased caspase activity and tumor lysis results in an increase in free serum amino levels. High amino acid levels, however, are not associated with the formation of renal stones.

5. Correct: A. Pyridoxine.

Supplementation with vitamin B_6 is beneficial for some patients with an ALA synthase deficiency. δ-Aminolevulinic acid synthase catalyzes the first step in heme synthesis and requires pyridoxal phosphate (PLP) as a cofactor, as illustrated on the following page which shows the pathway for heme synthesis. PLP is derived from vitamin B_6 (pyridoxine).

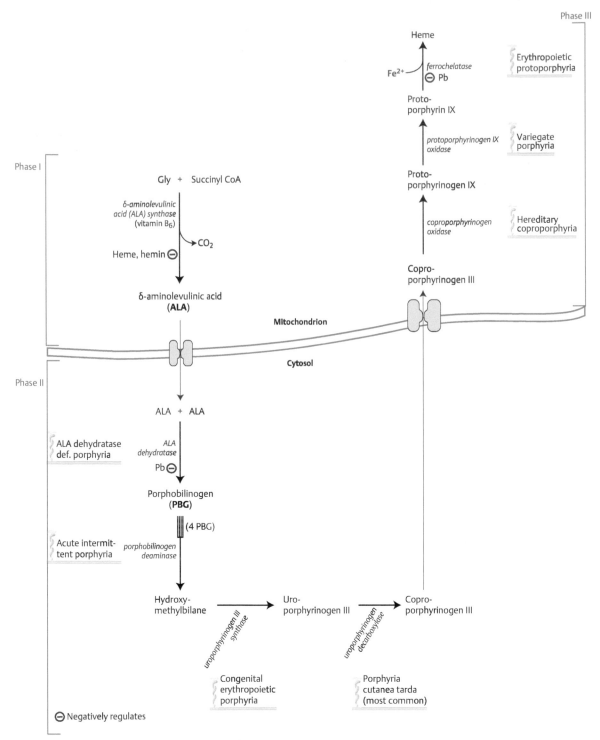

Source: Panini S. Medical Biochemistry - An Illustrated Review. 1st Edition. Thieme; 2013.

B is incorrect. Folic acid does not provide the cofactor associated with ALA synthase.

C is incorrect. Cobalamin does not provide the cofactor associated with ALA synthase.

D is incorrect. Ascorbic acid does not provide the cofactor associated with ALA synthase.

E is incorrect. Cholecalciferol does not provide the cofactor associated with ALA synthase.

6. Correct: B. Consumption of a diet high in seafood and alcohol.

This patient has gouty arthritis, which can be aggravated by diets high in seafood or alcohol consumption. The diagnosis is confirmed by the observation of sharp, needle-like crystals that are highly birefringent, and is consistent with the self-resolving nature of his episodes. Gout is caused by accumulation of urate crystals in the joints; urate is the product of purine degradation. Seafood often has a high purine content, thus increasing the levels of serum uric acid. Consumption of alcohol is linked to impaired renal secretion of uric acid. These two dietary components together will thus increase the probability of hyperuricemia and formation of urate crystals in the joints.

A is incorrect. Consumption of a diet high in saturated fats, as described here, does not adversely affect serum urate levels.

C is incorrect. Increased release of pyrophosphate from chondrocytes may contribute to the accumulation of calcium pyrophosphate crystals, which are observed in pseudogout. Attacks of pseudogout, however, tend to last for several days, and polarized microscopy of synovial fluid usually reveals shorter rhomboid crystals that are not highly birefringent.

D is incorrect. Bacterial infections do not produce the urate crystals observed in this patient's synovial fluid.

E is incorrect. A genetic deficiency in tyrosine metabolism, such as a deficiency in homogentisate dioxygenase, can cause painful accumulation of ochronotic pigment in joints. However, the joint pain is long-lasting, and the ochronotic pigment does not form needle-like crystals in the synovial fluid.

7. Correct: C. Serum ferritin.

Serum ferritin is the most appropriate marker for monitoring the treatment of this individual who has hemochromatosis. The most common form of hemochromatosis is due to missense mutations in the *HFE* (*H*igh serum *Fe*) gene, which encodes a protein that stimulates the production and secretion of hepatic hepcidin. Decreased hepcidin production results in increased stability of ferroportin, and thus increased transport of iron from enterocytes into the blood and organs of the body, even when iron stores are adequate. (Normally, hepatocytes increase their production of hepcidin in response to increased iron stores. See the figure in Answer 1.) The result is iron overload, which can lead to irreversible oxidative damage to several organs, including the liver, pancreas, and heart. The goal of the phlebotomy treatment is to reduce his body iron stores by frequent removal of iron (in erythrocytes and bound to transferrin). Analysis of serum ferritin is the best measure of body iron stores. Recall that iron is stored in various tissues (liver, spleen, and bone marrow, primarily) bound to ferritin, a small amount of which leaks from these tissues into serum. The serum ferritin concentration reflects the size of the body's iron stores, and should decrease as this patient's treatment continues.

A is incorrect. This individual has a problem with iron overload. Although his hemoglobin concentration may change slightly during this therapy, it is not the most sensitive and reliable measurement of body iron stores.

B is incorrect. Mutations in *HFE* have no effect on mean corpuscular volume, neither will phlebotomy.

D is incorrect. Total iron binding capacity (TIBC) is a measure of the amount of transferrin in the serum. Although it is sensitive to the level of body iron stores (it decreases with iron overload, and increases with iron deficiency), which we want to monitor in this patient, it is not the *most* sensitive measure of iron stores.

E is incorrect. Total serum iron measurement is not specific enough to allow the physician to accurately follow the progress of this patient's treatment; the goal is to specifically follow body iron stores, and total serum iron can be affected by several other factors.

8. Correct: C. Porphobilinogen.

The urinalysis most likely revealed the presence of porphobilinogen. This individual's symptoms and treatment with glucose and hematin are consistent with a diagnosis of acute intermittent porphyria (AIP). In AIP, a deficiency in porphobilinogen deaminase results in accumulation of porphobilinogen (BPG) and δ-aminolevulinic acid (ALA), both of which are eventually eliminated in the urine, under conditions where hepatic heme synthesis is stimulated. (See the figure in Answer 5 for a review of the heme biosynthetic pathway.) In this patient's case, the precipitating factor was excessive alcohol consumption, which stimulated hepatic expression of cytochrome P450 2E1 and thus increased demand for heme. ALA is a neurotoxin and is most likely the cause of this patient's neurologic symptoms (pain and psychosis). Treatment with glucose and hematin (an analog of heme) inhibits the activity of ALA synthase and thus decreases the levels of accumulated ALA and BPG.

A is incorrect. The presence of β-hydroxybutyrate in the urine would be indicative of ketosis. Although excessive alcohol consumption can trigger hypoglycemia and ketosis, the symptoms of ketosis do not include psychosis, and hematin is not used in treatment of ketosis.

B is incorrect. The presence of lactate in the urine would be indicative of lactic acidosis. Although excessive alcohol consumption can trigger hypoglycemia and lactic acidosis, the symptoms of hypoglycemia and lactic acidosis do not include psychosis, and hematin is not used in treatment of lactic acidosis.

D is incorrect. The presence of elevated levels of uric acid in the urine is indicative of hyperuricemia, a condition that does not cause the symptoms experienced by this patient. Although hyperuricemia can be triggered by alcohol consumption, the cause in that case is impaired renal excretion of uric acid due to inhibition by lactic acid; hence, urinary uric acid levels would not be elevated. Furthermore, treatment of acute hyperuricemia does not include parenteral glucose and hematin.

E is incorrect. Urinary uroporphyrin is elevated in individuals afflicted with porphyria cutanea tarda, an acquired or inherited deficiency in the activity of uroporphyrinogen decarboxylase. Symptoms include photosensitivity, and blistering of skin exposed to sunlight, and do not include abdominal pain or psychosis.

9. Correct: D. Cytidine monophosphate.

Cytidine monophosphate will be produced at lower concentrations in this patient's cells. Dihydroorotate reductase catalyzes a key step in pyrimidine synthesis, which is summarized in the figure below. Inhibition of this enzyme will thus result in decreased levels of the pyrimidine nucleotides: cytidine, uridine, and thymidine monophosphates.

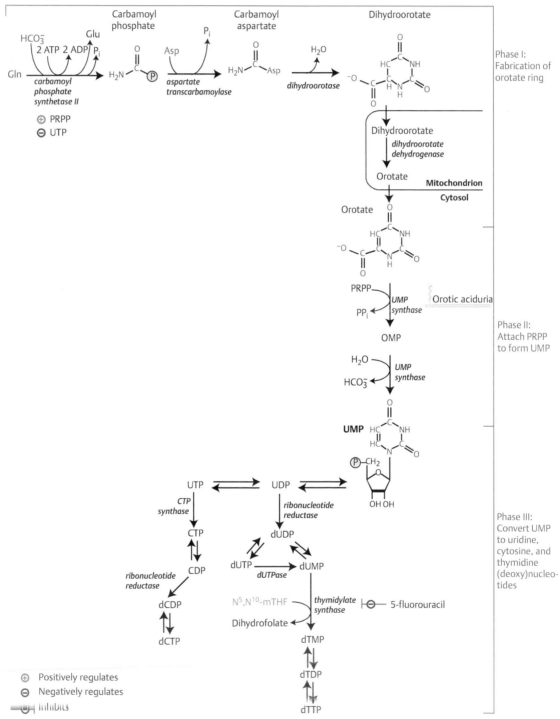

Source: Panini S. Medical Biochemistry - An Illustrated Review. 1st Edition. Thieme; 2013.

A is incorrect. Uric acid is produced as a product of purine nucleotide catabolism. Dihydroorotate reductase is involved in the synthesis of pyrimidine nucleotides; its inhibition will not reduce purine nucleotide or uric acid levels.

B is incorrect. Carbamoyl phosphate is a precursor of dihydroorotate, the substrate for dihydroorotate reductase. Inhibition of dihydroorotate reductase would cause an increase in carbamoyl phosphate levels, if it affected carbamoyl phosphate levels at all.

C is incorrect. Guanosine monophosphate is a purine nucleotide; its synthesis will not be affected by inhibition of dihydroorotate dehydrogenase.

E is incorrect. Dihydroorotate dehydrogenase is not involved in glutathione synthesis, nor would its inhibition cause oxidative stress. Therefore, a decrease in glutathione levels would not be expected.

10. Correct: B. A mutation in the promotor region of bilirubin UDP-glucuronyltransferase.

This individual most likely has Gilbert's syndrome, a genetic deficiency in which expression of bilirubin UDP-glucuronyltransferase is approximately one-third of normal levels. This disorder results from inherited mutations (autosomal recessive) in the promoter region of bilirubin UDP-glucuronyltransferase, and is seen in approximately 10% of the population. It presents as mild hyperbilirubinemia (total bilirubin < 3mg/dL) during periods of illness, physiologic stress (such as fasting), and after alcohol consumption. Because the deficiency is in conjugation of bilirubin, the hyperbilirubinemia will be primarily indirect, other liver function test will be normal, and there will be no indication of hemolysis. Note that inherited missense mutations in bilirubin UDP-glucuronyltransferase itself are the cause of Crigler–Najjar syndrome. This is a much more severe disease; some patients die from kernicterus within a few years, while others with milder forms may develop kernicterus only episodically during periods of trauma.

A is incorrect. An inactivating mutation in cholesterol 7α-hydroxylase will impair synthesis of bile salts and could eventually result in obstruction of the bile ducts. In this case, any hyperbilirubinemia that developed would be primarily direct. Furthermore, the hyperbilirubinemia would not be dependent on physiologic stress.

C is incorrect. Heme oxidase catalyzes the first step in heme degradation. A mutation in this enzyme would impede the generation of bilirubin; symptoms would not include hyperbilirubinemia.

11. Correct: E. Deoxyuridine triphosphate (dUTP).

This patient most likely has impaired ability to form deoxythymidine triphosphate (dTTP) from dUTP and will thus have elevated dUTP concentrations and impaired DNA synthesis in her bone marrow. Methotrexate is a folate analog inhibitor of dihydrofolate reductase. See the figure below. Treatment with methotrexate decreases cellular levels of tetrahydrofolate, thus decreasing cellular *de novo* purine nucleotide synthesis and interfering with the activated methyl cycle. More importantly, the decreased level of available methylene tetrahydrofolate slows the activity of thymidylate synthase, and accumulated dihydrofolate also inhibits thymidylate synthase by product inhibition. The net effect is decreased cellular dTTP, and increased dUTP. The combination of low dTTP and high dUTP results in a high rate of base misincorporation during DNA synthesis in rapidly dividing cells, thus impairing replication. Note that patients who take low doses of methotrexate to treat autoimmune disorders such as psoriasis or rheumatoid arthritis are frequently also prescribed a low dose of folinic acid (N^5-formyl-tetrahydrofolate) in order to reduce side effects. Patients who are given high doses of methotrexate to treat neoplasms are sometimes given folinic acid a few days later in order to "rescue" noncancerous cells from the effects of methotrexate and thus prevent some cytotoxicity.

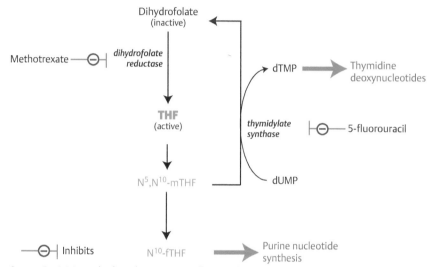

Source: Panini S. Medical Biochemistry - An Illustrated Review. 1st Edition. Thieme; 2013.

D is incorrect. A mutation in hemoglobin, as is seen in several hemoglobinopathies including sickle cell anemia, could result in hemolysis. The hyperbilirubinemia observed in this case would be primarily indirect. However, the CBC would be expected to show some abnormalities, which are not observed with this patient.

E is incorrect. Multidrug resistance–associated protein 2 is the transporter responsible for excreting conjugated bilirubin from hepatocytes. Deficiency in this transporter is the cause of Dubin–Johnson syndrome, and results in direct hyperbilirubinemia with no other abnormalities in liver function tests.

D is incorrect. Protoporphyrin is the last intermediate in the heme biosynthetic pathway. Its concentration may be elevated in cases of iron deficiency or lead poisoning, thus leading to microcytic anemia. However, this patient also has low white cell and platelet counts, and methotrexate is not known to directly interfere with heme synthesis.

12. Correct: B. Divalent metal transporter-1.

This patient's anemia is most likely attributable to decreased activity of divalent metal transporter-1 due to indirect inhibition by omeprazole. A combination of frequent iron loss via blood donations, decreased iron uptake via the divalent metal transporter-1, and lack of dietary heme iron from meat products makes this individual particularly susceptible to iron deficiency anemia. Recall that the divalent metal transporter cotransports divalent metals, including Fe^{+2} and a proton from the intestinal lumen into enterocytes. Individuals who utilize H^+/K^+-ATPase inhibitors to reduce stomach acid production will have slightly higher duodenal pH and are thus at higher risk of developing iron deficiency anemia if they have additional contributing factors. See the figure below for a review of various forms of anemia, and the figure in Answer 1 for a review of iron metabolism.

A is incorrect. ALA synthase catalyzes the first step in heme biosynthesis. Deficiency in this enzyme will, indeed, cause microcytic hypochromic anemia, as observed in this patient. However, deficiencies are quite rare and are either inherited or acquired due

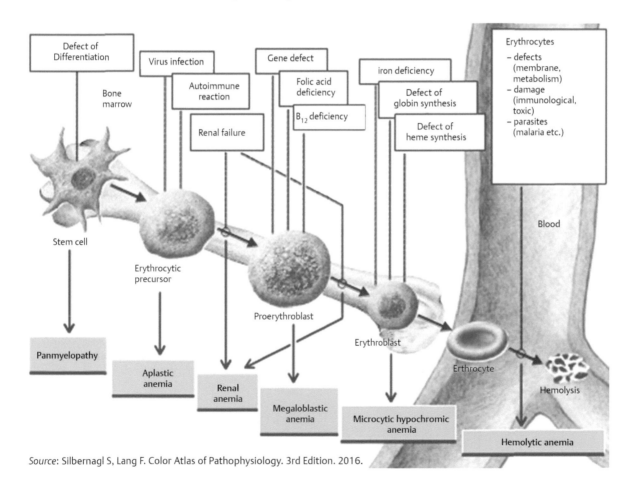

Source: Silbernagl S, Lang F. Color Atlas of Pathophysiology. 3rd Edition. 2016.

to vitamin B$_6$ deficiency. This patient's history is not consistent with either of these.

C is incorrect. Frataxin is a chaperone protein that facilitates incorporation of iron into iron–sulfur proteins. Individuals who are homozygous (or compound heterozygous) for a mutation in the frataxin gene develop Friedreich's ataxia; progressive degeneration of tissues with high mitochondrial energy demand. Symptoms include muscle weakness, ataxia, and impaired hearing, speech, and vision.

D is incorrect. Heme oxidase catalyzes the first step in heme degradation. A deficiency in this enzyme would not result in anemia.

E is incorrect. Hepcidin is a small peptide, released from hepatocytes, that regulates the activity of ferroportin. Decreased hepcidin activity would result in increased release of dietary iron from enterocytes via the ferroportin transporter. This patient's hepcidin activity is most likely *increased*, as his liver senses iron deficiency and is increasing hepcidin secretion.

13. Correct: C. Hydroxyurea.

This patient most likely received treatment with hydroxyurea. Hydroxyurea inhibits ribonucleotide reductase, the enzyme that reduces ribonucleoside diphosphates to deoxyribonucleoside diphosphates. See the figure below. The resulting decline in cellular deoxyribonucleoside triphosphate concentrations impairs DNA replication and has been shown to be effective in the treatment of some forms of cancer, as well as polycythemia vera. Hydroxyurea is also used in the treatment of sickle cell anemia. In that case, however, the mechanism of action most likely involves alteration of globin chain synthesis (favoring hemoglobin F) due to hydroxyurea-induced oxidative stress.

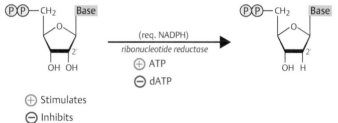

Nucleotide diphosphate

2′-deoxynucleotide diphosphate

(req. NADPH)
ribonucleotide reductase

⊕ ATP
⊖ dATP

⊕ Stimulates
⊖ Inhibits

Source: Panini S. Medical Biochemistry - An Illustrated Review. 1st Edition. Thieme; 2013.

A is incorrect. 5-Fluorouracil is an irreversible inhibitor of thymidylate synthase. Treatment with 5-fluorouracil impairs DNA replication by directly decreasing cellular concentrations of dTTP (only).

B is incorrect. Folinic acid is a highly bioavailable form of tetrahydrofolic acid. It is most frequently used to "rescue" cells following treatment or accidental poisoning with methotrexate, which inhibits recycling of tetrahydrofolate.

D is incorrect. Methotrexate inhibits dihydrofolate reductase, and thus the recovery of tetrahydrofolate that is consumed in the reaction catalyzed by thymidylate synthase. In effect, methotrexate inhibits the activity of thymidylate synthesis, resulting in decreased cellular concentrations of dTTP (only).

E is incorrect. Zidovudine (AZT; 3′-azido-2′,3′-deoxythymidine) is an antiviral drug used to treat acquired immune deficiency syndrome (AIDS). It is a thymidine analog that inhibits viral reverse transcriptases.

14. Correct: B. *De novo* purine synthesis.

This child most likely has elevated *de novo* purine synthesis, leading to hyperuricemia. This child's hypotonia, poor muscle control, and (probable) nephrolithiasis are all consistent with a diagnosis of either classic or variant Lesch–Nyhan disease. The "orange sand" in the child's diaper is most likely uric acid crystals tinged with a small amount of blood due to microhematuria. Lesch-Nyhan disease and its variants are caused by X-linked mutations in the hypoxanthine guanine phosphoribosyl transferase (*HGPRT*) gene. *HGPRT* catalyzes the addition of guanine or hypoxanthine to 5-phosphoribosyl-1-pyrophosphate (PRPP), the activated form of ribose-5-phosphate, to form guanosine monophosphate (GMP) or inosine monophosphate (IMP), respectively, in the purine salvage pathway, which is illustrated in the figure below. The inability to salvage hypoxanthine and guanine results in increased uric acid production as hypoxanthine and guanine are catabolized. In order to generate purine nucleotides for proper cell function, then, the *de novo* purine synthesis pathway must be activated. (Under normal conditions the great majority of purine nucleotide synthesis occurs via the salvage pathway, and a small minority occurs via *de novo* synthesis.) Patients with HGPRT deficiency develop pronounced hyperuricemia in childhood and are prone to attacks of gouty arthritis or, more commonly, uric acid kidney stones. HGPRT deficiency is also associated with neurologic problems including mental retardation, motor disability, and self-mutilation. The appearance and severity of symptoms varies along a spectrum from variant to classic Lesch–Nyhan disease, with individuals afflicted with the classic form experiencing all associated symptoms.

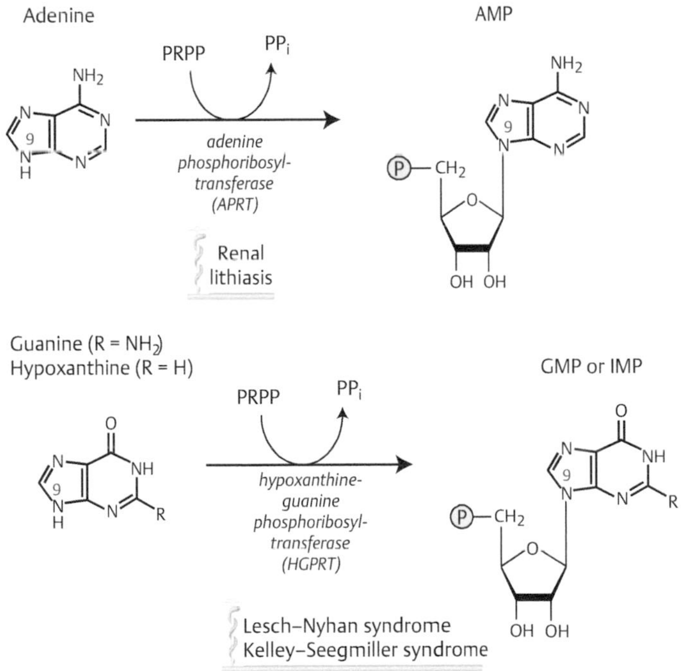

Source: Panini S. Medical Biochemistry - An Illustrated Review. 1st Edition. Thieme; 2013.

A is incorrect. This patient's symptoms are not associated with any disorders involving significantly increased rates of protein synthesis, or biosynthesis of compounds that require methylation by *S*-adenosylmethionine. Also, there is no reason to suspect elevated homocysteine levels. Hence, there is no reason to expect that the activated methyl cycle would be hyperactivated.

C is incorrect. This patient's disorder most likely involves purine metabolism; there is no reason to expect that pyrimidine metabolism will also be affected.

D is incorrect. The purine salvage pathway will run at a *decreased* rate in this patient.

E is incorrect. This patient's disorder most likely involves purine metabolism; pyrimidine metabolism will not be significantly affected.

F is incorrect. Flux through the urea cycle increases under conditions of either high muscle proteolysis and amino acid catabolism or a very high protein diet. This may result in elevated blood urea nitrogen (BUN) and will certainly result in elevated urinary urea levels. It does not cause hyperuricemia, as seen in this patient.

---

15. Correct: D. 5-Phosphoribosyl-1-pyrophosphate.

This patient has a deficiency in HGPRT; thus, the substrates for that enzyme (PRPP, guanine, and hypoxanthine) will accumulate. Guanine and hypoxanthine are oxidized to uric acid. PRPP, however, will accumulate. When the PRPP concentration gets high enough, the activity of glutamine phosphoribosyl pyrophosphate amidotransferase, the committed and rate-limiting step of *de novo* purine biosynthesis, will be stimulated. (See the figure below for a review of de novo purine biosynthesis.) Glutamine phosphoribosyl pyrophosphate amidotransferase is an allosteric enzyme that exhibits cooperativity and a much lower affinity for PRPP than does HGPRT. Under normal circumstances, PRPP is utilized by HGPRT and the salvage pathway, but with HGPRT deficiency, PRPP becomes available at high enough concentrations for use by the amidotransferase. (Note that elevated PRPP levels also have potential to activate the pyrimidine *de novo* pathway, as cytosolic carbamoyl phosphate synthetase is allosterically activated by PRPP. However, carbamoyl phosphate synthetase is also allosterically inhibited by UTP; thus, the pathway will not be stimulated much beyond normal levels, as UTP concentrations will not be affected by the HGPRT deficiency.]

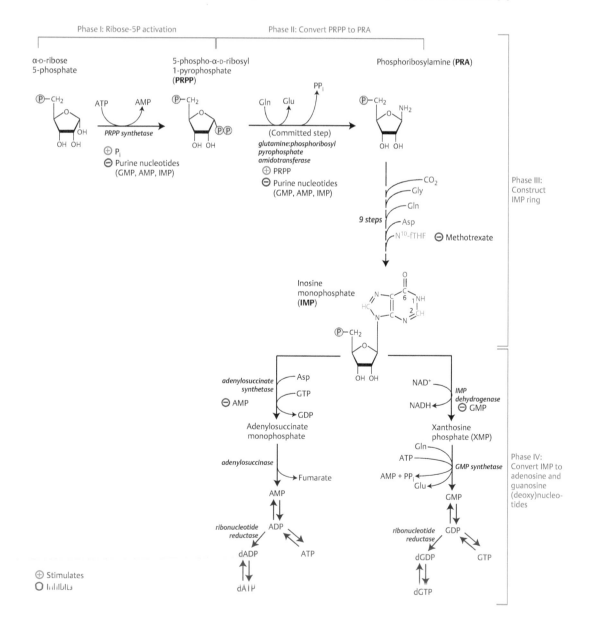

A is incorrect. Although AMP levels may be slightly elevated in this patient due to increased availability of PRPP for use by adenosine phosphoribosyl transferase (APRT), the change will most likely not be significant. Furthermore, elevated AMP levels would inhibit, rather than stimulate, *de novo* purine synthesis.

B is incorrect. Because this patient's disorder does not involve either the urea cycle or *de novo* pyrimidine synthesis, there is no reason to expect elevated carbamoyl phosphate levels. Furthermore, carbamoyl phosphate levels will not influence the rate of *de novo* purine synthesis.

C is incorrect. Hypoxanthine levels will certainly be elevated in this patient. However, *de novo* purine synthesis is not regulated by hypoxanthine.

E is incorrect. Ribose-5-phosphate is produced in the nonoxidative phase of the pentose phosphate pathway and is used "as needed" by PRPP synthetase. Its concentration will not increase in response to HGPRT deficiency.

16. Correct: D. Sunlight-triggered formation of reactive oxygen species.

This patient's blistering is most likely caused by sunlight-triggered formation of reactive oxygen species. He displays the classic symptoms of porphyria cutanea tarda: wine or tea-colored urine, and photosensitivity with blisters, scarring, and hypertrichosis. Porphyria cutanea tarda, due to deficiency in the activity of uroporphyrinogen decarboxylase (see the figure in Answer 5), can be inherited or acquired. The acquired form is frequently associated with hepatitis, iron overload, or chronic alcohol abuse. Accumulated uroporphyrinogen leaks from hepatocytes into the bloodstream where it spontaneously oxidizes to form various porphyrin species. These porphyrins accumulate in cutaneous tissue, or are eliminated in the urine, giving it a red or purple color. In the skin, the porphyrins give rise to reactive oxygen species (ROS) upon exposure to light. These ROS damage cells, causing the formation of blisters that often take up to 1 month to heal. Scarring is common, as is excessive hair growth.

A is incorrect. The production of antibodies to type VII collagen occurs in epidermolysis bullosa acquisita. Blistering occurs after minor trauma and is not limited to sun-exposed areas. Furthermore, this disorder is not associated with changes in urine color, and its acquisition is associated with liver pathology.

B is incorrect. Impaired synthesis of ATP in cutaneous tissue, as observed in niacin deficiency, can result in dermatitis. However, it is not associated with blistering, hypertrichosis, or changes in urine color.

C is incorrect. Niacin deficiency, or pellagra, causes dermatitis of the face, neck, hands, and feet. It is not associated with blistering, hypertrichosis, or changes in urine color.

E is incorrect. Some viral infections of the skin do cause blistering, or even scarring. However, they are not associated with hypertrichosis or changes in urine color.

Chapter 11

Nutrition and Integrated Metabolism

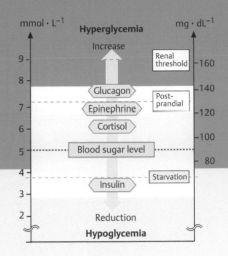

LEARNING OBJECTIVES

▶ Define calorie, basal metabolic rate, respiratory quotient, and daily energy expenditure; estimate and use these values where appropriate.

▶ List major dietary sources of macro- and micronutrients, as well as fiber, and know approximate dietary recommendations for macronutrient intake.

▶ Interpret presenting symptoms and medical or dietary history with deficiencies or toxicity of macronutrients, micronutrients, fiber, or trace elements.

▶ Apply knowledge of multiple biochemical concepts, pathways, and processes to solve integrated, clinically based problems.

▶ Recommend appropriate dietary therapies for various metabolic conditions.

11.1 Questions

Easy	Medium	Hard

Consider the following vignette for questions 1 to 3.

In an attempt to improve his athletic performance, a competitive bicyclist begins a new fad diet. The new diet consists of daily consumption of 75% of calories from fat, 20% protein, and 5% carbohydrates, with enough calories to sustain his daily energy expenditure. The only supplement he consumes is carnitine. He follows the diet closely for 3 months and then visits his physician complaining of joint pain, fatigue, and shortness of breath. Physical examination reveals inflammation of his gums and a small cut on his upper arm, which the patient explains has been there for 3 weeks and keeps reopening.

1. What should the physician advise this patient to do if he insists on continuing the diet?

A. Replace some of the grains that he is consuming with fresh fruits and vegetables

B. Replace some of the fresh fruits and vegetables that he is consuming with whole grains

C. Replace some of the meat that he is consuming with eggs

D. Increase the ratio of unsaturated to saturated fats in his diet

E. Increase his consumption of vegetable oil in order to meet his dietary fat intake goals

2. The insulin/glucagon ratio in this patient's serum results in activation of which of the following enzymes?

A. Lipoprotein lipase in adipocytes

B. Acetyl-CoA carboxylase in hepatocytes

C. Protein kinase B in all tissues

D. Phosphoenolpyruvate carboxykinase in hepatocytes

E. Glucose transporter 4 in adipocytes and myocytes

3. Which of the following most likely describes the primary sources of fuel for energy production in this patient's myocytes, neurons, and erythrocytes after 2 months on this diet?

	Myocytes	Neurons	Erythrocytes
A	Ketone bodies	Ketone bodies	Ketone bodies
B	Fatty acids	Ketone bodies	Glucose
C	Fatty acids	Glucose	Fatty acids
D	Glucose	Ketone bodies	Glucose
E	Fatty acids	Glucose	Glucose

4. The newborn screening results for a 2-day-old infant indicate that the child has classical galactosemia; consumption of dietary galactose could result in severe liver damage and death. For which of the following disorders should this patient be monitored in the future?

A. Beriberi

B. Pellagra

C. Pernicious anemia

D. Rickets

E. Scurvy

5. Hepatocellular carcinomas primarily utilize glutamine, rather than glucose, as a precursor for lipid biosynthesis. Which of the following enzymes could be downregulated or inhibited without affecting the rate of fatty acid synthesis in these cells?

A. Citrate lyase

B. Fumarase

C. Glutaminase

D. Isocitrate dehydrogenase

E. Malic enzyme

6. A healthy 38-year-old man who was recently diagnosed with mild hypercholesterolemia following a routine physical examination prefers to try to bring his low-density lipoprotein (LDL) cholesterol levels down by lifestyle modifications rather than medication. His physician proposes increased exercise, a lower-fat diet, and increased consumption of fiber and phytosterols. What are the primary mechanisms by which fiber and phytosterols may benefit this individual?

	Fiber	Phytosterols
A	Slows intestinal absorption of bile salts	Inhibit *de novo* cholesterol synthesis
B	Slows intestinal absorption of bile salts	Inhibit intestinal absorption of dietary cholesterol
C	Slows intestinal absorption of dietary cholesterol	Inhibit *de novo* cholesterol synthesis
D	Slows intestinal absorption of glucose	Inhibit intestinal absorption of dietary cholesterol
E	Slows intestinal absorption of glucose	Inhibit *de novo* cholesterol synthesis

7. A 4-year-old child of Sudanese descent who has been living in a Ugandan refugee camp for the last 2 years is brought to the health clinic by his mother. She states that he has been extremely lethargic for the last several days, and has been suffering with diarrhea for the last several weeks. Physical examination reveals that the child is underweight, has very sparse hair with a reddish tinge, and that his skin is dry and scaly. His abdomen is distended, he has a palpable liver, and edema is noted in his lower extremities. Although not obtained at the camp, a biopsy of this child's liver would produce hepatocytes similar to those shown in the figure below. This child's hepatomegaly is most likely due to which of the following hepatic biochemical alterations?

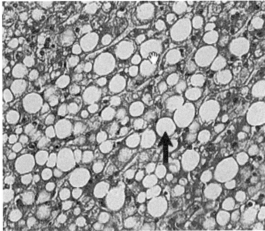

Source: Riede U, Werner M. Color Atlas of Pathology: Pathologic Principles · Associated Diseases · Sequela. 1st Edition. 2004.

A. Decreased activity of glucose-6-phosphatase
B. Decreased synthesis of apolipoprotein B-100
C. Decreased synthesis of serum albumin
D. Increased NADH:NAD⁺ ratio
E. Increased synthesis of LDL receptors

Consider the following scenario when answering questions 8 and 9.

A 65-year-old homeless man with a decade's long history of alcohol abuse was admitted to the emergency department complaining of dizziness and severe nausea. He was hyperventilating, and reported having recently consumed a significant volume of wood alcohol in addition to his usual daily consumption of beer. Laboratory results indicated that he was acidotic and severely hypoglycemic. Intravenous glucose was administered, along with bicarbonate, fomepizole, and folic acid.

8. In addition to folic acid, which of the following vitamins or minerals should also be administered to this patient?

A. Calcium
B. Cobalamin
C. Iron
D. Niacin
E. Thiamine

9. Administration of folic acid will most likely have which of the following beneficial effects for this patient?

A. Increased renal generation of serum bicarbonate
B. Increased nucleotide synthesis
C. Inhibition of the production of a toxic metabolite
D. Removal of homocysteine from his serum
E. Removal of a toxic metabolite from his serum

10. An 8-year-old girl with a history of frequent episodes of weakness, sweating, and pallor that is relieved by eating is brought to the emergency department with a 2-day history of fever, vomiting, and diarrhea. Blood was drawn and the following plasma laboratory results were obtained:

	Patient	Normal
pH	7.26	7.35–7.45
Glucose	50 mg/dL	60–105 mg/dL
Lactate	7.1 mM	0.5–2 mM
Total ketones	400 mg/L	30 mg/L
Triglycerides	4 g/L	1.5 g/L
Uric acid	10 mg/dL	2–7 mg/dL

Which of the following is the most likely cause of this patient's hyperuricemia?

A. Elevated hepatic adenosine monophosphate (AMP) concentrations
B. Consumption of shellfish
C. Hypoxanthine guanine phosphoribosyl transferase (HGPRT) deficiency
D. Extensive lysis of hepatocytes
E. Vitamin B_6 deficiency

11. A 4-year-old girl child who was rescued from a house fire is brought to the emergency department due to smoke inhalation. She is extremely lethargic and complains of dizziness and stomach pain. She is acidotic and her serum lactate level is 10 mM (normal, .<2 mM). Her oral temperature is 37.5°C. The attending physician administers hydroxycobalamin. Which of the following is most likely the cause of this patient's hyperlactatemia?

A. Systemic tissue hypoxia
B. Inhibition of oxidative phosphorylation
C. Uncoupling of oxidative phosphorylation
D. Inhibition of gluconeogenesis

Consider the following vignette when answering questions 12 to 14.

A 40-year-old woman who weighs 220 pounds (100 kg) and is 5 feet, 8 inches (1.73 m) tall (body mass index [BMI] = 33.4) visits her primary care physician for her annual physical examination. At her last appointment, it was determined that she has metabolic syndrome and is at risk for developing diabetes and/or cardiovascular disease. She reports that she has been struggling to lose weight for the last few months and has recently obtained about 100 tablets of fen-phen (see structures in the figure below), a mixture of two weight loss drugs that was popular in the 1990s but is now scarcely available. Knowing that fen-phen has been linked to the development of potentially fatal pulmonary hypertension and heart valve problems, her physician advised her not to use the tablets, but rather to adopt some sustainable lifestyle changes that will help her to lose weight and keep it off.

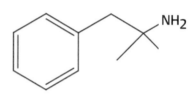

"Fen"   "Phen"

12. In which portion of the gastrointestinal tract, the stomach or the intestine, will "fen" and "phen" more readily cross cell membranes via passive diffusion?

	"Fen"	"Phen"
A	Stomach	Intestine
B	Intestine	Stomach
C	Stomach	Stomach
D	Intestine	Intestine

13. While discussing appropriate lifestyle changes with her physician, the patient asked how much protein she should be consuming daily. Which of the following is the most nutritionally sound answer?

A. About 50% of her calorie intake

B. Less than 10% of her calorie intake

C. At least 176 g

D. At least 80 g

E. As much as 100% of her calorie intake

14. During the discussion regarding lifestyle modifications, the physician told this patient that her basal metabolic rate is approximately 2,400 kcal/d. The physician estimated this using the 24 kcal/d/kg body weight rule of thumb that was developed based on physiologic studies of young, male subjects who had an average body weight of 70 kg. Is this most likely an over- or underestimate of this patient's calorie needs, and why?

	Overestimate or underestimate	Reason for error in estimate
A	Overestimate	Differences in relative adiposity
B	Overestimate	Differences in plasma insulin levels
C	Overestimate	Differences in dietary habits
D	Underestimate	Differences in relative adiposity
E	Underestimate	Differences in plasma insulin levels
F	Underestimate	Differences in dietary habits

15. A 25-year-old woman is referred to a neurologist regarding complaints of general fatigue and muscle weakness. She participated on her college track team until age 20, at which time she stopped because her race times were no longer competitive. During the last 2 years, she has noticed that she tires easily while climbing stairs. She sometimes requires assistance to get out of her car. Physical examination indicates slightly impaired lung function, and the patient indicates that she does not experience muscle pain. If this patient's condition is attributable to a metabolic disorder, which of the following laboratory or biopsy results would most likely be observed?

A. Abnormally low α-glucosidase activity in muscle biopsy samples

B. Elevated plasma carnitine

C. Elevated plasma medium-chain acylcarnitines and dicarboxylic acids

D. Large cytoplasmic glycogen granules in muscle biopsy samples

E. Ragged red fibers in muscle biopsy samples

Consider the following vignette for questions 16 to 18.

A 50-year-old man visited his physician for an annual physical examination. He fasted for 12 hours prior to the examination, during which blood was drawn for a comprehensive metabolic panel and lipid profile. Some of the results of those tests are shown here:

	Patient	Normal or recommended
Glucose	135 mg/dL	70-110 mg/dL
Triglycerides	240 mg/dL	< 150 mg/dL
Total cholesterol	210 mg/dL	< 200 mg/dL
LDL cholesterol	125 mg/dL	< 100 mg/dL
HDL cholesterol	35 mg/dL	> 40 mg/dL

A review of the patient's medical records indicated that this was the first time an elevated fasting glucose level had been recorded. The physician ordered another fasting glucose measurement, obtained 2 weeks later. That test yielded a serum glucose concentration of 140 mg/dL. The physician subsequently prescribed lifestyle modifications, along with metformin.

16. The physician's medical plan for this patient included measurements of glycosylated hemoglobin (HbA1c) every 4 months. HbA1c measurements may not provide an accurate indication of the success of the medical treatment plan if the patient also has which of the following conditions?

A. Glucokinase deficiency

B. Ankyrin-1 deficiency

C. Hemochromatosis (untreated)

D. Familial hypercholesterolemia

E. Type AB negative blood

17. Increased activity of which of the following enzymes, directly resulting from this patient's disease, is most likely contributing to his hypertriglyceridemia?

A. Acetyl-CoA carboxylase

B. HMG-CoA reductase

C. Hormone-sensitive lipase

D. Lipoprotein lipase

E. Phosphoenolpyruvate carboxykinase

18. After 12 years of treatment with metformin, this patient presented to his physician with complaints of fatigue and shortness of breath. The physician ordered a complete blood count, the results of which are shown below. The physician suspected that the abnormalities revealed by the report may be due to a micronutrient deficiency that has recently been identified as a side effect of metformin treatment. Analysis of which of the following plasma metabolites or proteins would most conclusively determine the cause of this patient's presenting symptoms?

	Patient	Normal
Leukocytes (10^9/L)	6.5	4–15.5
Erythrocytes (10^{12}/L)	5.2	4.3–5.9
Hemoglobin (g/dL)	7.4	13.5–17.5
Hematocrit (%)	32.5	41–53
Mean corpuscular volume (fL)	134	80–100

A. Ferritin

B. Homocysteine

C. Methionine

D. Methylmalonate

E. Transferrin

Consider the following vignette for questions 19 and 20.

A 32-year-old woman who was diagnosed with Crohn's disease at age 23 received total parenteral nutrition (TPN) following extensive resection of her small bowel. Prior to the surgery, she was anorexic and her weight dropped from 73 kg to 60 kg over a 2-month period. The TPN consisted of 340 g carbohydrate, 80 g protein, and 50 g fat, and was supplemented with vitamins and trace elements. A few days after the initiation of TPN, it was noted that her plasma triglyceride levels were slightly elevated. Two weeks later, while the patient was still on TPN, physical examination was indicative of hepatomegaly, and a dry, scaly skin rash was noted on her axilla, elbows, and groin.

19. How many kilocalories (i.e., food calories) were supplied by the TPN solution this patient received?

A. 1,880

B. 2,130

C. 2,370

D. 2,620

20. The symptoms this patient developed while on TPN were linked to a nationwide disruption in the supply of a particular TPN component. Which of the following nutrients was most likely inadequate in the TPN solution?

A. Carnitine

B. Linoleic acid

C. Methionine

D. Phylloquinone

E. Thiamine

Consider the following plasma laboratory values obtained from patients A, B, C, D, and E when answering questions 21 to 23.

	Normal value	A	B	C	D	E
Plasma glucose (mg/dL)	65–110	230	170	750	100	75
Plasma free fatty acids (mM)	0.2–1.1	3	2.5	1.0	0.4	1.0
Urinary ketones	0	+4	0	+1	0	0
Urinary nitrogen (g/d)	4–20	16	30	18	6	25

21. Which of the five patients is most likely recovering from a severe burn?

A. Patient A

B. Patient B

C. Patient C

D. Patient D

E. Patient E

22. Regarding patients A and C, which one most likely has a serum pH below 7.3, and which one is *least* likely to have measureable amounts of C-peptide in his plasma?

	Serum pH < 7.3	No measurable C-peptide
A	Patient A	Patient A
B	Patient C	Patient C
C	Patient A	Patient C
D	Patient C	Patient A

23. Which of the four patients most likely has the highest respiratory quotient (RQ)?

A. Patient A

B. Patient B

C. Patient C

D. Patient D

E. Patient E

24. A 16-year-old adolescent girl, who had no prenatal medical care, gave birth at 32-weeks' gestation to a boy. Physical examination of the infant revealed cleft palate and small, low-set ears. Subsequent testing was indicative of ventricular septal defects. Upon questioning, the boy's mother admitted that prior to and during her pregnancy she had sporadically been taking some medication that was prescribed for a friend. The medication she took is most likely a derivative of which of the following vitamins?

A. Cobalamin

B. Folate

C. Pyridoxine

D. Riboflavin

E. Retinol

Consider the following vignette for questions 25 and 26.

A 30-year-old insulin-dependent engineer traveling for business developed a severe case of gastroenteritis and was found several hours later, unconscious in his hotel room, by his business partner. In the emergency department, the attending physician found that the man had severe hyperglycemia and ketoacidosis, with a serum pH of 7.07.

25. In an attempt to compensate for metabolic acidosis, the man's respiratory pattern changed. Which of the following statements most accurately explains how his altered respiration influences the serum bicarbonate buffering system?

A. It decreases the dissociation of $H_2CO_3 \rightarrow H_2O + CO_2$

B. It decreases association of $H^+ + HCO_3^- \rightarrow H_2CO_3$

C. It decreases the pK_a of carbonic acid

D. It decreases the dissociation of $H_2CO_3 \rightarrow H^+ + HCO_3^-$

E. It decreases expression of carbonic anhydrase in erythrocytes

26. In order to correct this patient's hyperglycemia and ketosis, the attending physician administered insulin. Following the administration of insulin, which of the following sets of changes in the activity of hepatic proteins is most likely?

	Protein phosphatase 1	Acetyl-CoA carboxylase	Protein kinase A
A	↑	↑	↑
B	↑	↑	↓
C	↑	↓	↓
D	↓	↓	↓
E	↓	↓	↑
F	↓	↑	↑

11.2 Answers and Explanations

Easy	Medium	Hard

1.   Correct: A. Replace some of the grains that he is consuming with fresh fruits and vegetables.

The physician should advise this patient to increase his consumption of fresh fruits and vegetables. The patient's symptoms of joint pain, fatigue, shortness of breath, gum inflammation, and a recalcitrant wound are consistent with a vitamin C (ascorbic acid) deficiency. His diet, which is very low in carbohydrates could result in a vitamin C deficiency if he is not getting his carbohydrates from fresh fruits and vegetables, the primary sources of dietary ascorbic acid. (Milk and very fresh fish and meat also provide a small amount of ascorbic acid but given the relatively low protein content of his diet, it's extremely unlikely that this individual would be obtaining adequate vitamin C from these sources.) Ascorbic acid is required for collagen synthesis, a deficiency results in improper connective tissue synthesis which can cause bleeding, joint pain, poor wound healing, and

poor skeletal growth. Ascorbic acid deficiency can also result in iron deficiency anemia, as ascorbic acid facilitates intestinal absorption of dietary iron.

B is incorrect. The patient's symptoms are consistent with a vitamin C deficiency; whole grains are not a significant dietary source of vitamin C, unlike fresh fruits and vegetables.

C is incorrect. Eggs are a good source of several B vitamins, as well as vitamin D. However, the symptoms this patient exhibits are not indicative of a deficiency in either B or D vitamins.

D is incorrect. Although a very-high-fat diet will probably contain a high ratio of saturated to unsaturated fat if the patient is consuming primarily animal fats, the consequences of a diet high in saturated fats and low in unsaturated fats (i.e., cardiovascular disease) do not result in the symptoms described here.

E is incorrect. Although this patient's bleeding gums could be symptomatic of a vitamin K deficiency, which could be corrected by increased consumption of plant oils, his other symptoms make it more likely that he suffers from a vitamin C deficiency, which would not be corrected by this dietary change.

2.   Correct: D. Phosphoenolpyruvate carboxykinase in hepatocytes.

Phosphoenolpyruvate carboxykinase will be activated in this patient's hepatocytes. His extremely low-carbohydrate diet will result in a very low insulin/glucagon ratio. Thus, his metabolic state will be very similar to that of a fasting person, although he is daily ingesting an adequate number of calories. Of the enzymes listed here, only phosphoenolpyruvate carboxykinase (PEP carboxykinase) is stimulated by a low insulin/glucagon ratio. Activation of PEP carboxykinase will stimulate gluconeogenesis in this patient's hepatocytes, thus providing glucose to maintain proper glucose homeostasis.

A is incorrect. Lipoprotein lipase activity in adipocytes is stimulated by a high insulin/glucagon ratio and facilitates the transfer of fatty acids from chylomicrons and very-low-density lipoproteins (VLDL) into adipocytes for storage.

B is incorrect. Acetyl-CoA carboxylase activity in hepatocytes is stimulated by a high insulin/glucagon ratio and catalyzes the committed and rate-limiting step in fatty acid synthesis.

C is incorrect. Protein kinase B is stimulated in the signaling pathway that is initiated by binding of insulin to its receptor; it will be active when the insulin/glucagon ratio is high.

E is incorrect. Glucose transporter 4 activity in adipocytes and myocytes is stimulated by a high insulin/glucagon ratio, and facilitates the transport of glucose from the serum into fat and muscle tissue.

3. Correct: B. Myocytes = Fatty acids; Neurons = Ketone bodies; Erythrocytes = Glucose.

This individual's myocytes will be utilizing fatty acids, his neurons will rely primarily on ketone bodies, and his erythrocytes will utilize glucose. Although his calorie intake is sufficient, his extremely low dietary carbohydrate intake will result in a very low insulin/glucagon ratio. Hence, his metabolic state will reflect that of someone in an extended state of fasting. Muscle tissue will rely on fatty acids for fuel, as the GLUT4 transporter is not actively taking in glucose. The ketone body concentration will be high enough to allow neurons to utilize ketone bodies for much (but not all) of their energy needs. Erythrocytes lack mitochondria, so will require glucose for energy production via anaerobic glycolysis regardless of the body's metabolic state.

A is incorrect. After 3-5 days in the fasting metabolic state, muscle tissue stops utilizing ketone bodies and relies more on fatty acids. Furthermore, erythrocytes lack mitochondria and thus cannot oxidize ketone bodies.

C is incorrect. When serum ketone body levels are high, as will be the case in this individual, neurons prefer to oxidize ketones over glucose. Furthermore, erythrocytes lack mitochondria and thus cannot oxidize fatty acids.

D is incorrect. In the fasting state, myocytes do not have adequate GLUT4 activity to take in glucose. Hence, they will utilize fatty acids, or in the early stages of a fast, ketone bodies for energy production.

E is incorrect. When serum ketone body levels are high, as will be the case in this individual, neurons prefer to oxidize ketones over glucose.

4. Correct: D. Rickets.

This child should be monitored for symptoms of rickets. Lactose is the primary source of dietary galactose and is found in milk and dairy products, which also provide a significant source of dietary calcium and are fortified with vitamin D. Individuals, such as those diagnosed with galactosemia, who do not consume milk or dairy products may be at risk for calcium and/or vitamin D deficiency, which can lead to rickets in children and osteomalacia in adults. Galactosemic individuals, especially children, should consult regularly with a dietician to ensure that dietary intake of calcium and vitamin D is sufficient. If intake is not sufficient, dietary supplementation is recommended.

A is incorrect. Beriberi is associated with dietary deficiency in thiamine. Galactosemic individuals do not need to restrict dietary intake of thiamine-rich foods such as pork, whole grains, and fortified grain products. Furthermore, thiamine is present in moderate amounts in most nutritious foods.

B is incorrect. Pellagra is associated with dietary deficiencies in niacin or tryptophan. Galactosemic individuals do not need to restrict dietary intake of protein, which provides tryptophan, or thiamine-rich foods such as eggs, meat, poultry, fish, whole grains, and fortified grain products.

C is incorrect. Pernicious anemia is associated with dietary deficiencies in cobalamin or folate. Galactosemic individuals do not need to restrict dietary intake of meat, poultry, eggs, or fish, which are all good sources of cobalamin. They also are able to consume adequate amounts of dietary folate sources such as leafy green vegetables, legumes, and fortified grains.

E is incorrect. Scurvy is associated with dietary deficiency in ascorbate. The primary sources of dietary ascorbate are fruits and vegetables, most of which are not restricted in the diet recommended for galactosemic individuals.

5. Correct: D. Isocitrate dehydrogenase.

Decreased isocitrate dehydrogenase activity would have no effect on the ability to generate lipids from glutamine. Fatty acid synthesis requires citrate, nicotinamide adenine dinucleotide phosphate, reduced (NADPH), and adenosine triphosphate (ATP). (For a review of fatty acid synthesis, see the figure on the next page) Metabolism of glutamine can generate all three of these reactants. Initially, glutamine is converted to glutamate, using the enzyme glutaminase. Then, glutamate is converted in an anaplerotic reaction to α-ketoglutarate via the activity of either a transaminase or glutamate dehydrogenase. α-Ketoglutarate enters the citric acid cycle, where some of the subsequent reactions generate NADH for ATP synthesis in the electron transport chain. Some of the α-ketoglutarate will be converted to malate, which leaves the mitochondria to undergo oxidative decarboxylation by malic enzyme, forming pyruvate and NADPH. That pyruvate can reenter the mitochondria and be used as a substrate for citrate synthase, which requires the cosubstrate oxaloacetate, also generated from the α-ketoglutarate that was produced from glutamine. The citrate generated in this reaction is transported to the cytosol for fatty acid synthesis. During this process, all of the citric acid cycle enzymes that catalyze the reactions that occur between the intermediates α-ketoglutarate and citrate are used. The only citric acid cycle enzymes that are *not* used are aconitase and isocitrate dehydrogenase.

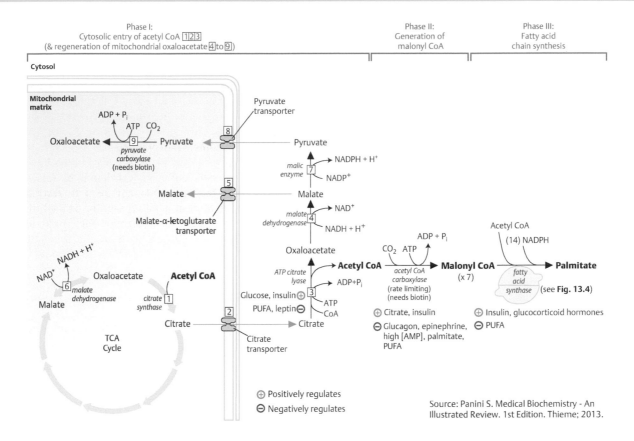

Phase I:
Cytosolic entry of acetyl CoA [1][2][3]
(& regeneration of mitochondrial oxaloacetate [4] to [9])

Phase II:
Generation of
malonyl CoA

Phase III:
Fatty acid
chain synthesis

Source: Panini S. Medical Biochemistry - An
Illustrated Review. 1st Edition. Thieme; 2013.

A is incorrect. Citrate lyase is required for fatty acid synthesis; it is used to generate cytosolic acetyl-CoA from citrate.

B is incorrect. Fumarase is required in order to convert α-ketoglutarate (generated from glutamine) to malate, which is exported from the mitochondria for production of NADPH via malic enzyme. Fumarase is also needed for synthesis of oxaloacetate for the citrate synthase reaction.

C is incorrect. Glutaminase catalyzes the first step in glutamine metabolism, regardless of which end products are produced.

E is incorrect. Malic enzyme is required for generation of NADPH for fatty acid synthesis from glutamine. It also produces pyruvate, which then provides acetyl-CoA for citrate synthesis.

6. Correct: B. Fiber = Slows intestinal absorption of bile salts; Phytosterols = Inhibit intestinal absorption of dietary cholestrol.

Fiber and phytosterols will slow intestinal absorption of bile salts and inhibit intestinal absorption of dietary cholesterol. Soluble dietary fiber, as found in oats, legumes, and the flesh of many fruits, binds to dietary glucose and to bile salts, thus slowing intestinal absorption of both of these substances. Slower intestinal absorption of bile salts results in increased elimination of them in the feces. The resulting reduced enterohepatic recirculation of bile salts forces the liver to consume more cholesterol to replace the lost bile salts, and thus helps to increase hepatic LDL receptor expression and decrease serum LDL cholesterol levels. (Recall also that *insoluble* dietary fiber, as found primarily in whole grains and the fibrous structures in vegetables in fruit skins, adds bulk to the stool and decreases transit time through the digestive tract thus providing protection against constipation and diverticular disease.) Phytosterols, on the other hand, are plant sterols that compete with dietary and biliary cholesterol for uptake by the Niemann–Pick C1-like protein 1 (NPC1L1) transporter on intestinal epithelial cells, thus inhibiting uptake of cholesterol. The epithelial cells expel most plant sterols, but not cholesterol. The phytosterols that do make it into circulation appear to provide additional protection against hypercholesterolemia and cardiovascular disease, although the mechanism of that protection is not well understood. Recall that ezetimibe, a prescription drug, is an inhibitor of NPC1L1.

A is incorrect. Phytosterols have no known effect on the rate of de novo cholesterol biosynthesis.

C is incorrect. The cholesterol-lowering effect of dietary fiber is linked primarily to its binding of bile salts, rather than cholesterol. Phytosterols have no known effect on the rate of de novo cholesterol biosynthesis.

D is incorrect. Although soluble dietary fiber does reduce the rate of intestinal glucose uptake, that is not the primary mechanism by which fiber decreases serum LDL levels.

E is incorrect. Although soluble dietary fiber does reduce the rate of intestinal glucose uptake, that is not the primary mechanism by which fiber decreases serum LDL levels. Furthermore, phytosterols are not known to inhibit de novo cholesterol biosynthesis.

7.   Correct: B. Decreased synthesis of apolipoprotein B-100.

The fatty deposits shown in the figure in Question 7 are due in large part to decreased hepatic synthesis of apolipoprotein B-100. This child exhibits classic symptoms of protein malnutrition (kwashiorkor), weight loss, diarrhea, edema, and changes in hair color and skin. His diet most likely provides adequate, or close-to-adequate, calories, but is extremely low in protein. Insufficient dietary protein intake results in loss of protein in the liver and other organs. Decreased synthesis of apolipoprotein B-100 for VLDL particles leads to hepatic retention of triglycerides, which under normal circumstances are constantly being circulated between the liver and adipocytes. This results in steatosis and hepatomegaly.

A is incorrect. A deficiency in glucose-6-phosphatase might cause similar fatty deposits in the liver due to increased synthesis of triglycerides from excess hepatic glucose and to increased transport of fatty acids to the liver from adipocytes due to a low insulin/glucagon ratio. However, this child's presentation is more consistent with that of protein malnutrition, which causes steatosis due to impaired synthesis of apolipoprotein B-100.

C is incorrect. The protein deficiency in this child's diet will result in decreased serum albumin synthesis. However, decreased serum albumin synthesis will not contribute to steatosis. Rather, it is more likely a contributing factor to this child's edema.

D is incorrect. An increased hepatic NADH:NAD$^+$ ratio, as seen in chronic alcoholism, can result in hepatic steatosis. (Recall that with chronic ethanol consumption, the inhibition of β-oxidation by the high NADH:NAD$^+$ ratio, coupled with a typically lower insulin/glucagon ratio, results in accumulation of fatty acids in the liver.) However, this child's presentation is more consistent with that of protein malnutrition, which causes steatosis due to impaired synthesis of apolipoprotein B-100. His hepatic NADH:NAD$^+$ ratio should be close to normal.

E is incorrect. There is no reason to expect that this child's LDL receptor expression level will increase.

8.   Correct: E. Thiamine.

This patient should also receive thiamine. Chronic alcohol consumption is known to cause thiamine deficiency; poor dietary habits often accompany alcohol dependency, and ethanol impairs intestinal thiamine absorption. Thiamine is utilized by enzymes in both the tricarboxylic acid (TCA) cycle and the nonoxidative phase of the pentose phosphate pathway. Individuals who are deficient in thiamine thus have impaired ability to metabolize glucose aerobically and to generate ribose-5-phosphate for nucleotide synthesis. These deficiencies result in impaired energy production, accumulation of certain metabolic intermediates such as lactate and pentose phosphate pathway intermediates, and decreased synthesis of the neurotransmitter γ-aminobutyric acid (GABA) which is generated from α-ketoglutarate, a TCA cycle intermediate. These deficiencies are particularly detrimental to the nervous system and the heart, sometimes leading to Wernicke's encephalopathy, Wernicke's cardiomyopathy, or Wernicke–Korsakoff syndrome. Administration of glucose to a thiamine-deficient individual may significantly exacerbate the problems caused by thiamine deficiency by rapidly increasing the flux of glucose through pathways that are blocked due to the thiamine deficiency.

A is incorrect. Although his diet may result in inadequate calcium intake, absorption, and processing, there is no need to administer calcium as a calcium deficiency will not impair glucose metabolism or the treatment of methanol toxicity.

B is incorrect. There is no reason to expect that this patient would be deficient in cobalamin, as cobalamin deficiency is not associated with chronic alcohol consumption. The most common deficiencies associated with chronic alcohol consumptions are folate, pyridoxine, thiamine, and vitamin A. Furthermore, cobalamin is not required for effective utilization of glucose.

C is incorrect. Although his diet may result in inadequate iron intake and absorption, there is no need to administer iron as an iron deficiency will not impair glucose metabolism or the treatment of methanol toxicity.

D is incorrect. The most common deficiencies associated with chronic alcohol consumptions are folate, pyridoxine, thiamine, and vitamin A. Niacin deficiency is also sometimes observed, but does not lead to rapidly emergent conditions such as encephalopathy upon administration of glucose.

9. Correct: E. Removal of a toxic metabolite from his serum.

Administration of folic acid will facilitate the removal of formic acid, a metabolite of methanol, from this patient's serum. Recall that methanol is oxidized to formaldehyde and then formic acid, which is quite toxic. (See the figure on the next page for a review of alcohol metabolism.) Formate reacts slowly with tetrahydrofolate, forming N^{10}-formyl tetrahydrofolate. Therefore, folic acid or folinic acid is sometimes administered in the treatment of methanol poisoning. This is generally done in addition to administration of ethanol or fomepizole to inhibit the alcohol dehydrogenase-catalyzed oxidation of methanol to formaldehyde, and bicarbonate to correct metabolic acidosis. In some cases, it is necessary to perform hemodialysis in order to remove methanol and formic acid from the serum.

A is incorrect. Tetrahydrofolate, which is generated from folic acid, is not required in the metabolic pathways required for generation of renal bicarbonate. Recall that tetrahydrofolate is used primarily in nucleotide and methionine synthesis.

B is incorrect. Although tetrahydrofolate is utilized for nucleotide biosynthesis, increased nucleotide biosynthesis will not facilitate the detoxification of methanol or alleviate this patient's symptoms.

C is incorrect. The toxic metabolite generated upon methanol ingestion is formic acid (see the figure above). Fomepizole or ethanol are used to prevent oxidation of methanol by alcohol dehydrogenase; folic acid does not play a role in this process.

D is incorrect. Although treatment with folic acid can reverse homocysteinemia (by increasing the activity of methionine synthase) in some patients, the presence of homocysteine in his serum is not of primary concern for this patient.

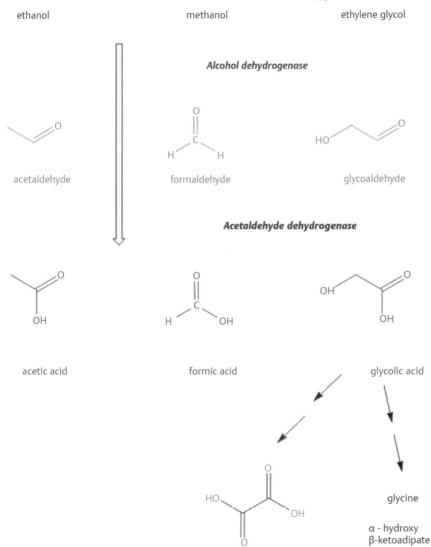

10. Correct: A. Elevated hepatic adenosine monophosphate (AMP) concentrations.

This patient's hyperuricemia is most likely due to elevated hepatic AMP concentrations resulting from impaired glucose-6-phosphatase activity (von Gierke's disease). The girl's history of weakness, sweating, and pallor that is relieved by eating is consistent with a disorder in fasting metabolism. Her hypoglycemia coupled with hyperlactatemia suggests that the problem is with gluconeogenesis, and hyperketosis indicates that the problem is *not* with fatty acid oxidation and the production of ATP and NADH to support gluconeogenesis. Of the various disorders that can impair gluconeogenesis (hyperinsulinemia, hypocortisolism, and deficiencies in glucose 6-phosphatase or fructose 2,6-bisphosphatase), only glucose-6-phosphatase deficiency is associated with hyperlipidemia and hyperuricemia. Increased transport of fatty acids to the liver from adipocytes, stimulated by hypoglycemia and a decreased insulin/glucagon ratio, coupled with increased synthesis of glycerol 3-phosphate from accumulated hepatic glucose-6-phosphate, results in increased synthesis of triglycerides in the liver and leads to hypertriglyceridemia. The accumulation of glucose-6-phosphate caused by the glucose-6-phosphatase deficiency "ties up" cellular phosphate, thus impairing the synthesis of ATP by ATP synthase. Cellular concentrations of adenosine diphosphate (ADP), and then AMP, begin to rise. Accumulated AMP becomes a substrate for the purine degradation pathway, thus generating large quantities of uric acid.

B is incorrect. Consumption of shellfish meat, which contains large amounts of purine nucleotides, can result in a rise in serum urate level and aggravate gout in some individuals. However, it is not associated with hyperuricemia in children.

C is incorrect. HGPRT deficiency does cause hyperuricemia. However, the symptoms of HGPRT deficiency do not include fasting hypoglycemia with lactic acidosis, ketosis, and hypertriglyceridemia. HGPRT deficiency is known as Lesch–Nyhan disease; its symptoms include motor and cognitive handicaps as well as behavioral problems including self-mutilation.

D is incorrect. Extensive cell lysis, especially in the case of tumor lysis upon treatment with chemotherapeutic agents, can cause hyperuricemia. However, this patient is unlikely to be experiencing extensive cell lysis, even though her liver is clearly not functioning with a normal capacity regarding its role in fasting metabolism.

E is incorrect. Vitamin B_6 deficiency is not associated with hyperuricemia, or any of the other symptoms and laboratory results described for this patient.

11. Correct: B. Inhibition of oxidative phosphorylation.

This child most likely has been exposed to cyanide, which inhibits oxidative phosphorylation. Smoke from a house contains both carbon monoxide, which binds tightly to hemoglobin and impairs delivery of oxygen to tissues, and cyanide, which binds tightly to complex IV of the electron transport chain and inhibits oxidative phosphorylation. Generally, the greatest concern from smoke inhalation is cyanide poisoning. A key indication that toxicity is due to cyanide, rather than carbon monoxide, is a serum lactate concentration higher than 10 mmol/L in cases of smoke inhalation. An antidote for cyanide poisoning is injection with hydroxycobalamin. In the serum, the hydroxyl group bound to the cobalt ion in hydroxycobalamin readily exchanges for a cyanide ion. Cyanocobalamin is then eliminated in the urine.

A is incorrect. Carbon monoxide poisoning results in hyperlactatemia due to systemic hypoxia, as carbon monoxide binds tightly to hemoglobin and impairs delivery of oxygen. However, the very high serum lactate concentration in this child, along with the administration of hydroxycobalamin as an antidote, indicate that she suffers from cyanide, rather than carbon monoxide, poisoning.

C is incorrect. Smoke does not generally contain toxins that uncouple oxidative phosphorylation. Furthermore, uncoupling of oxidative phosphorylation at levels that would produce acute illness generally results in a significantly increased body temperature.

D is incorrect. Although inhibition of gluconeogenesis causes hyperlactatemia in fasting individuals, administration of hydroxycobalamin would not correct the problem, and smoke does not contain toxins that inhibit gluconeogenesis.

12. Correct: D. Fen = Intestine; Phen = Intestine.

Both "fen" and "phen" will be less positively charged at the higher pH of the intestine as compared to the stomach and will thus more readily cross cell membranes in the intestine. Recall that the pK_a values of amines, such as "fen" and "phen" are generally close to 9. Thus, around pH 9, they will be 50% protonated, at pH values higher than 9, they will be mostly deprotonated, and at pH values less than 9, they will be mostly protonated. The structures shown in the figure above represent the deprotonated forms of these drugs. Protonated amines carry a positive (+1) charge and do not cross nonpolar cell membranes readily, unless that transport is mediated by a protein transporter. Intestinal pH ranges from 6 to 7.4, while the stomach pH ranges from 1.5 to 3.5. While the majority of both "fen" and "phen" molecules will be protonated, and thus positively charged, at intestinal pH, significantly *more* molecules will be protonated at stomach pH.

A is incorrect. Both molecules will be more positively charged in the stomach than the intestine. Therefore, both molecules will passively diffuse across cell membranes at a *slower* rate in the stomach than in the intestine.

B is incorrect. Both molecules will be more positively charged in the stomach than the intestine. Therefore, both molecules will passively diffuse across cell membranes at a *slower* rate in the stomach than in the intestine.

C is incorrect. Both molecules will be more positively charged in the stomach than the intestine. Therefore, both molecules will passively diffuse across cell membranes at a *slower* rate in the stomach than in the intestine.

13. Correct: D. At least 80 g.

This patient's daily protein intake should be at least 80 g. The USDA recommendation for daily protein intake for adult females who are not pregnant or lactating is 0.8 g protein per kilogram body mass, so this patient's intake should be 0.8 g x 100 kg = 80 g. (The recommended daily protein intake for adult males is also 0.8 g per kg body mass. Recommended protein intake increases for athletes and pregnant or lactating women.) Consumption of this recommended level of protein ensures that body protein lost daily due to turnover and loss of tissue will be replaced; individuals who consume less than this recommended amount may lose body protein. Protein consumed in excess of this amount is used for energy production or storage.

A is incorrect. The USDA recommendation for protein intake is not expressed as a percentage of total calorie consumption, as the amount of protein needed in one's diet is largely dependent on body mass. However, some reputable organizations recommend protein intake at 10 to 35% of daily calorie consumption.

B is incorrect. The USDA recommendation for protein intake is not expressed as a percentage of total calorie consumption, as the amount of protein needed in one's diet is dependent on body mass. (The < 10% calorie consumption is the recommended daily intake of saturated fat.) However, some reputable organizations recommend protein intake at 10 to 35% of daily calorie consumption.

C is incorrect. The calculation for recommended protein intake is based on body mass in kilograms, not pounds.

E is incorrect. Although there may be health benefits provided from eating a high-protein diet, it is not true that there are no risks associated with consumption of extremely high-protein diets. High-protein diets may result in dietary fiber deficiency, overconsumption of saturated fat, or renal complications.

14. Correct: A. Overestimate or underestimate = Overestimate; Reason for error in estimate = Differences in relative adiposity.

Approximately 2,400 kcal/d is an overestimate of this woman's basal metabolic rate because the woman has higher body fat composition than an average 70-kg male. The basal metabolic rate is proportional to the amount of metabolically active tissue in the body; major organs and lean muscle are metabolically active, but fat is not. This woman's large BMI, coupled with the recent determination that she has metabolic syndrome, suggests that she has a significant amount of adipose tissue. In general, the 24 kcal/d/kg body weight estimate is accurate only for younger males with a fairly muscular build. It is an underestimate for muscular individuals, who have disproportionately more metabolically active body weight, and for children, who require additional energy for growth. It is an overestimate for women, who normally have higher relative adiposity than men, and for overweight and obese individuals. As an individual ages, they tend to lose muscle mass and gain fat mass, so the estimate becomes less accurate. Other factors that affect the basal metabolic rate are body temperature (increased with fever), environmental temperature (increased with cold temperatures), thyroid activity (increased with hyperthyroidism), and pregnancy and lactation (increased).

B is incorrect. Although it is correct that 2,400 kcal/d is an overestimate, the error is not attributable to differences in plasma insulin levels. This woman most likely has higher serum insulin levels than the average 70-kg young male, as she has metabolic syndrome. Higher serum insulin levels have been linked to increased, rather than decreased, resting energy expenditure in some studies.

C is incorrect. Although it is correct that 2,400 kcal/d is an overestimate, the error is not attributable primarily to dietary habits. Although the energy required to digest, absorb, transport, and store nutrients (i.e., diet-induced thermogenesis [DIT]), does change slightly with dietary patterns, the contribution of this to variations in basal metabolic rate between individuals is not significant.

D is incorrect. Approximately 2,400 kcal/d is an overestimate, not an underestimate of this woman's basal metabolic rate.

E is incorrect. Approximately 2,400 kcal/d is an overestimate, not an underestimate of this woman's basal metabolic rate.

F is incorrect. Approximately 2,400 kcal/d is an overestimate, not an underestimate of this woman's basal metabolic rate.

15.   Correct: A. Abnormally low α-glucosidase activity in muscle biopsy samples.

If this disorder is, indeed, due to a metabolic disease, the most likely laboratory result will be low α-glucosidase activity in muscle tissue. This patient's symptoms are consistent with late-onset Pompe's disease (type II glycogen storage disease), in which deficient lysosomal α-glucosidase activity results in lysosomal accumulation of glycogen. The late-onset form of Pompe's disease causes progressive limb girdle muscle weakness, especially of the pelvic muscles, and eventually respiratory insufficiency. Infantile Pompe's disease presents in the first few months of life with generalized muscle weakness (babies are "floppy") and cardiomyopathy, in addition to respiratory insufficiency.

B is incorrect. Elevated plasma carnitine levels would be indicative of a deficiency in carnitine palmitoyltransferase I (CPTI), which initiates the transport of long-chain fatty acids into mitochondria for β-oxidation. (For a review of fatty acid transport, see the figure below.) Deficiencies in CPTI affect both liver and muscle fatty acid metabolism and cause hypoketotic hypoglycemia during states of fasting and illness. Progressive muscle weakness is not associated with this disorder.

C is incorrect. Elevated plasma medium-chain acylcarnitines and dicarboxylic acids are indicative of a problem with β-oxidation, most likely a deficiency in medium-chain acyl-CoA dehydrogenase, resulting in hypoketotic hypoglycemia during states of fasting and illness. Progressive muscle weakness is not associated with this disorder.

D is incorrect. The presence of large cytoplasmic glycogen granules in myocytes is consistent with a muscle glycogen phosphorylase deficiency (McArdle's disease) or, if the glycogen structure is unusually large, a debranching enzyme deficiency (Cori's disease). Muscle glycogen phosphorylase deficiency presents with muscle cramps during exercise, and rhabdomyolysis; it is not associated with progressive muscle weakness. Debranching enzyme deficiency affects both the liver and muscle tissue, or just the liver, and generally presents in early childhood or infancy with hepatomegaly, ketotic hypoglycemia, and cardiomyopathy.

E is incorrect. The presence of ragged red fibers in muscle tissue is indicative of some mitochondrial disorders including myoclonic epilepsy with ragged red fibers (MERRF syndrome). Although these disorders are progressive, and often present in childhood or early adulthood, as is the case with this individual, the symptoms generally include uncontrolled muscle movement, seizures, and loss of vision and hearing.

Transport of long-chain fatty acids (13-20 C) into mitochondrial matrix

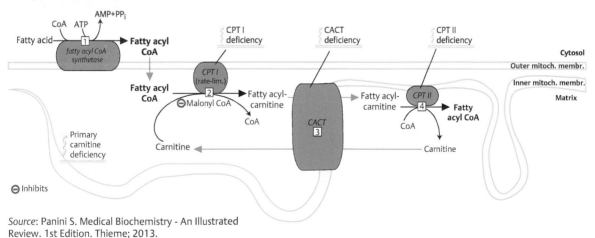

Source: Panini S. Medical Biochemistry - An Illustrated Review. 1st Edition. Thieme; 2013.

16. Correct: B. Ankyrin-1 deficiency.

HbA1c measurements can be misleading in individuals with mutations in ankyrin-1, a cystoskeletal protein that plays a key role in maintaining erythrocyte structure and stability. Ankyrin-1 deficiency results in hereditary spherocytosis, a disorder in which erythrocyte lifetime is significantly decreased due to hemolysis. The measurement of Hb1Ac is a useful tool for monitoring average serum glucose levels over periods of weeks to months. However, in individuals with hemolytic anemias, including some hemoglobinopathies and hereditary spherocytosis, those measurements will be falsely low because of the resulting shorter-than-normal hemoglobin lifespan.

A is incorrect. Deficiency in glucokinase, which catalyzes the first step in glycolysis in hepatocytes and pancreatic β-cells, results in a higher set point for glucose-induced pancreatic insulin secretion. Individuals who are heterozygous for loss-of-function mutations in glucokinase are diagnosed with maturity-onset diabetes of the young, type II (MODY-2), and are generally hyperglycemic from birth. HbA1c levels will still provide accurate estimates of long-term serum glucose concentrations in these individuals.

C is incorrect. Hemochromatosis will not affect hemoglobin lifespan, and thus should not alter the accuracy of HbA1c levels. The exception would be if the patient is treating his hemochromatosis by regular phlebotomy, in which case HbA1c levels may be falsely low.

D is incorrect. Familial hypercholesterolemia will not affect hemoglobin lifespan, or cause random, non–insulin-related alterations in serum glucose.

E is incorrect. Blood type has no influence on hemoglobin lifespan and will not affect HbA1c measurements.

17. Correct: C. Hormone-sensitive lipase.

The hypertriglyceridemia associated with inadequate insulin activity, due to either type I or type II diabetes, results in part from increased hormone-sensitive lipase activity. Recall that hormone-sensitive lipase regulates the release of free fatty acids from adipose tissue; the lipase is inhibited by insulin and thus is more active in individuals with impaired insulin production or insulin response. (See the figure on the following page for a review of adipocyte lipolysis.) The increased flux of free fatty acids to the liver, coupled with increased hepatic concentrations of glycerol 3-phosphate (also a result of poor insulin control) results in increased hepatic triglyceride synthesis and production of VLDL particles.

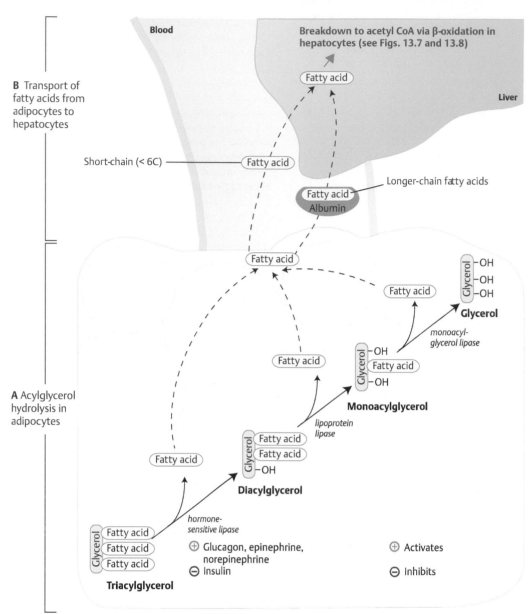

B Transport of fatty acids from adipocytes to hepatocytes

Breakdown to acetyl CoA via β-oxidation in hepatocytes (see Figs. 13.7 and 13.8)

Blood

Liver

Short-chain (< 6C) — Fatty acid

Fatty acid
Albumin

Longer-chain fatty acids

Fatty acid

A Acylglycerol hydrolysis in adipocytes

Glycerol —OH —OH —OH
Glycerol

Fatty acid

monoacyl-glycerol lipase

Glycerol —OH
Fatty acid
—OH
Monoacylglycerol

Fatty acid

lipoprotein lipase

Glycerol
Fatty acid
Fatty acid
—OH
Diacylglycerol

Fatty acid

hormone-sensitive lipase

Glycerol
Fatty acid
Fatty acid
Fatty acid
Triacylglycerol

⊕ Glucagon, epinephrine, norepinephrine
⊖ Insulin

⊕ Activates
⊖ Inhibits

Source: Panini S. Medical Biochemistry - An Illustrated Review. 1st Edition. Thieme; 2013.

A is incorrect. Acetyl-CoA carboxylase catalyzes the regulated step in fatty acid synthesis. This enzyme is activated by insulin, and thus has decreased catalytic function in diabetic individuals.

B is incorrect. HMG-CoA reductase catalyzes the regulated step in cholesterol synthesis. This enzyme is activated by insulin, and thus has decreased catalytic function in diabetic individuals.

D is incorrect. Lipoprotein lipase activity *decreases* in individuals with poor insulin control. Recall that lipoprotein lipase is located on the capillary walls in muscle and adipose tissue, and that its migration from those tissues to the capillary walls is stimulated by insulin. Thus, diabetics have lower capillary lipoprotein lipase activity, and are thus less able to move triglycerides carried in chylomicrons and VLDL from the plasma into myocytes, cardomyocytes, and adipocytes. This, in addition to other factors influencing lipid metabolism, contributes to hypertriglyceridemia.

E is in correct. Phosphoenolpyruvate carboxykinase catalyzes a key regulated step in gluconeogenesis. Its activity is stimulated by glucagon and inhibited by insulin and will thus increase in diabetic individuals. However, the increased activity of this enzyme contributes only to the hyperglycemia observed in diabetics, and not to hypertriglyceridemia.

18. Correct: D. Methylmalonate.

An abnormally high plasma concentration of methylmalonate will confirm that this patient's megaloblastic anemia is caused by cobalamin deficiency. The abnormally high mean corpuscular volume indicates that this patient's anemia could be due to a deficiency in either folate or cobalamin; a deficiency in either of these micronutrients can impair nucleotide biosynthesis in erythroid cells, thus producing megaloblasts. In addition, inhibition of the activated methyl cycle due to deficiencies in either of these micronutrients will results in homocysteinemia. (For a review of the activated methyl cycle, see the figure below.) However, a deficiency in cobalamin will result in elevated plasma methylmalonate levels, while a folate deficiency will not. Studies indicate that as many as 30% of individuals who take metformin for an extended period develop cobalamin deficiency.

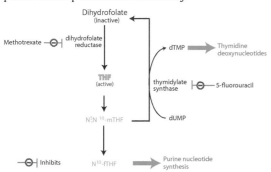

Source: Panini S. Medical Biochemistry - An Illustrated Review. 1st Edition. Thieme; 2013.

A is incorrect. This patient has a macrocytic anemia, and therefore is not likely to be iron-deficient. Analysis of serum ferritin will not be informative.

B is incorrect. This patient has a macrocytic anemia, possibly caused by a deficiency in either folate or cobalamin. Measurement of serum homocysteine levels will not provide evidence that would distinguish between these two possibilities, as either deficiency may cause homocysteinemia.

C is incorrect. This patient has a macrocytic anemia, possibly caused by a deficiency in either folate or cobalamin. Measurement of serum methionine levels will not provide evidence that would distinguish between these two possibilities, as either deficiency could cause a decrease in methionine synthesis.

E is incorrect. This patient has a macrocytic anemia, and therefore is not likely to be iron-deficient. Analysis of serum transferrin will not be informative.

19. Correct: B. 2,130.

The TPN solution supplied 2,130 kcal of nutritional energy. This can be determined using the standard energy values associated with each micronutrient: carbohydrates and protein each contain 4 kcal/g, and fat contains 9 kcal/g. (Recall also that ethanol provides on average 7 kcal/g.)

340 g carbohydrate × (4 kcal/g) = 1,360 kcal from carbohydrates.

80 g protein × (4 kcal/g) = 320 kcal from protein.

50 g fat × (9 kcal/g) = 450 kcal from fat.

Total sum of kcal: 1,360 + 32 + 450 = 2,130 kcal.

20. Correct: B. Linoleic acid.

This patient's hypertriglyceridemia, hepatomegaly, and xerosis cutis are most likely attributable to a deficiency of linoleic acid (LA) in the TPN solution. Deficiencies in the essential fatty acids, linoleic acid,

and α-linolenic acid, are quite rare and tend to occur only in infants who are fed formula that is not supplemented with the essential fatty acids, and individuals with severe fat malabsorption or who are on TPN that is not adequately supplemented. This particular patient had additional risk for LA deficiency due to her anorexia prior to surgery; approximately 10% of adipose stores are LA, thus individuals on TPN who lack adipose tissue are more likely to develop LA deficiency. Symptoms of essential fatty acid deficiency include altered lipid metabolism resulting in hypertriglyceridemia and hepatic steatosis, as well as a dry, scaly skin rash.

A is incorrect. A deficiency of carnitine in the TPN solution would produce symptoms more consistent with inadequate calorie intake, such as significant weight loss, due to impaired ability to oxidize fatty acids.

C is incorrect. A deficiency in methionine or any other essential amino acid in the TPN solution would produce symptoms more consistent with protein malnutrition, such as edema and changes in hair color or texture. Although protein malnutrition can cause hepatic steatosis and hepatomegaly, it would result in *hypo-*, rather than hypertriglyceridemia.

D is incorrect. A deficiency in phylloquinone, one of the variants of vitamin K, in the TPN solution would result in bruising, petechiae, or hematomas, symptoms suggestive of a deficiency in blood clotting.

E is incorrect. A deficiency of thiamine in the TPN solution would produce cardiac symptoms (Wernicke's cardiomyopathy; enlarged heart, shortness of breath, and fatigue) or neurologic symptoms including peripheral neuropathy or Wernicke's encephalopathy.

21. Correct: B. Patient B.

Patient B is most likely recovering from a severe burn or other major physiologic trauma. Physiologic trauma such as infection, moderate-to-severe injury, surgery, cancer, and severe burns results in significant and sustained increased release of all of the stress hormones: epinephrine, norepinephrine, and cortisol (in the case of a severe burn, e.g., catecholamine concentrations increase by as much as 20-fold). Epinephrine and cortisol both stimulate pancreatic secretion of glucagon, and the hyperglycemia induced by high levels of glucagon, epinephrine, and cortisol results in increased insulin secretion. Thus, all five of the major regulatory hormones of metabolism are elevated in cases of trauma. These individuals become hypermetabolic. Epinephrine, cortisol, and glucagon all stimulate the release of fatty acids from adipose tissue, resulting in elevated serum free fatty acid concentrations. Cortisol stimulates muscle proteolysis, and decreases insulin sensitivity in muscle tissue; this results in a significant increase in serum amino acid concentrations. This, coupled with stimulation of hepatic gluconeogenesis

203

by epinephrine, glucagon, and cortisol, results in increased urinary nitrogen output. Finally, stimulation of hepatic gluconeogenesis and glycogenolysis (by epinephrine and glucagon), coupled with decreased insulin sensitivity, results in moderate hyperglycemia. Ketosis is generally not observed, as the insulin levels are high enough to prevent it.

A is incorrect. This patient does not exhibit signs of hypermetabolism, as his urinary nitrogen output is not extremely elevated. Furthermore, his hyperglycemia is indicative of poor insulin control.

C is incorrect. This patient does not exhibit signs of hypermetabolism, as his urinary nitrogen output is not extremely elevated. Furthermore, his hyperglycemia is indicative of poor insulin control.

D is incorrect. This patient does not exhibit signs of hypermetabolism, as his urinary nitrogen output is not extremely elevated. Furthermore, he is not hyperglycemic, and his plasma free fatty acids are within normal range.

E is incorrect. This patient most likely has not eaten in the last 2 or 3 days. His serum glucose level in on the low end of normal, and his free fatty acids are on the high end of normal, indicating that his insulin:glucagon ratio is low. His urinary nitrogen excretion is moderately high, as he is relying on amino acids to provide carbon for gluconeogenesis. If he continues to fast, the urinary nitrogen excretion will drop back to the normal range as his neural tissues begin to use more ketone bodies for fuel, thus decreasing the hepatic demand for gluconeogenic amino acids.

22. Correct: A. Serum pH < 7.3 = Patient A; No measurable C-peptide = Patient A.

Patient A most likely suffers from diabetic ketoacidosis, and thus will have both a low serum pH and no measurable C-peptide. Hyperglycemia coupled with urine ketones indicates diabetic ketoacidosis, which usually presents in individuals with type I diabetes. In these individuals, pancreatic β-cells produce very little or no insulin. Thus, the plasma will not have measurable levels of C-peptide ("connecting peptide), which is cleaved from proinsulin during the process of pancreatic insulin maturation. C-peptide is released to the serum along with insulin and is a more accurate indicator of pancreatic insulin production and secretion than is insulin itself. The severe hypoinsulinemia in uncontrolled type I diabetes results in ketosis, which is not seen as frequently in uncontrolled type II diabetes. The reason for this is that insulin levels and insulin response in type II diabetes is usually adequate enough to prevent the extensive lipolysis that is triggered by a very low insulin:glucagon ratio.

B is incorrect. Patient C most likely suffers from a hyperosmolar hyperglycemic state, and thus will have a normal or only mildly acidic serum pH and will be likely to have measureable C-peptide levels. The severe hyperglycemia (> 600 mg/dL) coupled with the absence of urine ketones indicates hyperosmolar glycemic state, which usually presents in individuals with type II diabetes. In these individuals, pancreatic β-cells produce insulin; early in the disease process, insulin secretion is greater than normal, although later in the disease process insulin secretion may decline. Thus, C-peptide, which is released along with insulin from the pancreas, will be present in the plasma. Ketosis, and thus metabolic acidosis, is not generally observed in uncontrolled type II diabetes because adipocytes are responsive enough to insulin to prevent extensive lipolysis, and the insulin:glucagon ratio is high enough to prevent it.

C is incorrect. Although patient A will most likely have a low serum pH, patient C will most likely have measureable levels of C peptide.

D is incorrect. Patient C is not likely to have a low serum pH; the lack of urinary ketones implies that he does not have ketoacidosis.

23. Correct: D. Patient D.

Patient D most likely has the highest RQ value. Of the five patients, this is the only one who is not relying significantly on fat or protein for energy production; his serum fatty acid and urinary nitrogen levels are on the low end of the normal range. His serum glucose is on the higher end of the normal range, suggesting that he *may* be in the fed metabolic state, and thus be relying primarily on carbohydrate, or a mixture of carbohydrate, lipid, and protein for energy production. Recall that the RQ is the ratio of CO_2 produced to O_2 used in metabolism and is measured with a respirometer. A value of 0.7 indicates that lipids are being metabolized, 0.8 for proteins, and 1 for carbohydrates. The RQ of a mixed diet is approximately 0.8. The RQ value is highest for carbohydrate metabolism because carbohydrates are partially oxidized (i.e., they have several carbon–oxygen bonds), and thus utilize stoichiometrically less oxygen for complete oxidation to CO_2 than do lipids, which have fewer carbon–oxygen bonds.

A is incorrect. Patient A has very high serum fatty acid levels, suggesting that he is primarily metabolizing lipids, which produce a lower RQ value. Furthermore, his very high serum glucose levels are indicative of insulin resistance, which disfavors carbohydrate oxidation.

B is incorrect. Patient B has very high serum fatty acid levels and is excreting large quantities of nitrogen, suggesting that he is metabolizing primarily lipids and protein. The hyperglycemia indicates some degree of insulin resistance, which would disfavor carbohydrate metabolism. His RQ value will most likely be somewhere between 0.7 and 0.8.

C is incorrect. Patient C has very high serum fatty acid levels, suggesting that he is primarily metabolizing lipids, which produce a lower RQ value.

Furthermore, his very high serum glucose levels are indicative of insulin resistance, which disfavors carbohydrate oxidation.

E is incorrect. This patient most likely has not eaten in the last 2 or 3 days. His serum glucose level is on the low end of normal, and his free fatty acids are on the high end of normal, indicating that his insulin:glucagon ratio is low. His urinary nitrogen excretion is moderately high, as he is relying on amino acids to provide carbon for gluconeogenesis. His RQ value will most likely be somewhere between 0.7 and 0.8.

---

24.   Correct: E. Retinol.

This individual was most likely taking isotretinoin, a derivative of retinol (vitamin A) that is used to treat acne. Retinoids are involved in the expression of *Hox* genes, which function in signaling pathways that regulate the patterning of embryonic structures. Consumption of excess vitamin A or derivatives such as isotretinoin interferes with proper patterning and disrupts genetic control of body shape (axial patterning) during the embryo's development. Such disruptions can lead to developmental defects such as cleft lip and cleft palate, malformations of the eyes, ear, and jaw, and heart defects. Affected infants may also experience significant delays in intellectual development. For these reasons, standard medical practice is that pregnancy should be excluded in female patients prior to commencement of isotretinoin treatment, and they should use two simultaneous forms of effective contraception during treatment.

A is incorrect. Neither cobalamin, nor its pharmaceutical derivatives, are known teratogens.

B is incorrect. Neither folate, nor its pharmaceutical derivatives, are known teratogens. Antifolates, such as methotrexate, however, are contraindicated during pregnancy as they may produce folate deficiency, which is associated with neural tube defects (spina bifida and anencephaly).

C is incorrect. Neither pyridoxine, nor its pharmaceutical derivatives are known teratogens.

D is incorrect. Neither riboflavin, nor its pharmaceutical derivatives are known teratogens.

---

25.   Correct: D. It decreases the dissociation of $H_2CO_3 \rightarrow H^+ + HCO_3^-$.

Respiratory compensation will decrease the dissociation of $H_2CO_3 \rightarrow H^+ + HCO_3^-$. In response to metabolic acidosis, the respiratory system will compensate by hyperventilating. This response is known as Kussmaul breathing. Hyperventilation causes more CO_2 gas to be blown out of the lungs, thus resulting in less retention of CO_2 and a decrease in carbonic acid concentration (See the figure below; the equilibrium shifts to the left when $p\text{Co}^2$ increases). This decreased carbonic acid concentration results in decreased dissociation of carbonic acid to produce bicarbonate ions and protons (or, conversely, one can say it results in increased association of protons and bicarbonate ions) which helps to increase the serum pH.

$$CO_2 + H_2O \rightleftharpoons H_2CO_3 \rightleftharpoons H^+ + HCO_3^-$$

A is incorrect. Loss of CO_2 gas during hyperventilation would *increase* the dissociation of $H_2O + CO_2 \rightarrow H_2CO_3$; the reverse of what is stated here.

B is incorrect. Loss of CO_2 gas during hyperventilation would *increase* the association of $H_2CO_3 \rightarrow H^+ + HCO_3^-$; the reverse of what is stated here.

C is incorrect. The pK_a of a weak acid is not affected by changes in the concentrations of reactants or products of the equilibrium reaction involving the weak acid. The pK_a can only be changed by altering the chemical structure of the acid in question, or by changing the temperature.

E is incorrect. Mature erythrocytes lack nuclei, and therefore are unable to alter the level of carbonic anhydrase by regulating its expression.

---

26. Correct: B. Protein phosphatase 1 = Increases; Acetyl-CoA carboxylase = Increases; Protein kinase A = Decreases.

Administration of insulin will stimulate the activities of protein phosphatase 1 and acetyl-CoA carboxylase and will inhibit the activity of protein kinase A. Binding of insulin to its receptor initiates a signaling cascade that activates protein phosphatase 1 (PP1).

PP1, in turn, dephosphorylates many of the proteins that are phosphorylated by protein kinase A, which is activated by glucagon. In this way, insulin reverses many of the effects of glucagon. Among this group of proteins that are activated by dephosphorylation is acetyl-CoA carboxylase, the rate-limiting enzyme in fatty acid biosynthesis. Finally, the insulin signaling pathway also activates protein kinase B, which in turn phosphorylates and activates an isoform of cyclic adenosine monophosphate (cAMP) phosphodiesterase, thus facilitating the decline of cytosolic cAMP and inactivating protein kinase A.

A is incorrect. Insulin stimulates the hydrolysis of cAMP, and thus the inactivation of protein kinase A, which is activated by cAMP.

C is incorrect. Insulin stimulates the activation of acetyl-CoA carboxylase via dephosphorylation.

D is incorrect. Insulin stimulates the activity of protein phosphatase 1 and acetyl-CoA carboxylase.

E is incorrect. Insulin stimulates the activity of protein phosphatase 1 and acetyl-CoA carboxylase and inhibits protein kinase A.

E is incorrect. Insulin stimulates the activity of protein phosphatase 1 and inhibits protein kinase A.

Chapter 12

Cellular Signaling and Posttranslational Modifications

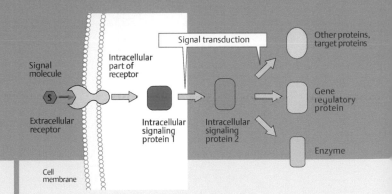

LEARNING OBJECTIVES

▶ List the major types of posttranslational protein modifications and the amino acid modified by each and discuss how these modifications can alter protein structure, activity, and localization.

▶ Describe the cellular signaling events that occur with receptor tyrosine kinases, cytokine receptors, serine-/threonine-linked receptors, G-protein–coupled receptors, cytoplasmic/nuclear receptors, and channel-associated receptors.

▶ Describe how alterations in signal transduction pathways can lead to human disease.

▶ List the various types of second messenger molecules and their downstream effectors.

▶ Describe how signal transduction pathways can be used as targets for disease therapy.

12.1 Questions

Easy	Medium	Hard

1. Congenital disorders of *N*-linked glycosylation are most likely to affect the posttranslational modification of proteins that ultimately reside in which cellular location?

A. Cell membrane

B. Cytosol

C. Lysosome

D. Mitochondria

E. Nucleus

2. A 4-year-old child arrives in the emergency department with a 2-day history of vomiting and diarrhea. Her mother has been treating her with over-the-counter oral electrolyte solution, but the child has had difficulty keeping anything down. Her mother does not know the last time the child has urinated. The child is lethargic and upon examination you find her pulse weak and thready. Which of the following is the first intracellular signaling event that is currently occurring in the patient's cardiomyocytes, in response to activation of sympathetic discharge by the baroreceptor response?

A. Activation of protein kinase A

B. Activation of the tyrosine kinase activity of the receptor

C. Exchange of guanosine triphosphate (GTP) for guanosine diphosphate (GDP) by the heterotrimeric G-protein complex

D. Receptor dimerization and translocation to the nucleus

E. Synthesis of cyclic adenosine monophosphate (cAMP)

3. A variant allele of the β1-receptor gene (*ADRB1*) has a variant allele with a specific amino substitution at position 389. The presence of the variant allele is fairly uniform among racial group populations, though it is slightly more common in African-Americans (frequency of variant allele: Caucasians ~ 30%; African-Americans ~ 42%; Hispanics ~ 30%; Asians ~ 25%). The figure below shows the effect of agonist activation of the β1-receptors with the amino acid substitution of the variant allele and a receptor with the more common allele on adenylyl cyclase activity. In cardiac cells sunder stimulation of the sympathetic nervous system, which of the following would be present in an individual who is homozygous for the variant allele, compared to an individual who is homozygous for the common allele?

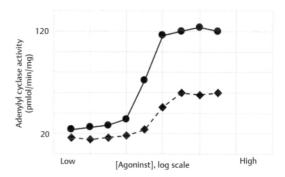

A. Elevated free G-β/G-γ subunits

B. Elevated protein kinase C activity

C. Reduced binding of epinephrine to the receptor

D. Reduced cAMP levels

E. Reduced GTP-bound G_s-α subunit

4. A 72-year-old Chinese-American immigrant with a 40-pack-year history of cigarette smoking showed a strong response when treated for non–small-cell lung cancer (NSCLC) using the epidermal growth factor receptor (EGFR) inhibitor gefitinib. Eighteen months later, he returned with recurrence of the NSCLC. Following biopsy and genotyping, the recurrent tumor was found to contain a mutation in *EGFR* gene that leads to substitution of methionine for threonine at position 790 (T790M) of the EGFR protein, producing resistance to EGFR inhibitor drugs. Which of the following effects could this amino acid substitution have on EGFR protein which would potentially create resistance to EGFR inhibitor drugs?

A. Increased affinity of ATP binding by EGFR

B. Increased ubiquitylation of EGFR

C. Increased transport of EGFR to the nucleus

D. Reduced enzymatic activity of EGFR

E. Reduced phosphorylation of EGFR

5. A rare, congenital immunodeficiency has been found to be caused by a mutation in the *STAT1* gene, encoding the signal transducer and activator of transcription 1 (STAT1) protein. The mutation results in the substitution of phenylalanine for tyrosine at a specific location, resulting in an inactive protein. The mutant protein localizes solely to the cytoplasm. Which of the following is most likely the biochemical mechanism for the loss of STAT1 function?

A. Loss of an acetylation site on the STAT1 protein

B. Loss of a farnesylation (prenylation) site on the STAT1 protein

C. Loss of kinase activity by the STAT1 protein

D. Loss of ligand (hormone) binding site by the STAT1 protein

E. Loss of a phosphorylation site on the STAT1 protein

6. A 77-year-old long-time patient of yours comes to see you about her debilitating rheumatoid arthritis that has progressed to the proliferative inflammatory phase. Physical examination reveals multiple rheumatoid nodules on both hands (as shown in the figure below). You decide to prescribe adalimumab (Humira), a monoclonal antibody that binds and sequesters tumor necrosis factor α (TNF-α). Which of the following biochemical changes occur in the inflammatory cells resident in your patient's joints following treatment with adalimumab?

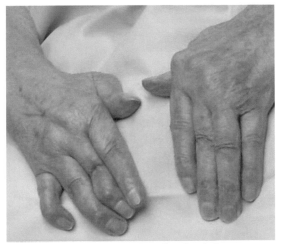

Source: Riede U, Werner M. Color Atlas of Pathology: Pathologic Principles · Associated Diseases · Sequela. 1st Edition. 2004.

A. Increased tyrosine phosphorylation of STAT proteins

B. Increased activation of apoptotic effectors (caspases)

C. Reduced cAMP levels

D. Reduced hydrolysis of GTP

E. Reduced transcription factor nuclear factor kappa B (NF-κB) in nuclei

7. Mutations in a *RAS* gene resulting in amino acid substitutions are common in many types of cancer, altering the protein's function. *RAS* gene mutations most likely have which of the following effects on RAS protein function?

A. Decreased rate of GDP-GTP exchange

B. Decreased rate of GTP hydrolysis

C. Decreased release of regulatory G-protein subunits

D. Increased GDP binding

E. Increased kinase activity

8. Treatment of cancer cell lines dependent on mutant RAS signaling for cell division with a farnesyl transferase inhibitor (FTI) demonstrated significant inhibition of cell growth. Which of the following subcellular compartments/organelles would much of the RAS protein reside or be associated with in cells treated with an FTI?

A. Cell membrane

B. Cytoplasm

C. Endoplasmic reticulum

D. Mitochondria

E. Nucleus

9. On a medical mission to Haiti, you treat a patient diagnosed with cholera using appropriate antibiotics and aggressive rehydration. With respect to cellular signaling, which of the following events is occurring within cells infected by *Vibrio cholerae*?

A. Decreased internalization of G-protein–coupled receptors

B. Decreased levels of GTP

C. Decreased phosphorylation of protein kinase A (PKA) targets

D. Increased levels of cyclic adenosine monophosphate (cAMP)

E. Increased protein kinase A (pK_a) protein levels

10. A 58-year-old man comes to your clinic for a well-man visit. His blood pressure is mildly elevated and he has a body mass index (BMI) of 40 (normal = 18–25). You order a fasting metabolic panel and the results show increased glucose levels, increased insulin, increased levels of triglycerides and low-density lipoprotein (LDL) cholesterol, and decreased concentrations of high-density lipoprotein (HDL) cholesterol. In comparison to a healthy individual, which of the following events is likely to be occurring in the skeletal muscle of this patient?

A. Increased cytosolic/plasma membrane ratio for GLUT4 glucose transporters

B. Increased insulin receptor expression

C. Increased production of phosphatidylinositol 3,4,5-triphosphate (PIP_3)

D. Increased protein kinase B (PKB) activation

E. Increased RAS activation

11. The G-protein–coupled receptor melanocortin 1 receptor (MC1R) activates adenylyl cyclase upon binding of its ligand amelanocyte-stimulating hormone (α-MSH). Expression of eumelanin is increased following MC1R activation. Some individuals with red hair, freckles, and increased risk of melanoma have an allele of MC1R with cysteine at position 151 compared to the more common allele with arginine at the same position. In the melanocytes of these individuals, which of the following molecules would be expected to be produced at lower levels compared to melanocytes harboring the more common allele, following α-MSH stimulation?

A. Adenosine 5'-triphosphate (ATP)

B. Arachidonic acid

C. Cyclic adenosine monophosphate

D. Guanosine 5'-triphosphate (GTP)

E. Inositol triphosphate (IP_3)

12. A 51-year-old woman was recently diagnosed with chronic myelogenous leukemia (CML). The pathology report from a bone marrow biopsy indicates that blasts make up less than 10% of her bone marrow. Her induction therapy is 400 mg/d imatinib (Gleevec), which targets the fusion protein produced by the chromosomal translocation associated with CML. Biochemical analysis of her leukemia cells treated with imatinib would show reduced levels of which of the following posttranslational modification, on specific target proteins?

A. Acetylation

B. ADP-ribosylation

C. Methylation

D. Phosphorylation

E. Farnesylation

13. A 19-year-old woman attending a local university comes to your clinic to discuss options for contraception. During your physical examination, you notice extensive freckling with scattered, light brown macules (as shown in the figure below). When questioned about these markings, she said they had increased in size and number over the years, but never caused her discomfort or concern. No other medical practitioner had asked her about them, and she has always been in general good health. You suspect that these markings are caused by a mutation in a tumor-suppressor gene. The patient consents to genetic testing which confirms the presence of a mutation in the neurofibromatosis 1 (*NF1*) gene. The activity of which of the following signaling factors is excessive in this patient, due to the NF1 mutation, resulting in the epidermal melanocytic hyperplasia responsible for the macules?

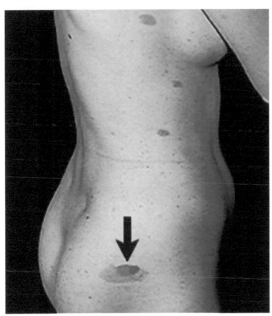

Source: Riede U, Werner M. Color Atlas of Pathology: Pathologic Principles · Associated Diseases · Sequela. 1st Edition. 2004.

A. Epidermal growth factor receptor

B. Estrogen receptor

C. Protein kinase A

D. Protein kinase C

E. RAS signaling

14. A 68-year-old man who has been your patient for many years presents in your clinic for an annual check-up. After greeting him, he immediately tells you his main reason for his visit is that he is "having difficulty in the bedroom." He reports that he and his wife of 41 years were generally engaging in intercourse "a couple times a month, or so" but in the past 6 months he has had difficulty achieving an erection and when he does have an erection, it is not sufficiently turgid. After a review of systems that shows him to be in good general health, you prescribe sildenafil (Viagra). Which of the following second messenger molecule is increased by the action of sildenafil?

A. Calcium

B. Cyclic adenosine monophosphate (cAMP)

C. Cyclic guanosine monophosphate (cGMP)

D. Inositol triphosphate (IP_3)

E. Nitric oxide (NO)

15. Cowden's syndrome (CS; also known as multiple hamartoma syndrome) is a congenital syndrome that includes multiple cutaneous and mucocutaneous lesions, involvement of different organs that results in a very significant cumulative lifetime risk of cancer. The genetic basis of CS is a homozygous or heterozygous loss-of-function mutation in a single gene that results in excessive intracellular signaling following receptor activation by growth factors. Biochemical analysis of mammary epithelial cells from a CS patient specifically identified persistent and elevated activation of mechanistic target of rapamycin (mTOR) following growth factor stimulation. Which of the following proteins, in the affected signaling pathway, has lost its function in patients with CS?

A. Mitogen activated protein kinase (MEK)

B. Phosphatase and tensin homolog (PTEN)

C. Phosphoinositol-3-kinase (PI3K)

D. Protein kinase B (PKB; AKT)

E. RAS

16. A 56-year-old woman had a routine screening mammography that revealed a small group of microcalcifications in the upper/inner quadrant of her left breast. On a visit to discuss these results, she had palpable masses but denied nipple discharge or other symptoms. Subsequent work-up, including biopsy, leads to a diagnosis of ductal carcinoma in situ that was positive for estrogen and progesterone receptor but negative for HER2. Following surgical excision of the lesion, she was prescribed the selective estrogen receptor (ER) modulator, tamoxifen. Binding of tamoxifen to the ER leads to which of the following downstream signaling events in ER-positive mammary epithelium?

A. Activation of tyrosine kinase activity

B. Binding of the estrogen receptor to DNA

C. Exchange of GDP for GTP on a heterotrimeric G-protein

D. Increased cAMP synthesis

E. Increased phosphorylation of ER

17. A 62-year-old man presents in your clinic 1 month after you performed total knee arthroplasty on his right leg. He complains of pain and swelling of his replaced knee of 3 days duration, partially relieved by 400-mg ibuprofen every 4 hours. Physical examination reveals edema and erythema. His temperature is 37.9°C, pulse is 90/min, respiration 24/min, blood pressure 128/85 mmHg. As part of your work-up of his infection, you order plasma interleukin-6 (IL-6) which is 9.3 pg/mL (normal range: 0.31–5 pg/mL). Which of the following events is most directly responsible for the elevated IL-6 in this patient's circulation?

A. Phosphorylation of a heterotrimeric G-protein

B. Phosphorylation of glucocorticoid receptor

C. Phosphorylation of inhibitor of kappa B (IκB)

D. Phosphorylation of pK_a

E. Phosphorylation of RAS protein

18. A 48-year-old woman recently diagnosed with stage IIA breast cancer is scheduled for neoadjuvant therapy prior to surgery. The biopsy of her tumor was positive for HER2 and trastuzumab (Herceptin) in combination with pertuzumab (Perjeta) were prescribed by her oncologist. Radiologic studies following the course of anti-HER2 therapy and prior to surgery showed a modest response to the drugs. Following surgery, analysis of the excised tumor indicated a gain-of-function mutation that led to constitutive activation of a specific enzyme that could potentially explain the weak response to the anti-HER2 therapies. Which of the following genes most likely harbors a gain-of-function mutation in her breast cancer, contributing to the poor response to the prescribed neoadjuvant chemotherapy?

A. Adenylyl cyclase

B. Guanylyl cyclase

C. Phosphatase and tensin homolog (PTEN)

D. Phosphoinositol-3-kinase (PI3K)

E. Protein kinase A

19. A 6-year-old girl is brought to your clinic by her father with a chief complaint of "runny nose, some coughing, and fever." The child's temperature was 37.5°C, and her father reported that the symptoms has worsened over a 3-day period. Physical examination revealed nasal mucosal erythema and edema, though the child's lungs sounded clear and she reported only a mild, unproductive cough. In response to the likely rhinovirus infection, T cells are actively secreting cytokines to coordinate an immune response. One such factor leads to the translocation of factors known as signal transducer and activator of transcription (STATs) from the cytoplasm to the nucleus of cells exposed to one of the T-cell–derived cytokines. Which of the following is responsible for the observation that the levels of STAT proteins are elevated in the nucleus?

A. Insulin-like growth factor 1 (IGF-1)

B. Interferon γ (IFN-γ)

C. Interleukin-1 (IL-1)

D. Tumor necrosis factor α (TNF-α)

E. Transforming growth factor β (TGF-β)

12.2 Answers and Explanations

Easy	Medium	Hard

1. Correct: A. Cell membrane.

Secreted and cell surface proteins typically have *N*-linked glycosylation, with the sugar residues attached via the amino group of the aspara-gine amino acid side chain. Two major forms of *N*-linked glycosylation occur: mannose-rich and complex. *O*-linked glycosylation, which occurs on the hydroxyl groups of serine and threonine is not associated with secreted proteins (as shown in the figure below).

B is incorrect. Proteins with *N*-linked glyco-sylation are targeted to the cell surface or are secreted.

C is incorrect. Proteins with *N*-linked glyco-sylation are targeted to the cell surface or are secreted.

D is incorrect. Proteins with *N*-linked glyco-sylation are targeted to the cell surface or are secreted.

E is incorrect. Proteins with *N*-linked glycosyl-ation are targeted to the cell surface or are secreted.

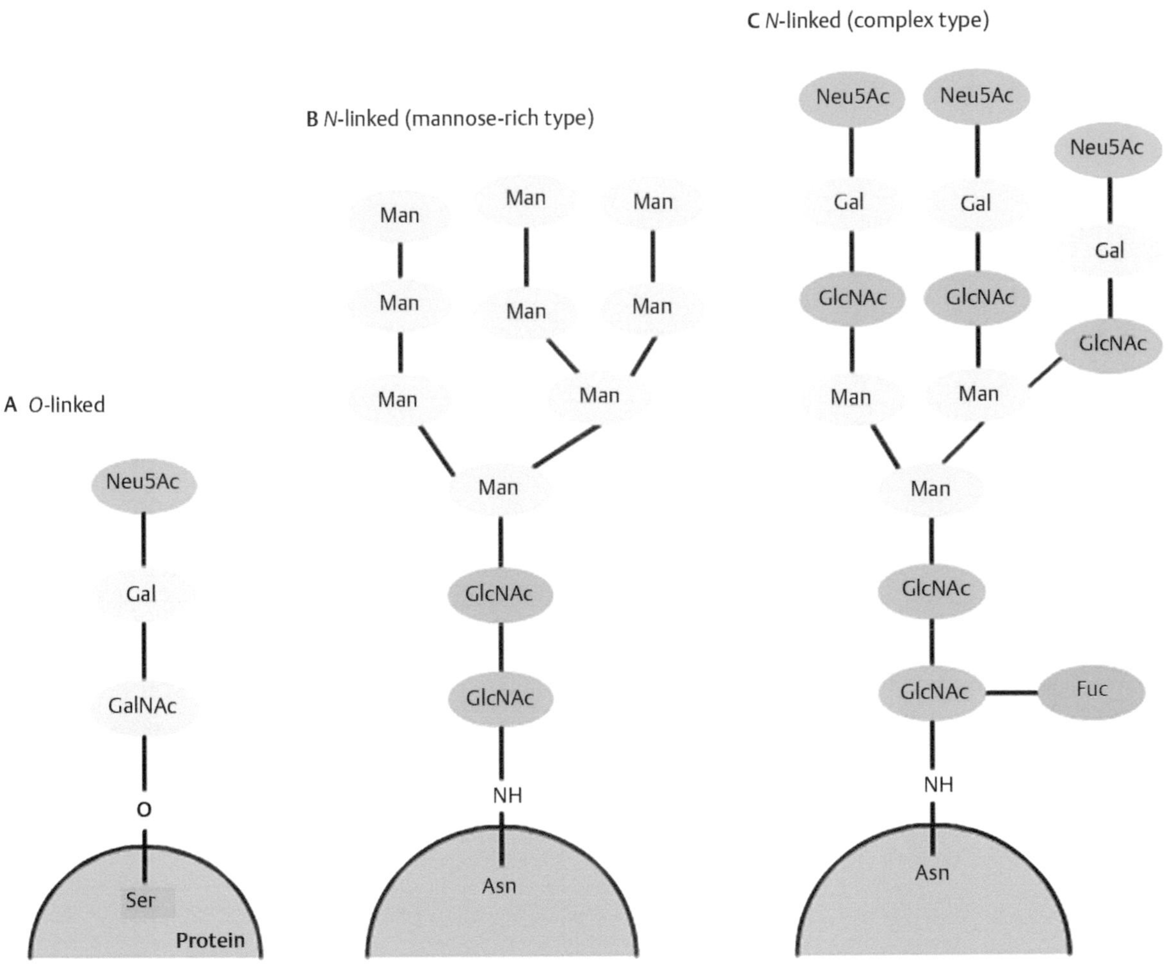

Source: Panini S. Medical Biochemistry - An Illustrated Review. 1st Edition. Thieme; 2013.

2. Correct: C. Exchange of guanosine triphosphate (GTP) for guanosine diphosphate (GDP) by the heterotrimeric G-protein complex.

The sympathetic nervous system releases epinephrine and norepinephrine which activate β1-adrenergic receptors in the heart. This receptor activation leads to exchange of GDP for GTP by receptor-bound heterotrimeric G protein. This in turn causes the G-α subunit to dissociate from the G-γ/G-β subunits. GTP-bound G-α activates adenylyl cyclase which makes cAMP from adenosine triphosphate (ATP). The cAMP activates protein kinase A which phosphorylates downstream effector proteins (as shown in the figure below).

A is incorrect. Protein kinase A activation is not the most immediate event following receptor activation.

B is incorrect. The β1-adrenergic receptor does not have intrinsic tyrosine kinase activity.

D is incorrect. The β1-adrenergic receptor does not dimerize or translocate to the nucleus (nuclear hormone receptors are activated in this manner).

E is incorrect. Synthesis of cyclic adenosine monophosphate is not the most immediate event following receptor activation.

3. Correct: A. Elevated free G-β/G-γ subunits.

Receptor activation leads to the swapping of GDP for GTP bound to the G_s-α subunit of the tripartite G-protein complex and release of G-β/G- – subunits. GTP–G_s-α interacts with and stimulates the adenyl cyclase enzyme. From the figure in Question 3, it can be concluded that the common allele has higher basal and agonist-simulated adenylyl cyclase activity than the variant allele and therefore the events upstream must be occurring at higher rates, resulting in elevated free G-β/G-γ subunits.

B is incorrect. Adenyl cyclase converts ATP to cAMP which activates protein kinase A enzyme. This pathway does not directly activate protein kinase C.

C is incorrect. Reduced binding of epinephrine to the receptor would lead to lower adenyl cyclase activity, which is not the case.

D is incorrect. The common allele, which is associated with elevated adenyl cyclase, would lead to elevated cAMP levels.

E is incorrect. The common allele is associated with greater activation of the signaling pathways and therefore higher levels of GTP-bound G_s-α subunit would be expected.

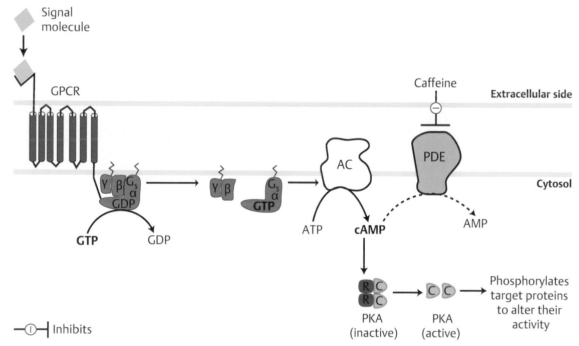

Source: Panini S. Medical Biochemistry - An Illustrated Review. 1st Edition. Thieme; 2013.

4. Correct: A. Increased affinity of ATP binding by EGFR.

The growth of the NSCLC tumor is dependent on constitutive signaling by the EGFR receptor tyrosine kinase. The T790M substitution leads to increased affinity of the EGFR receptor for ATP, reducing the ability of ATP-competitive reversible EGFR tyrosine kinase inhibitors (e.g., gefitinib) to bind to EGFR.

B is incorrect. Increased ubiquitylation would most likely lead to lower levels of the EGFR protein thus would not support tumor growth.

C is incorrect. EGFR is a transmembrane receptor protein and is not found in the nucleus.

D is incorrect. Reduced enzymatic activity would inhibit the ability of EGFR to support tumor growth.

E is incorrect. While threonine residues can be phosphorylated, there is no evidence that threonine-790 is phosphorylated nor has phosphorylation of that residue ever been reported to affect the binding or activity of the EGFR inhibitors.

5. Correct: E. Loss of a phosphorylation site on the STAT1 protein.

STAT1 proteins are phosphorylated on tyrosine residues by cytokine and growth factor receptor kinases. Phosphorylation results in dimerization, translocation to the nucleus and DNA binding, altering transcription of specific genes.

A is incorrect. Acetylation of proteins occurs on lysine residues. For a list of the most common post-translational protein modifications, see the table below.

Modification		Functional Group	Residue Affected
Acylation	N-terminus bonded to acetyl or long-chain acyl residue thioesterification with a long-chain acyl group	Amine($-NH_3^+$) Sulfhydryl (-SH)	N-terminus Cys
Acetylation	Covalent linkage to amine	Amine($-NH_3^+$)	Lys
Glycosylation	O-glycosylation	Hydroxyl (–OH)	Ser, Thr
	N-glycosylation	Acid-amide ($-CONH_2$)	Asn, Gln
Phosphorylation	Phosphate linked via esterification	Hydroxyl (–OH)	Ser, Tyr, Thr; also Asp and His
g-carboxylation	Addition of –COOH group	g-carbon	Glu
Ubiquitination	Covalent modification with ubiquitin	Amine($-NH_3^+$)	Lys
Hydroxylation	Addition of –OH group	C-4	Pro and Lys
Disulfide bonds	Oxidation to achieve covalent linkage of cysteine residues	Sulfhydryl (-SH)	Cys
prenylation	An isoprenoid group such as farnesyl or geranyl geranyl in C-terminal CAAX or CC motifs		Cys

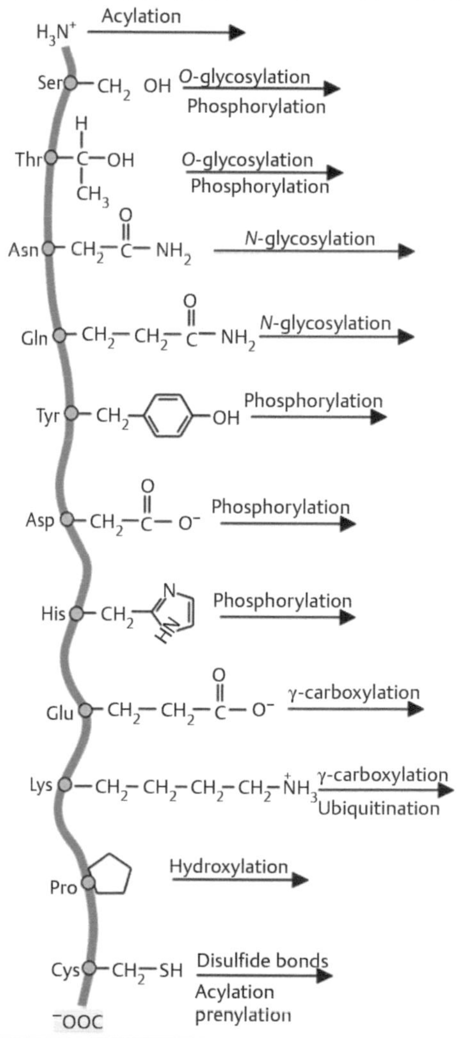

Source: Panini S. Medical Biochemistry - An Illustrated Review. 1st Edition. Thieme; 2013.

B is incorrect. Farnesylation occurs on cysteine residues. Farnesylation is associated with anchoring proteins to the inner leaflet of the plasma membrane. For a list of the most common posttranslational protein modifications, see the table on the previous page.

C is incorrect. STAT1 is substrate for kinases but is not, itself, a kinase.

D is incorrect. STAT1 does not bind hormone ligands.

6.   Correct: E. Reduced transcription factor nuclear factor kappa B (NF-κB) in nuclei.

Signal transduction cascades from activated TNF-α receptors directly result in the translocation of NF-κB to the nucleus which activates transcription of proinflammatory genes. Blockade of TNF-α signaling results in a decline in NF-κB in the nucleus.

A is incorrect. TNF-α signaling does not directly affect signaling through the Janus kinase (JAK)-signal transducer and activator of transcription (STAT) pathway.

B is incorrect. TNF-α signaling generally promotes caspase activation. Blockade of TNF-α signaling would result in less caspase cleavage/activation.

C is incorrect. TNF-α signaling does not directly affect protein kinase A activity, the enzyme that converts ATP to cAMP.

D is incorrect. TNF-α signaling does not directly affect G-protein activity or GTP hydrolysis.

7.   Correct: B. Decreased rate of GTP hydrolysis.

RAS signaling is activated by numerous growth factors and promotes cell division. RAS is activated by swapping GDP for GTP; it is active in the GTP-bound form. Hydrolysis of GTP to GDP by RAS ends the signaling event (as shown in the figure below). The most common mutations of RAS reduce the intrinsic GTPase activity, resulting in persistent signaling from RAS.

A is incorrect. Decreased GDP-GTP exchange would reduce RAS signaling, since the GDP-bound RAS is inactive (as shown in the figure below).

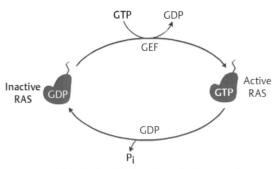

Source: Panini S. Medical Biochemistry - An Illustrated Review. 1st Edition. Thieme; 2013.

C is incorrect. RAS is a monomeric G-protein, in contrast to trimeric G-proteins which have catalytic and regulatory subunits (as shown in the figure on the left).

D is incorrect. Increased GDP binding would result in reduced signaling from RAS since it is active in the GTP-bound form (as shown in the figure on the left).

E is incorrect. RAS protein has no kinase activity.

8.   Correct: B. Cytoplasm.

Farnesylation of RAS protein is necessary for normal activity. The lipid-soluble farnesyl group (a 15-carbon isoprenoid) added by the farnesyl transferase enzyme embeds in the inner leaflet of the plasma membrane, associating RAS protein with this location. Inhibition of farnesylation results in RAS protein being primarily associated with the cytoplasm, losing its specific association with the plasma membrane and significantly reducing RAS-dependent signal transduction.

A is incorrect. RAS protein would be farnesylated in untreated cells and the lipid-soluble farnesyl group (a 15-carbon isoprenoid) would embed in the inner leaflet of the plasma membrane, associating RAS protein with this location.

C is incorrect. RAS protein associates with the cytosolic leaflet of the endoplasmic reticulum only after it has been farnesylated by cytosolic farnesyl transferase. Inhibition of this enzyme would prevent association of RAS with the endoplasmic reticulum.

D is incorrect. RAS protein does not specifically associated with mitochondria, in the presence or absence of FTI.

E is incorrect. RAS protein is not found in the nucleus, in the presence or absence of FTI.

9.   Correct: D. Increased levels of cyclic adenosine monophosphate (cAMP).

Cholera toxin ADP-ribosylates the G_s-α subunit of the tripartite G-protein complex, inhibiting its GTPase activity such that it remains in the active, GTP-bound form longer. The GTP-bound G-α subunit interacts with and activates adenylyl cyclase (AC) which catalyzes the synthesis of cAMP from ATP. The net result is extended production of cAMP.

A is incorrect. Internalization of G-protein–coupled receptors following activation can occur, but the events regulating this are independent of G-protein signaling. Therefore, cholera toxin will not have an effect on receptor levels.

B is incorrect. Cholera toxin ADP-ribosylates the G_s-α subunit of the tripartite G-protein complex, inhibiting its GTPase activity such that it remains in the active, GTP-bound form longer. Although G-protein signaling is unlikely to significantly alter cellular GTP pools, if anything, the net outcome of these events would be to increase GTP levels.

C is incorrect. ADP-ribosylates the G_s-α subunit of the tripartite G-protein complex, inhibiting its GTPase activity such that it remains in the active, GTP-bound form longer. The GTP-bound G-α subunit interacts with and activates adenylyl cyclase (AC) which catalyzes the synthesis of cAMP from adenosine triphosphate (ATP). The cAMP generated by adenylyl cyclase binds to the regulatory (R) subunit of PKA, releasing the catalytic (C) subunit which phosphorylates downstream effector proteins. Given the extended activation of G_s-α as a result of ADP-ribosylation, more cAMP is present in the cell and PKA enzyme will be more active resulting in increased phosphorylation of PKA target proteins.

E is incorrect. The levels of the PKA protein itself do not change during extended G-protein signaling, only the activity of the enzyme is increased.

10. Correct: A. Increased cytosolic/plasma membrane ratio for GLUT4 glucose transporters.

The patient likely is insulin resistant which, despite elevated circulating insulin, results in deficient insulin signaling within cells. One key activity of insulin on skeletal muscle cells is increased transport of GLUT4 glucose transporter from the cytoplasm to the plasma membrane, resulting in increased glucose transport (as shown in the figure below). Since the patient is insulin resistant, this event is likely not occurring efficiently and therefore the cytosolic/plasma membrane ratio of GLUT4 is elevated.

B is incorrect. Insulin receptor protein levels have not been observed to be altered in insulin resistance.

C is incorrect. All downstream signaling events are inefficient, to varying degrees, in patients with insulin resistance. Production of phosphatidylinositol 3,4,5-triphosphate (PIP_3) following insulin receptor activation is likely reduced in this patient.

D is incorrect. All downstream signaling events are inefficient, to varying degrees, in patients with insulin resistance. Activation of PKB following insulin receptor activation is likely reduced in this patient.

E is incorrect. All downstream signaling events are inefficient, to varying degrees, in patients with insulin resistance. Activation of RAS following insulin receptor activation is likely reduced in this patient.

11. Correct: C. Cyclic adenosine monophosphate.

When activated, adenylyl cyclase converts ATP to the second messenger cyclic adenosine monophosphate (cAMP). cAMP activates protein kinase

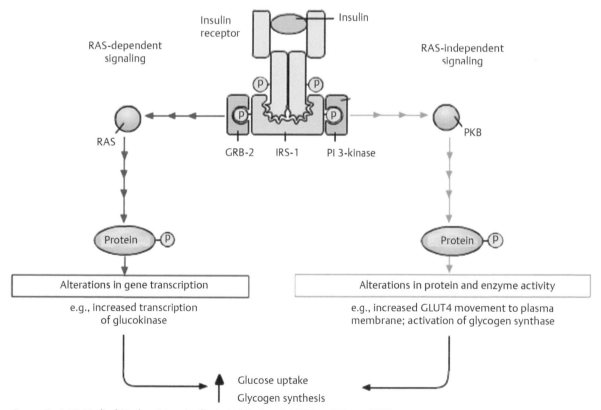

Source: Panini S. Medical Biochemistry - An Illustrated Review. 1st Edition. Thieme; 2013.

A, which has many downstream effectors including transcription factors that alter gene expression. One such target gene of this pathway is the protein eumelanin, which is photoprotective by virtue of absorbing ultraviolet light as well as acting as a scavenger for reactive oxygen species. The individuals with the MC1R cysteine-151 variant have reduced pigmentation and elevated melanoma risk from lowered expression of eumelanin. Therefore, the cysteine-151 variant of MC1R must not be as catalytically active, resulting in less cAMP being produced upon activation by α-melanocyte-stimulating hormone, in comparison to the more common arginine-151 variant.

A is incorrect. ATP is not a second messenger for any G-protein–coupled receptor. Production of cAMP from ATP would not have an appreciable effect on cellular ATP pools.

B is incorrect. Arachidonic acid is a second messenger for some G-protein–coupled receptors; however, arachidonic acid does not directly affect adenylyl cyclase activity.

D is incorrect. Guanosine 5'-triphosphate (GTP) is not a second messenger for any G-protein–coupled receptors.

E is incorrect. Inositol triphosphate (IP_3) is a second messenger for some G-protein–coupled receptors; however, IP_3 does not directly affect adenylyl cyclase activity.

12. Correct: D. Phosphorylation.

Imatinib inhibits the kinase activity of the BCR-Abl fusion protein that is produced by the translocation between chromosome 9 (which has the Abl gene) and chromosome 22 (which has the *BCR* gene) which produces the so-called Philadelphia chromosome (as shown in the figure on the right). Imatinib binds the substrate binding pocket of the Abl kinase moiety, preventing entry by and subsequent phosphorylation of protein substrates.

A is incorrect. The BCR-Abl fusion protein, which is inhibited by imatinib is a protein kinase, which transfers a phosphoryl group from ATP to specific serine and/or threonine amino acids on target proteins. It is incapable of acetylating proteins.

B is incorrect. The BCR-Abl fusion protein, which is inhibited by imatinib is a protein kinase, which transfers a phosphoryl group from ATP to specific serine and/or threonine amino acids on target proteins. It is incapable of ADP-ribosylation of proteins.

C is incorrect. The BCR-Abl fusion protein, which is inhibited by imatinib is a protein kinase, which transfers a phosphoryl group from ATP to specific serine and/or threonine amino acids on target proteins. It is incapable of methylating proteins.

E is incorrect. The BCR-Abl fusion protein, which is inhibited by imatinib is a protein kinase, which transfers a phosphoryl group from ATP to specific serine and/or threonine amino acids on target proteins. It is incapable of farnesylating proteins.

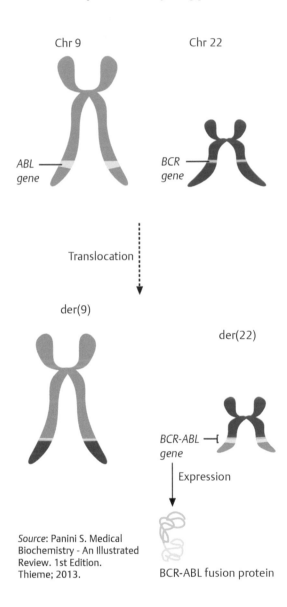

Source: Panini S. Medical Biochemistry - An Illustrated Review. 1st Edition. Thieme; 2013.

13. Correct: E. RAS signaling.

Café au lait spots are commonly associated with several genetic syndromes, in this instance neurofibromatosis. The NF1 tumor suppressor gene produces a protein that is a GTPase activating protein (GAP) for RAS. When present, NF1 activates the intrinsic GTPase activity of GTP-bound RAS, extinguishing signaling. In the absence of NF1, the GTPase activity of RAS is very slow, resulting in persistent signaling by GTP-RAS, which can lead to cellular proliferation.

A is incorrect. NF1 is a GTPase activating protein for RAS. It does not directly influence the activity of the EGFR.

B is incorrect. NF1 is a GTPase activating protein for RAS. It does not directly influence the activity of the estrogen receptor.

C is incorrect. NF1 is a GTPase activating protein for RAS. It does not directly influence the activity of protein kinase A.

D is incorrect. NF1 is a GTPase activating protein for RAS. It does not directly influence the activity of protein kinase C.

14. Correct: C. Cyclic guanosine monophosphate (cGMP).

NO is a potent vasodilator that activates guanylyl cyclase which converts GTP to cGMP. cGMP activates downstream effectors that leads to relaxation of vascular smooth muscle and vasodilation. Sildenafil inhibits the enzyme phosphodiesterase 5 (PDE5) which breaks down cGMP to guanosine monophosphate (GMP), potentiating the NO signaling and maintaining vasodilation. This vasodilation leads to greater blood flow into the spongy tissue of the penis, producing an erection. Sildenafil is also used to treat pulmonary arterial hypertension, based on the same vasodilatory activity.

A is incorrect. Calcium availability is reduced by the increased cGMP produced by inhibition of PDE5 by sildenafil, contributing to smooth muscle relaxation. cGMP is the second messenger that is directly increased by sildenafil.

B is incorrect. Cyclic adenosine monophosphate levels are not affected by sildenafil.

D is incorrect. Inositol triphosphate levels are not affected by sildenafil.

E is incorrect. NO initiates the signaling cascade that produces cGMP as a second messenger, but the levels of NO are not directly affected by sildenafil.

15. Correct: B. Phosphatase and tensin homolog (PTEN).

Binding of growth factor receptors by their ligand leads to intracellular signaling down two different pathways. One pathway is mediated by RAS signaling, resulting in mitogen activate protein kinase cascade and subsequent changes to transcription factor function. The other pathway is mediated by phosphoinositol-3-kinase, which increases phosphatidylinositol-3,4,5-triphosphate (IP_3) levels intracellularly, which activates downstream kinases including mTOR. *PTEN* is tumor suppressor gene that encodes a phosphatidylinositol-3,4,5-triphosphate 3-phosphatase, which dephosphorylates IP_3 to phosphatidylinositol-4,5-bisphosphate (IP_2). The dephosphorylation of IP_3 terminates the PI3K/AKT/mTOR signaling pathway initiated by growth factor receptor activation. Loss of function of PTEN would result in elevated and persistent levels of IP_3, activating that branch of growth factor signaling and leading to high level of mTOR activity.

A is incorrect. MEK is activated by growth factor receptors and is part of the RAS branch of signaling. A loss-of-function mutation leading to lost or decreased MEK activity would not lead to increased mTOR activation.

C is incorrect. Phosphoinositol-3-kinase (PI3K) increases IP_3 levels intracellularly, which activates downstream kinases including mTOR. Loss of PI3K activity would lead to reduced mTOR activity.

D is incorrect. PKB, also known as AKT, is activated by binding to IP_3. PKB phosphorylates and activates mTOR. Loss of PKB activity would lead to reduced mTOR activity.

E is incorrect. RAS proteins are activated by growth factor signaling and represent a signaling cascade that is activated in parallel to the IP_3 pathway. As such, a loss-of-function mutation in RAS would not lead to elevated mTOR activity.

16. Correct: B. Binding of the estrogen receptor to DNA.

Estrogen receptor (ER) is resident in the cytoplasm. The highly lipophilic ligands of ER (and other nuclear hormone receptors) diffuse through the plasma membranes of cells and into the cytoplasm. Upon binding of ligand, the ER dimerizes and translocates to the nucleus where it binds specific DNA sequences known as estrogen response elements (EREs). Once bound to EREs, the ER regulates transcription of associated genes, primarily increasing their transcription (as shown in the figure on the next page). Selective ER modulators like tamoxifen are not simple antagonists. When bound to ER, tamoxifen causes the same events to occur (e.g., dimerization, translocation, DNA binding to EREs) except that the qualitative and quantitative nature of gene regulation is different than with a pure ligand (e.g., estrogen).

A is incorrect. Estrogen does not bind to any receptor that has tyrosine kinase activity nor does the ER directly activate kinase activity.

C is incorrect. Estrogen does not bind to any G-protein–coupled receptor nor does the ER directly activate G-protein activity.

D is incorrect. Estrogen does not bind to any receptor that increases cAMP synthesis.

E is incorrect. ER can be phosphorylated but it is not a direct result of ligand binding.

219

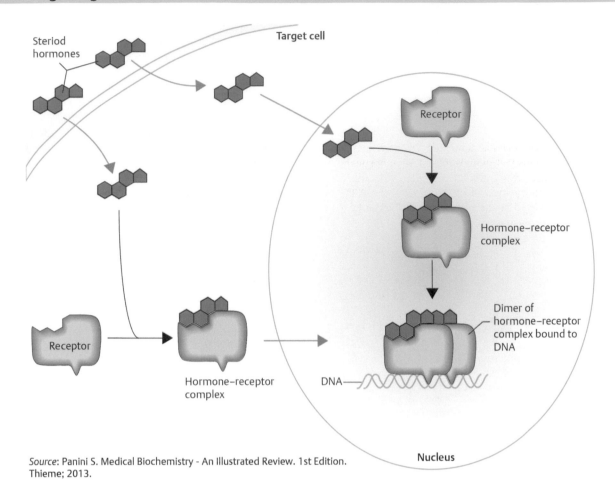

Source: Panini S. Medical Biochemistry - An Illustrated Review. 1st Edition.
Thieme; 2013.

17.   Correct: C. Phosphorylation of inhibitor of kappa B (IκB).

Transcription of the *IL-6* gene is induced under inflammatory conditions, via the action of the transcription factor NF-κB. Under noninduced conditions, NF-κB is retained in the cytoplasm bound to the IκB protein. Activation of cell surface inflammatory receptors (e.g., toll-like receptors, IL-1 receptor) leads to activation of IκB kinase (IKK) which phosphorylates IκB, leading to its ubiquitylation and subsequent degradation by the proteasome. This frees NF-κB to translocate to the nucleus and bind specific DNA sequences (NF-κB response elements) activating transcription of proinflammatory genes such as IL-6.

A is incorrect. Activation of heterotrimer G-proteins is via alteration in the structure of associated cell surface receptors upon ligand binding. It does not involve phosphorylation. G-proteins are not part of the primary signaling cascade that activates NF-κB.

B is incorrect. Glucocorticoid receptor can become phosphorylated, but not in response to the signaling events described. Glucocorticoid receptors are not part of the primary signaling cascade that activates NF-κB.

D is incorrect. PKA is activated by binding to the ligand cAMP, not by phosphorylation. PKA signaling is not part of the primary signaling cascade that activates NF-κB, though PKA can phosphorylate cAMP response element binding protein (CREB) which can cooperate with NF-κB to activate inflammatory genes such as *IL-6*.

E is incorrect. RAS can become phosphorylated, but not in response to the signaling events described. RAS is not part of the primary signaling cascade that activates NF-κB.

18.   Correct: D. Phosphoinositol-3-kinase (PI3K).

PI3K is part of a signaling cascade downstream of growth factors, including HER2. Blockade of HER2 by trastuzumab and pertuzumab would result in reduced PI3K kinase activity, since the initiating upstream signal would be diminished. However, if a mutation in the *PI3K* gene resulted in a gain of function, such that the PI3K kinase was constitutively active and independent of signals from ligand-activated HER2, it would render blockade of the HER2 ineffective in reducing downstream signals.

A is incorrect. Adenylyl cyclase is not part of the HER2 signaling pathway, so a gain-of-function mutation would not have any impact on the effectiveness of HER2 blockade.

B is incorrect. Guanylyl cyclase is not part of the HER2 signaling pathway, so a gain-of-function mutation would not have any impact on the effectiveness of HER2 blockade.

C is incorrect. *PTEN* is tumor suppressor gene that encodes a phosphatidylinositol-3,4,5-triphosphate 3-phosphatase, which dephosphorylates IP_3 to IP_2. The dephosphorylation of IP_3 terminates the PI3K/AKT/mTOR signaling pathway that is initiated by growth factor receptor (such as HER2) activation. A gain-of-function mutation in PTEN would reduce signaling initiated by HER2 activation and thus would be *additive* to blockade of HER2 by trastuzumab and pertuzumab.

E is incorrect. PKA is not part of the HER2 signaling pathway, so a gain-of-function mutation would not have any impact on the effectiveness of HER2 blockade.

19. Correct: B. Interferon γ (IFN-γ).

STAT proteins are transcription factors that are controlled by interferon signaling. The STAT proteins is regulated, primarily, by regulating subcellular localization; they are resident in the cytoplasm until interferon signaling induces their translocation to the nucleus. Interferons bind to cell surface receptors which dimerize and recruit Janus kinase (JAK) which phosphorylates the receptors on specific tyrosine residues. These phosphorylated tyrosines serve as docking sites STAT proteins. The STAT proteins, once docked, are themselves phosphorylated by JAK kinase, which leads to STAT dimerization and translocation to the nucleus. In the nucleus, STAT proteins bind to binds specific DNA sequences and regulates transcription of associated genes, primarily increasing their transcription.

A is incorrect. The signaling pathways activated by IGF-1 binding to receptors does not activate STAT proteins.

C is incorrect. The signaling pathways activated by IL-1 binding to receptors does not activate STAT proteins.

D is incorrect. The signaling pathways activated by TNF-α binding to receptors does not activate STAT proteins.

E is incorrect. The signaling pathways activated by TGF-β binding to receptors does not activate STAT proteins.

Chapter 13

DNA Replication and Cell Cycle

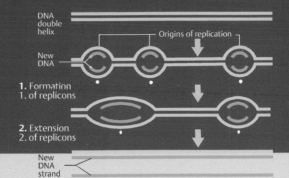

LEARNING OBJECTIVES

▸ Outline the basic steps and cellular machinery involved in DNA replication.

▸ Describe the basic chemical reaction catalyzed by DNA polymerase to join two nucleotides by a phosphodiester bond.

▸ Describe the double-stranded, helical, and antiparallel chain structure of DNA and how it relates to the processes of DNA replication, transcription, recombination, and repair.

▸ List the components of the DNA replication machinery and predict the outcome on DNA replication if they are lost or inhibited.

▸ Describe the role of telomerase in DNA replication and its contribution to aging and cancer.

▸ Describe the biochemical events that occur during each phase of the cell cycle.

▸ Explain the structure and function of chromatin in regulation of DNA transactions.

13.1 Questions

Easy   Medium   Hard

1. A patient brings a printout of a website for an out-of-state "antiaging" clinic she wishes to attend that requires a 1-week stay. She is particularly keen on their use of novel "antiaging" drugs, including a purported activator of an enzyme that "…is missing from most cells in the body, resulting in the shortening of chromosomes that contributes to organ failure with aging." To which of the following enzymes do you suspect the website is referring?

A. BRCA1

B. DNA polymerase

C. Histone acetyltransferase

D. RNA polymerase

E. Telomerase

2. A 67-year- old man presents with a chief complaint of "a lump on one testicle." He is diagnosed with testicular cancer (seminoma), which is treated with radical inguinal orchiectomy followed by a course of chemotherapy with etoposide. DNA replication is stalled in any residual cancer cells (and other replicating cells) due to which of the following biochemical events?

A. Accumulation of excess supercoils ahead of the replication fork

B. Chain termination of newly synthesized DNA strands

C. Direct inhibition of DNA polymerase delta and epsilon

D. Increased histone acetylation at origins of replication

E. Loss of primer synthesis

3. An investigator assembled a human DNA replication reaction in a test tube, including the required enzymes and protein factors, DNA template, deoxynucleotides, and adenosine triphosphate (ATP) as an energy source. However, the reaction does not proceed and no new DNA is synthesized. He troubleshoots the experiment and finds that although the helicase enzyme is consuming ATP, the DNA double helix does not appear to be unwinding, preventing the formation of the replicative complex. She concludes that she neglected to include one key factor. Which of the following components did she leave out of the reaction?

A. DNA polymerase delta/epsilon

B. DNA polymerase alpha/primase

C. DNA ligase

D. Single-stranded DNA binding protein (SSBP)

E. Topoisomerase II

4. During which phase of the cell cycle, illustrated in the figure below, does a cell that is normally diploid have a DNA complement somewhere between diploid and tetraploid?

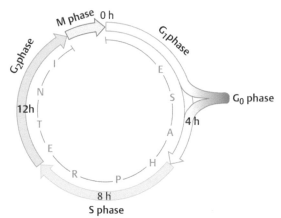

Source: Panini S. Medical Biochemistry - An Illustrated Review. 1st Edition. Thieme; 2013.

A. G0

B. G1

C. G2

D. M

E. S

5. In a diploid human cell, one copy of the tumor suppressor *TP53* gene, which encodes the p53 protein, has a base pair mismatch, with G (wildtype) on one strand and T (mutant) on the opposite strand of the double helix. If this is not repaired prior to DNA replication, what will the DNA sequence of the *TP53* gene be in the two daughter cells that result from a round of mitosis?

A. Both daughter cells will have one copy of mutated *TP53*

B. Both daughter cells will have two copies of mutated *TP53*

C. DNA replication cannot proceed with a mismatch in the DNA

D. One daughter cell will have one copy of mutated *TP53*

E. One daughter cell will have one copy of *TP53* that retains the mismatch and one copy with wild-type sequences

6. A pharmaceutical sales representative visits you in your office to tell you about a new drug for treatment of bladder cancer that targets DNA replication. This drug, he tells you, prevents DNA synthesis by inhibiting the activity of DNA polymerase alpha. You ask him specific details about its mechanism and he claims that the drug prevents initiation of DNA replication only at origins of replication, but has no effect on ongoing DNA replication. Which of the following reasons do you give him to refute his claim?

A. DNA polymerase alpha is necessary for both leading and lagging strand synthesis

B. DNA polymerase alpha is not present in the prereplicative complex

C. DNA polymerase alpha is the primary polymerase for synthesizing DNA during genome replication

D. DNA polymerase alpha is involved primarily in DNA repair mechanisms

7. A 72-year-old man presents in your clinic with a 3-day history of burning and itching on the left side of his chest and back accompanied by rash. He reports feeling "...tired, just no pep lately..." and has not been attending his weekly bridge club. Upon questioning, he explains that he felt an odd combination of tingling and numbness prior to onset of pain. Physical examination revealed a striking dermal efflorescence on the left side of his chest and extending toward his back (as shown in the figure below). You prescribe oral valacyclovir (Valtrex) to treat his condition. When this nucleotide analogue is incorporated into newly synthesized DNA, it prevents further elongation. Which of the following critical elements is missing from the valacyclovir molecule that results in the outcome described?

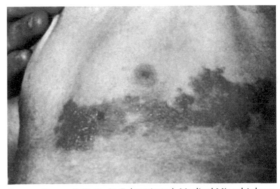

Source: Kayser F, Bienz K, Eckert J et al. Medical Microbiology. 1st Edition. 2004.

A. A chemical moiety that can form a phosphodiester bond with an incoming nucleotide

B. A chemical moiety that can form a phosphodiester bond with the terminal nucleotide of the DNA molecule being synthesized

C. A chemical moiety that can base-pair with the DNA template strand

D. A chemical moiety that has sufficient stored energy for formation of a phosphodiester bond

E. A chemical moiety that resembles a nucleic acid base

8. A 71-year-old woman discovered a mass in her breast which was diagnosed as ductal carcinoma and treated surgically. As part of a research study, sections of the excised tumor were stained with antibodies directed against the cyclin D protein. Cancer cells in the section stained intensely while surrounding normal ductal epithelium did not stain. Which of the following is mostly likely the direct result of elevated cyclin D expression in the cancer cells?

A. Decreased tumor suppressor protein expression

B. Increased DNA mutation rate

C. Increased local angiogenesis

D. Loss of immune system recognition

E. Loss of normal cell cycle control

225

Consider the following scenario for questions 9 and 10:

A patient with metastatic non–small-cell lung cancer (NSCLC) asks about enrolling in a clinical therapeutic trial he found through an online search. You determine that it is a phase III trial that is testing a peptide vaccine directed against the telomerase enzyme.

9. Which of the following best describes the rationale behind testing this therapeutic approach?

A. Cancer cells feature ongoing DNA synthesis

B. Cancer cells have defective cell cycle control

C. Cancer cells metastasize to distant organs

D. Cancer cells must evade the immune system

E. Cancer cells primarily utilize nonoxidative metabolism

10. If the patient is enrolled in the telomerase vaccine study, and the vaccine is effective in inducing an immune response directed against the enzyme, which of the following cell types would most likely be at risk for targeting by immune system effector cells activated by the vaccine?

A. Cardiomyocyte

B. Hematopoietic stem cell

C. Neuron

D. Neutrophil

E. Osteocyte

11. The following article was published in 2014 in the *New England Journal of Medicine*:

> "Helicase–Primase Inhibitor Pritelivir for HSV-2 Infection. Wald, A., et al. N Engl J Med 2014; 370: 201-210. Pritelivir, an inhibitor of the viral helicase–primase complex, exhibits antiviral activity in vitro and in animal models of herpes simplex virus (HSV) infection."

Based on the information in the article's title, which of the following events in the HSV viral DNA replication cycle do you think is *directly* blocked by pritelivir?

A. Ongoing synthesis of viral DNA

B. Packaging of the newly synthesized DNA into chromatin

C. Recognition of the viral DNA origin of replication

D. Removal of supercoils generated ahead of the replication fork

E. Unwinding of the double-stranded viral DNA

12. Exome sequencing of surgically excised colorectal cancers revealed a subset of these tumors with excessive, widespread single-nucleotide mutations in their DNA. Further analysis revealed that these tumors had in common a number of specific amino acid substitutions in the gene encoding DNA polymerase epsilon (gene *POLE*). Which of the following activities is likely defective in the DNA polymerase enzyme produced by these mutant alleles of *POLE*?

A. Binding to DNA

B. Catalysis of phosphodiester bond formation

C. DNA exonuclease activity

D. DNA helicase activity

E. Protein stability

13. A recent study revealed that melanoma cells with relatively higher levels of the protein PR70 had decreased growth rates in comparison to cells with lower levels of the same protein. Subsequent analysis revealed that PR70 interferes with DNA replication and cell cycle progression by stabilizing a protein found at origins of DNA replication at specific times during the cell cycle. Which of the following proteins is likely stabilized by the higher levels of PR70?

A. CDC6 licensing factor

B. DNA polymerase epsilon

C. MCM helicase

D. Origin recognition complex (ORC)

E. Replication protein A (RPA) SSBP

14. A 28-month-old boy presents your clinic after developing progressive left proptosis of 3 days duration. A family history delivered by his mother revealed cancer in multiple generations. One of two maternal half-siblings developed alveolar rhabdomyosarcoma of the tongue at age 3 years; the other child is in good health. Following extensive work-up, orbital rhabdomyosarcoma was diagnosed and chemotherapeutic protocols initiated. Genetic analysis of a peripheral blood samples from the boy revealed a mutation within the *p53* gene, which resulted in the substitution of histidine for arginine at amino acid position 175 (R175H), confirming that the boy had Li-Fraumeni syndrome. Which of the following cellular defects that result from the loss of p53 in the boy's cells likely contributed to the development of his rhabdomyosarcoma?

A. Excessive gene transcription from multiple oncogenes

B. Inability to induce apoptosis despite significant DNA damage

C. Inability to phosphorylate the retinoblastoma (RB) protein

D. Initiation of multiple rounds of DNA synthesis per cell cycle

E. Unregulated, continuous signaling of the RAS pathway

15. Analysis of global gene expression in more than 200, surgically excised glioblastoma multiforme (GM) tumors, identified a number of genes that are expressed differentially compared to cultures of normal glioblasts, the cell from which these tumors are thought to arise. In about 40% of the GM tumors analyzed, the gene *CDK4*, encoding the cyclin-dependent kinase 4 protein, was overexpressed several folds compared to glioblasts. Cells from six of the GM tumors used in the original gene expression study, that had elevated CDK4 expression, were cultured in vitro. Laboratory analysis of these cultured cells would be expected to reveal which of the following phenomenon?

A. Activating mutations in the RAS proto-oncogene

B. Cell cycle arrest after several rounds of cell division

C. Elevated expression of E2F target genes

D. Hyperphosphorylated p53 protein

E. Hypophosphorylated retinoblastoma (pRB) protein

16. You encounter a case report describing a young female patient with a complex syndrome that included growth retardation, severe immunodeficiency (hypoimmunoglobulinemia) and sun-sensitive facial erythema. She succumbed to a pulmonary infection at age 14 and upon autopsy, precancerous lesions were identified in numerous organs. The patient's parents and one older brother appeared to be in good health and were of normal stature. Following obtaining consent, perimortem fibroblasts were cultured in vitro and analysis of these cells revealed hypersensitivity to DNA damaging agents. Additionally, analysis of genomic DNA in cells within S phase revealed increased numbers of shorter DNA fragments, in comparison to what was observed in wild-type cells cultured in a similar manner. A deficiency in which of the following enzymatic activities would be consistent with these clinical and laboratory observations?

A. DNA helicase

B. DNA ligase

C. DNA polymerase epsilon

D. DNA polymerase alpha/primase

E. Single-stranded DNA binding protein

17. Homozygous deletion of *INK4* genes in pediatric acute lymphoblastic leukemia, which encode proteins that are inhibitors of CDKs, is associated with poorer clinical outcomes, with significantly elevated risk of relapse and death. These deletions would be predicted to be associated with increased activity of which of the following cell cycle regulatory factors?

A. Cyclin E–cyclin-dependent kinase 2

B. Cyclin A–cyclin-dependent kinase 1

C. E2F

D. p53

E. Retinoblastoma proteins (pRBs)

18. A 25-year-old man, who emigrated from Japan a few years earlier, presents in your clinic to complete a physical examination necessary for his application for permanent residence in the United States. Your examination reveals that he is in overall excellent health and he reports being an avid runner who competes in marathons. At the end of the visit, he confides that he is worried that his risk for developing leukemia is elevated, since he is sure he was exposed to radiation released following a nuclear power plant accident in Japan, that occurred near his hometown. When the patient was exposed to radiation from the accident, the stability and activity of which of the following proteins (or family of proteins) would have been increased, if significant DNA damage had occurred?

A. Cyclins

B. Cyclin-dependent kinases

C. E2F

D. p53

E. pRB

13.2 Answers and Explanations

Easy	Medium	Hard

1.   Correct: E. Telomerase.

The clinic's claim most likely refers to the shortening of chromosome ends or telomeres that occurs in most somatic cells with each round of DNA replication. Telomerase enzyme, a riboprotein complex, is required for replication of telomeres (as shown in the figure below). Most somatic cells lack telomerase, though it is found in stem and progenitor cells and is often present in cancer cells.

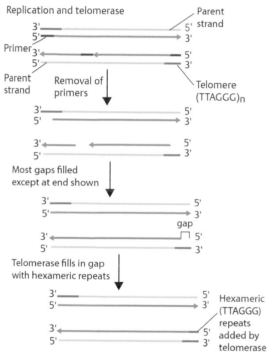

Source: Panini S. Medical Biochemistry - An Illustrated Review. 1st Edition. Thieme; 2013.

A is incorrect. BRCA1 is involved in specific DNA repair pathways but not telomere maintenance.

B is incorrect. DNA polymerases are involved in DNA repair and replication, including the replication of telomeres, but they are not "…missing from most cells in the body."

C is incorrect. Histone acetyltransferases are involved in many DNA transactions (transcription, replication, repair) but not specifically with telomere maintenance.

D is incorrect. Enzymes with RNA polymerase activity are involved in DNA replication but not specifically with telomere maintenance.

2.   Correct: A. Accumulation of excess supercoils ahead of the replication fork.

Etoposide inhibits the topoisomerase II enzyme which relaxes supercoils ahead of the replication fork, caused by the unwinding of the DNA double helix. The accumulation of overly supercoiled DNA eventually stalls the replication fork and can lead to DNA strand breakage.

B is incorrect. Etoposide is not incorporated into DNA.

C is incorrect. Etoposide does not directly inhibit DNA polymerase enzymes.

D is incorrect. Etoposide does not influence histone acetylation.

E is incorrect. Etoposide does not inhibit DNA primase.

3.   Correct: D. Single-stranded DNA binding protein (SSBP).

SSBP coats single-stranded DNA once it is unwound by the DNA helicase. In its absence, unwound DNA would quickly reanneal into a double helix (as shown in the figure below).

A is incorrect. DNA polymerase delta/epsilon synthesize DNA in a template-dependent manner and do not directly participate in DNA unwinding.

B is incorrect. DNA polymerase alpha/primase enzymes synthesize RNA-DNA primers to initiate DNA synthesis and do not directly participate in DNA unwinding.

C is incorrect. DNA ligase seals nicks in the DNA backbone by joining 3'-OH to 5'-phosphate groups in an ATP consuming reaction and does not directly participate in DNA unwinding.

E is incorrect. Topoisomerase II relaxes supercoils ahead of the replication fork and does not directly participate in DNA unwinding.

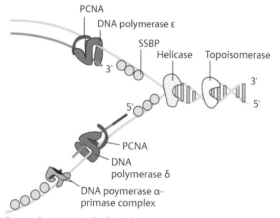

Source: Panini S. Medical Biochemistry - An Illustrated Review. 1st Edition. Thieme; 2013.

4.   Correct: E. S.

The genome is duplicated during the S phase (synthesis phase) so that its DNA complement is greater than diploid but still less than tetraploid. After S phase is complete, the cell is effectively tetraploid until completion of M phase (mitosis).

A is incorrect, cells in G_0 are diploid.

B is incorrect, cells in G_1 are diploid.

C is incorrect, cells in G_2 are effectively tetraploid.

D is incorrect, cells in M are effectively tetraploid until division is complete where they are diploid.

5. Correct: D. One daughter cell will have one copy of mutated *TP53*.

DNA replication is semiconservative: Each daughter cell gets one of the two strands of the parental cell double helix. Since only one strand of one copy of the *TP53* gene has a mutation (the T residue), DNA replication will produce four copies of the *TP53*: three wild-types and one mutant. Therefore, only one daughter cell will get one copy of the mutant *TP53* gene.

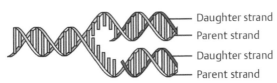

Daughter strand
Parent strand
Daughter strand
Parent strand

Source: Panini S. Medical Biochemistry - An Illustrated Review. 1st Edition. Thieme; 2013.

A is incorrect. This distribution is inconsistent with semiconservative replication.

B is incorrect. This distribution is inconsistent with semiconservative replication.

C is incorrect. While mismatched nucleotides are generally repaired prior to DNA replication, it is not a requirement for DNA replication to proceed.

E is incorrect. This distribution is inconsistent with semiconservative replication (as shown in the figure above).

6. Correct: A. DNA polymerase alpha is necessary for both leading and lagging strand synthesis.

DNA polymerase alpha, in a complex with the primase enzyme, synthesizes primers for DNA replication. DNA polymerase alpha–primase complex synthesizes short, RNA-DNA molecules using genomic DNA as a template. These short RNA-DNA molecules are used as primers for DNA synthesis by DNA polymerase delta and epsilon (see figure shown in Answer 3). It does so at origins of replication, and also about every thousand nucleotides on the lagging strand (given the semidiscontinuous nature of DNA synthesis; see the figure on the right). Therefore, the sales representative is wrong, since DNA polymerase alpha is active during ongoing DNA synthesis.

B is incorrect. DNA polymerase alpha is an important component of the prereplicative complex, responsible for adding 10 to 15 nucleotides of DNA to the RNA primer synthesized by the enzyme primase.

C is incorrect. DNA polymerase delta and epsilon and the two polymerases responsible for synthesizing the genome during DNA replication (as shown in the figure in Answer 3).

D is incorrect. DNA polymerase alpha is involved in some DNA repair pathways in addition to DNA replication, but that is not its primary role.

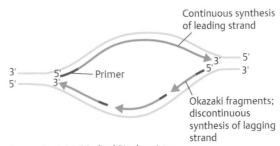

Continuous synthesis of leading strand

Primer

Okazaki fragments; discontinuous synthesis of lagging strand

Source: Panini S. Medical Biochemistry - An Illustrated Review. 1st Edition. Thieme; 2013.

7. Correct: A. A chemical moiety that can form a phosphodiester bond with an incoming nucleotide.

The patient has shingles from a reemergent varicella zoster virus infection. Valacyclovir (Valtrex) is a prodrug that is converted to acyclovir by the action of the valacyclovirase enzyme, a highly specific α-amino acid ester hydrolase found primarily in the liver and kidney. Acyclovir is a guanine base with a hemi acetyl group in place of deoxyribose. It is phosphorylated primarily in infected cells by the action of virally encoded thymidylate kinase, and then extended to the triphosphate form by cellular enzymes (as shown in the figure on the next page). The triphosphorylated acyclovir is incorporated into replicating viral DNA. Since it lacks deoxyribose, it does not have the 3'-hydroxyl group necessary to form a phosphodiester bond with the incoming nucleotide. It belongs to a class of drugs known as "chain terminators," since it terminates synthesis of new DNA chains.

B is incorrect. Triphosphorylated acyclovir has the necessary chemical moiety to form a phosphodiester bond with the terminal nucleotide of the DNA molecule being synthesized and indeed must do so to be incorporated into the growing DNA molecule as part of its mechanism of action.

C is incorrect. The guanine base in acyclovir can base-pair with cytosine on the template strand and indeed must do so to be incorporated into the growing DNA molecule as part of its mechanism of action.

D is incorrect. Acyclovir is triphosphorylated in cells and the energy contained in these phosphate groups is utilized to form a phosphodiester bond with the DNA molecule being synthesized.

E is incorrect. Acyclovir has a guanine base, identical to the base in guanosine triphosphate.

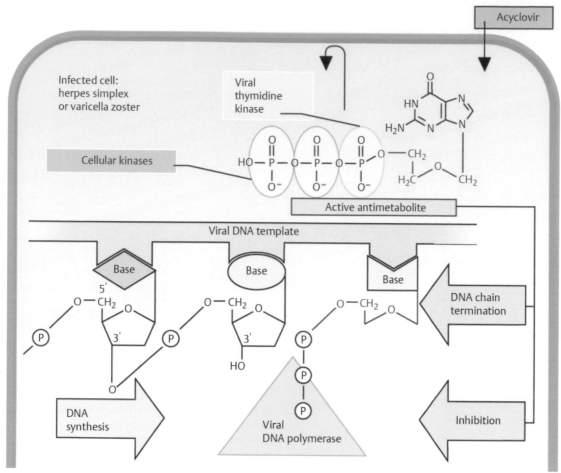

Source: Simmons M. Pharmacology—An Illustrated Review. 1st Edition. 2011.

8. Correct: E. Loss of normal cell cycle control.

Cyclins bind to cyclin-dependent kinases (CDKs) partially activating their kinase activity and participating in selection of target proteins (as shown in the figure below). In early G1 phase of the cell cycle, cyclin D binds both CDK4 and CDK6. The activity of these kinases allows the cell to transit the restriction point and enter S phase, after which cyclin D is quickly degraded. Elevated, sustained expression of cyclin D, as in breast cancer, allows cells to progress through the G1 restriction point, resulting in loss of a key aspect of normal cell cycle control.

A is incorrect. Cyclin D does not directly regulate expression of tumor suppressor genes.

B is incorrect. Cyclin D does not directly influence DNA repair mechanisms or affect mutation rates.

C is incorrect. Cyclin D does not directly affect the mechanisms responsible for angiogenesis.

D is incorrect. Cyclin D does not directly affect the mechanisms or protein factors involved immune system recognition of tumors.

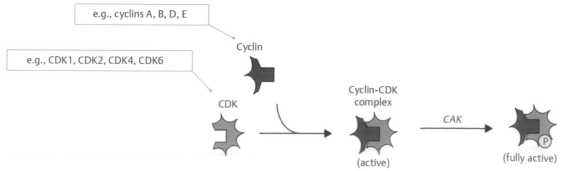

Source: Panini S. Medical Biochemistry - An Illustrated Review. 1st Edition. Thieme; 2013.

9. Correct: A. Cancer cells feature ongoing DNA synthesis.

DNA synthesis in humans requires the utilization of a specific enzyme, telomerase, to copy the ends of linear chromosomes (see the figure in Answer 1). In the absence of telomerase, each round of DNA synthesis (cell division) would result in progressive shortening of chromosomes which ultimately could trigger senescence or cell death. It has been reported that approximately 85% of cancers express telomerase; normal, somatic cells typically do not. Targeting telomerase with the body's immune system (following vaccination) could target cancer cells.

B is incorrect. Cancer cells do typically have defective cell cycle control, but telomerase is not directly involved in these mechanisms.

C is incorrect. Cancer cells can metastasize to distant organs, but telomerase is not directly involved in the mechanisms required to do this.

D is incorrect. Cancer cells typically must evade the immune system, but telomerase is not directly involved in the mechanisms required to do this.

E is incorrect. Cancer cells typically utilize non-oxidative metabolism (Warburg's metabolism), but telomerase is not directly involved in the mechanisms required to do so.

10. Correct: B. Hematopoietic stem cell.

Telomerase is expressed primarily in cells that have active, ongoing DNA synthesis and cell division, such as hematopoietic stem cells. Differentiated cells typically do not express telomerase.

A is incorrect. Cardiomyocytes are differentiated cells that typically do not express telomerase.

C is incorrect. Neurons are differentiated cells that typically do not express telomerase.

D is incorrect. Neutrophils are differentiated cells that typically do not express telomerase.

E is incorrect. Osteocytes are differentiated cells that typically do not express telomerase.

11. Correct: E. Unwinding of the double-stranded viral DNA.

The drug inhibits the viral helicase–primase complex. Helicase utilizes the energy in ATP to unwind double-stranded (dsDNA). Primase enzymes synthesize short primers onto which DNA polymerase adds nucleotides in a template-dependent manner, to copy the HSV genome. Only the activity of helicase, not primase, was an option.

A is incorrect. This is an activity necessary for DNA replication, but it is not carried out by "primase" or "helicase" enzymes.

B is incorrect. This is an activity necessary for DNA replication, but it is not carried out by "primase" or "helicase" enzymes.

C is incorrect. This is an activity necessary for DNA replication, but it is not carried out by "primase" or "helicase" enzymes.

D is incorrect. This is an activity necessary for DNA replication, but it is not carried out by "primase" or "helicase" enzymes.

12. Correct: C. DNA exonuclease activity.

DNA polymerases rarely will insert an incorrect nucleotide, that is, a nucleotide incapable of base-pairing with the opposing nucleotide on the template strand. DNA polymerase delta and epsilon, the enzymes responsible for the bulk of DNA synthesis during S phase of the cell cycle in human cells, have a proofreading activity that will repair such errors. The enzymes have 3' to 5' exonuclease activity, "backing up" and removing the incorrect nucleotide from the newly synthesized DNA. The DNA polymerase then restarts DNA synthesis. A number of single amino acid substitutions have been identified that reduce the 3' to 5' exonuclease activity of DNA polymerase epsilon, limiting the enzyme's ability to carry out its proofreading activity. As such, these cells accumulate an abnormally high level of single nucleotide mutations throughout the genome.

A is incorrect. A mutation that affected the ability of DNA polymerase epsilon to bind DNA would result in less efficient DNA synthesis but would not specifically cause widespread, single-nucleotide mutations in the genome.

B is incorrect. A mutation that affected the ability of DNA polymerase epsilon to catalyze phosphodiester bond formation would result in less efficient DNA synthesis but would not specifically cause widespread, single-nucleotide mutations in the genome.

D is incorrect. DNA polymerase epsilon does not have inherent DNA helicase activity. DNA unwinding is carried out by the minichromosome maintenance complex (MCM) complex which associates with DNA at replication forks.

E is incorrect. A mutation that affected the overall stability of DNA polymerase epsilon would result in less efficient DNA synthesis but would not specifically cause widespread, single-nucleotide mutations in the genome.

13. Correct: A. CDC6 licensing factor.

CDC6 is a DNA replication licensing factor that binds, along with the ORC to origins of DNA replication in late M/G1 phase of the cell cycle. Next, the MCM helicase and another licensing factor Cdt1 are recruited to origins. Following loading of MCM/Cdt1, the two licensing factors are released and exit the nuclease and/or are degraded. The removal of CDC6 and Cdt1 are necessary for the next events in DNA replication (e.g., binding of DNA polymerase, unwinding of DNA by MCM helicase) to occur. Regulation that limits the availability and activity of CDC6 (and Cdt1) during specific stages of the cell cycle ensures that only a single round of DNA replication can occur per cell cycle. Stabilization of CDC6 by PR70 slows progression of the replicative cycle, thereby slowing the rate at which the melanoma cells grow.

B is incorrect. DNA polymerase epsilon and delta are the primary DNA polymerases necessary for copying the genome during S phase of the cell cycle. Stabilizing either of these proteins would not slow cell growth.

C is incorrect. MCM helicase unwinds the DNA double helix at the origin of replication and moves with the replication machinery as it copies the genome. Stabilizing any of the proteins in the MCM complex would not slow cell growth.

D is incorrect. The ORC complex binds to the origins of replication and seeds the formation of the replicative complex. Stabilizing any of the proteins in the ORC complex would not slow cell growth.

E is incorrect. The RPA SSBPs bind to DNA once it has been unwound by the MCM helicase. Stabilizing RPA protein would not slow cell growth.

14.   Correct: B. Inability to induce apoptosis despite significant DNA damage.

Li-Fraumeni syndrome results from a heterozygous mutation of the *TP53* tumor suppressor gene and is characterized by patients developing cancer at a relatively young age (typically 30–40 years old) that can affect multiple tissues. p53 protein is sometimes referred to as the "guardian of the genome," responding to DNA damage and initiating cell cycle arrest and/or apoptosis in response.

A is incorrect. Loss of p53 would not directly lead to excessive gene transcription from multiple oncogenes.

C is incorrect. The RB protein is another important tumor suppressor gene and a downstream effector of p53. RB is the effector of the G1 checkpoint and must be phosphorylated by cyclin-dependent kinases for the cells to progress through G1 into S phase. Inability to phosphorylate RB would result in cell cycle arrest, the opposite of what occurs with loss of p53.

D is incorrect. Linkage of cell cycle and a single round of DNA synthesis involves mechanisms that do not involve the p53 protein.

E is incorrect. p53 does not directly influence signaling through the RAS pathway.

15.   Correct: C. Elevated expression of E2F target genes.

The pRB mediates the G1 cell cycle checkpoint, which regulates entry of cells into S phase and promotes terminal differentiation. pRB binds to a transcription factor known as E2F, preventing E2F from regulating gene transcription. Upon cells receiving signals to divide, cyclin proteins combine with CDKs to phosphorylate key regulators of cell division.

pRB is phosphorylated by CDK4/6-cyclin D which disrupts the interaction between pRB and E2F. E2F subsequently activates transcription of genes (regulatory proteins, metabolic enzymes, etc.) involved in cell cycle progression and cell growth (as shown in the figure below). Overexpression of CDK4 in the GM tumors results in elevated pRB phosphorylation and diminution of the G1 checkpoint, contributing to the uncontrolled growth associated with this aggressive tumor.

A is incorrect. Activating mutations in the RAS proto-oncogene are among the most common mutations found in human cancers. However, these mutations are independent of the observed increase in the expression of CDK4.

B is incorrect. The constitutive hyperphosphorylation of pRB by the overexpressed CDK$ removes a critical cell cycle checkpoint and contributes to the cells becoming fully transformed into neoplastic cells. Cancer cells typically are immortal and exit from cycling does not occur over time.

D is incorrect. CDK4 does not phosphorylate p53 protein.

E is incorrect. Overexpression of CDK4 is associated with the opposite phenomenon, hyperphosphorylation of pRB.

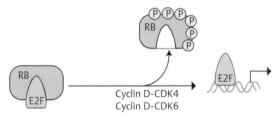

Source: Panini S. Medical Biochemistry - An Illustrated Review. 1st Edition. Thieme; 2013.

16.   Correct: B. DNA ligase.

The patient is homozygous for a defective (though not inactive) allele of DNA ligase. DNA ligase joins the ends of DNA molecules together, forming a phosphodiester bond between the 3'-OH and 5'-phosphate of adjacent molecules (as shown in the figure on the next page). Both the patient and the cells derived from her displayed a defect in DNA repair. DNA ligase is necessary to seal nicks following removal of damaged DNA and its replacement, in some types of DNA repair mechanisms. The increased numbers of shorter DNA fragments observed in the patient's cells during S phase is due to a reduced ability to join Okazaki fragments together. Okazaki fragments are the approximately 1,000 to 2,000 base pair stretches of newly synthesized DNA formed on the lagging strand, where discontinuous DNA synthesis occurs (as shown in the figure of Answer 6). Such a defect would have profound effects on genomic stability, likely leading to accumulation of mutations that contributed to the observed precancerous lesions identified in numerous organs of the patient.

A is incorrect. A defect in DNA helicase (in humans, the MCM) would also affect DNA repair and replication. However, it is not consistent with the observation of increased numbers of shorter DNA fragments observed in the patient's cells during S phase that results from a reduced ability to join Okazaki fragments together.

C is incorrect. DNA polymerase epsilon is responsible for synthesis of the leading strand during DNA replication. It is also involved in some types of DNA repair. However, a defective allele of this critical enzyme would not be consistent with the observation of increased numbers of shorter DNA fragments observed in the patient's cells during S phase that results from a reduced ability to join Okazaki fragments together.

D is incorrect. DNA polymerase alpha/primase is responsible for synthesizing primers during DNA replication, both to initiate synthesis on the leading strand and to initiate synthesis of each Okazaki fragment on the lagging strand. It is also involved in some types of DNA repair. However, a defective allele that inhibits the activity of DNA polymerase alpha/primase would not be consistent with the observation of increased numbers of shorter DNA fragments observed in the patient's cells during S phase that results from a reduced ability to join Okazaki fragments together.

E is incorrect. To prevent reannealing of DNA unwound by helicase, prior to synthesis of new strands, SSBP, also known as RPA, coats the single-stranded DNA. SSBP is involved in some types of DNA repair. However, a defective allele of this critical protein would not be consistent with the observation of increased numbers of shorter DNA fragments observed in the patient's cells during S phase that results from a reduced ability to join Okazaki fragments together.

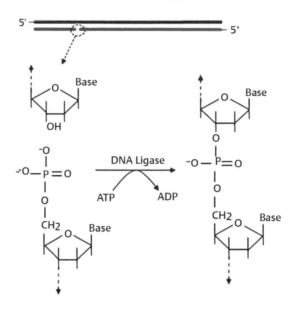

17. Correct: C. E2F.

Cyclin–CDK complexes are inhibited by specific CDK inhibitor (CKI) proteins, preventing the kinase from phosphorylating targets. There are two families of CKIs: CIP/KIP and INK4. The CIP/KIP family (p21, p27, and p57) inhibits G1-phase (cyclin D–CDK4 and cyclin D–CDK6) and S-phase (cyclin E–CDK2) complexes (as shown in the figure below). The INK4 family (p15, p16, p18, and p19) blocks the activity of the G_1-phase CDKs only. Loss of the INK4-encoded proteins would result in excess activity of the G1-phase CDKs which phosphorylate pRB. This disrupts the interaction between pRB and E2F. E2F is then free to bind DNA promoter elements of target genes, activating their transcription.

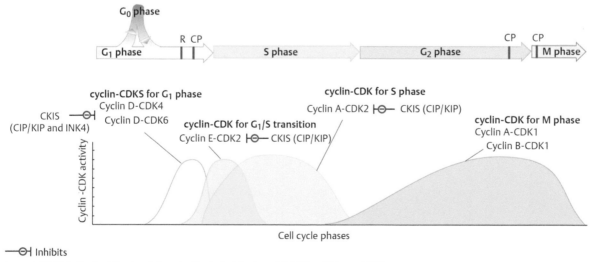

Source: Panini S. Medical Biochemistry - An Illustrated Review. 1st Edition. Thieme; 2013.

A is incorrect. The cyclin E–cyclin-dependent kinase 2 is inhibited by the CIP/KIP family of CKIs, not the INK4 family of CKIs (as shown in the figure on the previous page).

B is incorrect. The cyclin A–cyclin-dependent kinase 2 is inhibited by the CIP/KIP family of CKIs, not the INK4 family of CKIs (as shown in the figure on the previous page).

D is incorrect. Loss of the INK4 CKIs would not have a direct effect on p53 protein activity.

E is incorrect. The hyperphosphorylation of pRB that would result from loss of INK4 CKIs would inhibit the activity of pRB which is to bind to and prevent E2F from activating gene transcription.

18. Correct: D. p53.

p53 is often referred to as the "guardian of the genome" for its role in regulating cell cycle progression and survival following genome damage. When the genome is significantly damaged, the ataxia-telangiectasia mutated (ATM) kinase is activated which initiates a kinase cascade that ultimately results in p53 phosphorylation. Under nonstress conditions, p53 is associated with the E3 ubiquitin ligase Mouse double minute 2 homolog (MDM2) which ubiquitinates p53, resulting in the degradation of p53 by the proteasome. Phosphorylation of p53 causes it to dissociate from MDM2, preventing the degradation (i.e., stabilizing) the p53 protein. p53 translocates to the nucleus and binds to specific DNA sequences, activating transcription of target genes, suppressing cell cycle progression to allow DNA repair. If the genome is damaged to such a degree that repair is impossible, p53 activity will lead to apoptosis (as shown in the figure below).

A is incorrect. CKIs are induced by activated p53, preventing cell cycle progression. The activity (or stability) of cyclins is not increased.

B is incorrect. CKIs are induced by activated p53, preventing cell cycle progression. The activity of CDKs is therefore inhibited following significant DNA damage.

C is incorrect. Since CDKs are inhibited by p53 activation, the pRB is not phosphorylated and remains bound to and inhibits E2F.

E is incorrect. Since CDKs are inhibited by p53 activation, the pRB is not phosphorylated and remains bound to and inhibits E2F.

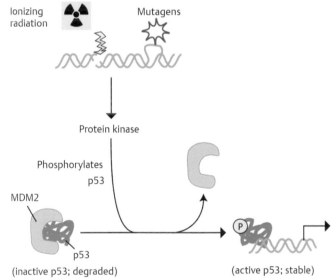

Ionizing radiation

Mutagens

Protein kinase

Phosphorylates p53

MDM2

p53
(inactive p53; degraded)

(active p53; stable)

Transcription of gene for p21 which leads to:

p21 binding to and inactivating cyclin-CDK complexes for G_1/S transition (cyclin E-CDK2), and S phase (cyclin A-CDK2). This keeps RB hypophosphorylated (and active), which sequesters E2F.

Source: Panini S. Medical Biochemistry - An Illustrated Review. 1st Edition. Thieme; 2013.

Chapter 14

DNA Mutation and Repair

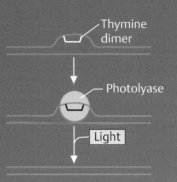

LEARNING OBJECTIVES

► Contrast frameshift, missense, nonsense, and silent mutations, and how such mutations might ultimately affect protein fate/function.

► List common physical and chemical agents that damage DNA and types of damage they produced.

► Explain how DNA damage and failure to repair can increase risk of diseases such as cancer.

► List the basic steps of DNA damage repair.

► Explain how different types of DNA repair mechanisms are employed for different types of DNA lesions.

► List the most common inherited syndromes involving defects in DNA repair and describe the pathology of each.

14.1 Questions

Easy	Medium	Hard

1. A 51-year-old man presents in your clinic complaining of fatigue, night sweats, and occasional low-grade fevers that began a month earlier but have recently been worsening. Physical examination is unremarkable except for tenderness around his sternum and moderate splenomegaly. Complete blood count reveals markedly elevated leukocytes with normal numbers of morphologically unremarkable red blood cells. Cytogenetic analysis of bone marrow aspirate reveals a chromosomal translocation pathognomonic for his disease (see figure below). Reviewing his social history, you note that he emigrated from Ukraine in 1992, 6 years after the Chernobyl nuclear power plant disaster. He tells you that he lived 20 miles downwind of the power plant at the time of the accident. The action of which of the following DNA repair mechanisms may have contributed to the development of his leukemia?

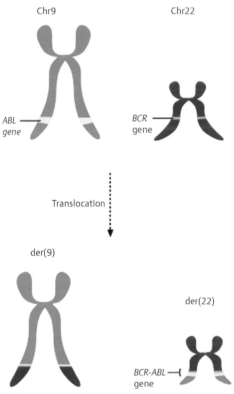

Source: Panini S. Medical Biochemistry - An Illustrated Review. 1st Edition. Thieme; 2013.

A. Base excision repair

B. Homologous recombination repair

C. Mismatch excision repair

D. Nonhomologous end-joining repair

E. Nucleotide excision repair

2. A 41-year-old, female patient presents with a chief complaint of fatigue. During your interview she also mentions she noticed her stools have been "odd," appearing very dark. Physical examination was unremarkable and laboratory tests revealed iron deficiency anemia. You order a colonoscopy which discovered a few, flat colonic adenomas that upon histological analysis display high-grade dysplasia. Following a family history that revealed a maternal grandmother who died at age 44 from ovarian cancer, you order a genetic analysis which showed the patient has gene mutations associated with hereditary nonpolyposis colorectal cancer/Lynch syndrome. On a follow-up visit, after the patient has read up on her genetic diagnosis, she says she will not allow any further diagnostic X-rays due to perceived risk. You tell her that her genetic background carries no increased risk from these imaging tests. Why are you justified in saying this?

A. DNA adducts are fixed primarily by nucleotide excision repair

B. Ionizing radiation causes primarily double-strand breaks

C. Lynch syndrome primarily affects DNA replication

D. Radiation from medical imaging carries only minor health risks

E. Ultraviolet radiation causes primarily thymidine dimers

3. Structural studies were performed on DNA exposed to a cross-linking cancer chemotherapeutic agent. Line drawings of an untreated DNA molecule and a treated DNA molecule are shown in the figure below. If cells were treated with this chemotherapeutic agent, which of the following mechanisms would most likely to repair this lesion?

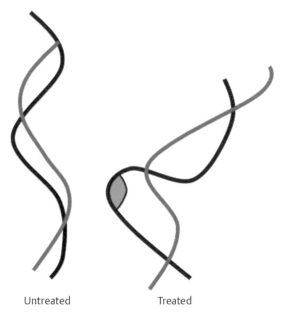

Untreated   Treated

A. Homologous recombination repair

B. Misincorporation repair by DNA polymerase epsilon

C. Mismatch repair

D. Nucleotide excision repair

E. Nonhomologous end-joining repair

4. A patient with a mixed glioma (oligoastrocytoma) is treated with surgical resection of as much tumor mass as possible followed by radiation treatment. Healthy, postmitotic neurons proximal to the glioma are also exposed to the therapeutic ionizing radiation. Which of the following pathways is likely to repair the major type of damage induced by ionizing radiation in these healthy neurons?

A. Base excision repair

B. Homologous recombination repair

C. Mismatch repair

D. Nucleotide excision repair

E. Nonhomologous end joining

5. Human DNA polymerase epsilon has a measured rate of incorrect nucleotide insertion during DNA replication of 1 in 10 million nucleotides. Much of this accuracy is due to DNA repair mechanisms. When the polymerase does incorporate an incorrect nucleotide during DNA synthesis, which of the following is the first mechanism to address this type of mistake?

A. Base excision repair

B. 3′ to 5′ exonuclease activity of DNA polymerase epsilon

C. Homologous recombination repair

D. Nucleotide excision repair

E. Postreplicative mismatch excision repair

6. Based on recent high-throughput sequencing studies of surgically excised cancer, approximately 7% of endometrial cancers were found to have mutations in the *POLE* gene encoding DNA polymerase epsilon. These mutations were found to disable the proofreading function of the enzyme. Analysis of the data from one such "proofreading negative" cell lines revealed a deletion of two nucleotides within the open reading frame of a gene involved in regulating cell division. Which of the following is the most likely functional outcome of this mutation on the protein encoded by this gene?

A. Production of elevated levels of the protein

B. Production of a protein with a single amino acid substitution

C. Production of a truncated, nonfunctional protein

D. Production of elevated levels of the messenger RNA (mRNA) transcript

E. Production of a truncated mRNA transcript

7. A 3-year-old boy was brought to the pediatric service with a chief complaint of abdominal pain and hematochezia. Review of his medical records revealed the child had previously reported pain in his perineal area, urinary urgency, and had pneumonia on three separate occasions. During your interview, it was revealed that he also suffers from epistaxis and easy bruising. Physical examination of the patient revealed curved fingers with short middle phalanges, café au lait spots on his legs and buttocks and short stature. Complete blood count revealed hemoglobin, platelet, and absolute neutrophil count consistent with mild bone marrow failure. Which of the following DNA repair syndromes is most consistent with the findings described for this child?

A. Ataxia-telangiectasia (A-T)

B. Cockayne's syndrome

C. Fanconi's anemia

D. Lynch syndrome

E. Xeroderma pigmentosum (XP)

8. A 39-year-old woman presents in your clinic with a chief complaint of, "A mole on my face has changed shape." Physical examination reveals a flat, brownish, pale, irregularly colored nevus on the zygomatic region of her face, proximal to her left ear (see the figure below). You suspect lentigo maligna melanoma and refer her to a plastic surgeon for removal of the nevus. Given the location of the lesion, which of the following types of DNA lesions likely contributed to the early events in the development of your patient's diseases?

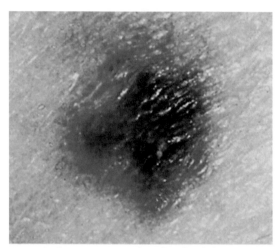

Source: Riede U, Werner M. Color Atlas of Pathology: Pathologic Principles · Associated Diseases · Sequela. 1st Edition. 2004.

A. DNA adduct formation
B. Double-stranded breaks
C. Interstrand cross-links
D. Pyrimidine dimers
E. Single-stranded breaks

9. A 68-year-old male patient presents to family medicine clinic with a chief complaint of "cough with some bloody mucus coming up." You determine his cough has a 4-month history with the hemoptysis starting 2 weeks prior to his appointment. A comparison of his chest radiograph obtained at presentation (see the figure below, (**b**)), to one the patient had 2 years prior (see the figure below (**a**)), results in you referring the patient to a specialist for further evaluation and treatment. The chemicals present in cigarette smoke likely had which of the following contributions to the development of the disease revealed on the patient's radiograph?

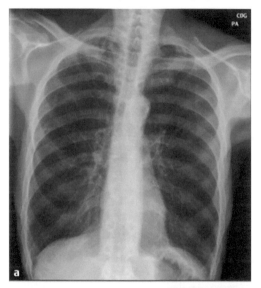

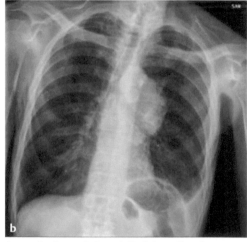

Source: Gunderman R. Essential Radiology. Clinical Presentation, Pathophysiology, Imaging. 3rd Edition. Thieme; 2014.

A. Binding of CO to hemoglobin in red blood cells
B. Activation of sympathetic neurotransmission
C. Elevated levels of plasma fibrinogen
D. Generation of DNA adducts
E. Poor nutrition due to loss of taste bud function

10. A 27-year-old woman comes to your clinic to discuss her concerns about elevated breast cancer risk. During your history, it is revealed that her mother died at age 34 from breast cancer. Her mother had no female siblings and her maternal grandmother died at age 77 from what your patient thinks was heart failure. Through a commercial genetic testing service, the patient discovered that she has an "elevated risk for breast and ovarian cancer." Which of the following pathways is most likely affected by the alleles the patient has which confer elevated risk of breast and ovarian cancer?

A. Base excision repair

B. Homologous recombination DNA repair

C. Mismatch repair

D. Nonhomologous end-joining repair

E. Nucleotide excision repair

11. While on a medical mission to Honduras, you encounter a 12-year-old boy who is brought to the clinic by his parents. On skin typically exposed to sunlight, he has a history of multiple skin tumors and currently has multiple, visible cancerous lesions on his face, hands, and lower arms. After obtaining consent, you collect skin biopsies from the patient and his apparently healthy mother, that you subsequently culture in the laboratory. Dermal fibroblasts cultured from the patient and his mother were exposed to a range of doses of UV light. Survival of the exposed cells was determined 48 hours later. The data from this experiment are shown in the graph below (Xp are the patient's cells; normal are the mother's cells). Based on these data, which of the following repair mechanisms is most likely deficient in this patient?

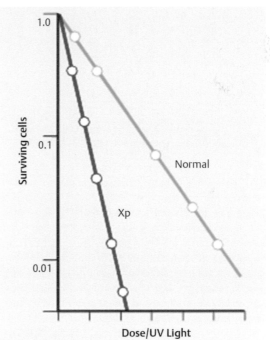

Source: Passarge E. Color Atlas of Genetics. 4th Edition. 2012.

A. Base excision repair

B. Homologous recombination DNA repair

C. Mismatch repair

D. Nonhomologous end-joining repair

E. Nucleotide excision repair

12. High-throughput exome sequencing of mRNA purified from a squamous cell carcinoma of the urinary bladder revealed a number of relevant mutations in key genes. The sequence of the 5′-end of the two alleles of the RAS gene from this sample are shown in the figure below. One allele was wild type, the other had a single-nucleotide substitution. Which of the following terms best describes the type of mutation in the mutated *RAS* gene?

Wildtype *h-ras* gene

| ATG | ACG | GAA | TAT | AAG | CTG | GTG | GTG | GTG | GGC | GCC | GGC | GGT... |
| MET | THR | GLU | TYR | LYS | LEU | VAL | VAL | VAL | GLY | ALA | GLY | GLY... |

Mutant, *h-ras* gene

| ATG | ACG | GAA | TAT | AAG | CTG | GTG | GTG | GTG | GGC | GCC | GTC | GGT... |
| MET | THR | GLU | TYR | LYS | LEU | VAL | VAL | VAL | GLY | ALA | VAL | GLY... |

A. Frameshift

B. Missense

C. Nonsense

D. Silent

E. Synonymous

13. You are working in the emergency department (ED) of the local hospital when a 28-year-old man is brought in by his supervisor, following exposure to an industrial chemical. The patient had been assigned a repair job on a length of industrial hose that was capped at both ends. On opening the hose, a small amount (~ 10 mL) of clear liquid spilled out, some of which got onto the patients' hand. He rinsed it off in the sink. About an hour later, he developed eye irritation with discomfort, lacrimation, and erythema which precipitated his visit to the ED. The supplying company was contacted by his supervisor and was told that the hose had been filled with dimethyl sulphate (DMS). You begin treatment by irrigating his eyes thoroughly with normal saline and then had him thoroughly shower with soap. The patient was admitted overnight for observation and was discharged the next day. One concern was DNA damage the skin of his hand from the DMS exposure, an agent known to methylate DNA nucleotides. It is quite likely that most methylation that occurred was repaired. Which of the following repair mechanisms was most likely responsible for the repair of the chemically methylated DNA nucleotides?

A. Base excision repair

B. Homologous recombination DNA repair

C. Mismatch repair

D. Nonhomologous end-joining repair

E. Nucleotide excision repair

14. A newly discovered chemical agent is being considered for development as a novel antifungal drug. In laboratory tests using *Candida albicans*, the agent specifically inhibited the 3′→5′ exonuclease activity of the DNA polymerase enzyme that replicates the yeast's genome, resulting in cytostasis and ultimately cell death. Studies performed in cultured human cells showed that the agent has a similar inhibitory effect on human DNA polymerases, though it required a higher dose to achieve lethal inhibition. While developing plans to test the agent in humans, a member of the research team noted that individuals with a specific defect in DNA repair should be barred from participating in clinical trials with the drug. Patients with which of the following conditions would be at particular risk of accumulating additional DNA mutations from inhibition of the 3′→5′ exonuclease activity of DNA polymerase?

A. Ataxia-telangiectasia

B. Disposition to cancers due to *BRCA1* or *BRCA2* mutations

C. Fanconi's anemia

D. Lynch syndrome/hereditary nonpolyposis colon cancer

E. Xeroderma pigmentosum

15. A retrospective study was performed to determine the effect of childhood computed tomography (CT) exposure on later development of cancer. A positive, linear relationship was observed between the estimated dose of radiation received by bone marrow from CT scans prior to age 22 and subsequent risk of developing leukemia in the subsequent 10-year window. One potential way to address this elevated risk is to develop a drug to be administered prior to CT that would heighten the activity of specific DNA repair pathways. Increased activity of which of the following DNA repair pathways might reduce the relative risk of cancers due to CT exposure?

A. Base excision repair

B. Homologous recombination repair

C. Mismatch excision repair

D. Nonhomologous end-joining repair

E. Nucleotide excision repair

16. You participated as an investigator in a clinical trial assessing a novel treatment for refractory small-cell lung cancer. The trial employed a single agent, a specific inhibitor of the enzyme poly (ADP-ribose) polymerase-1 (PARP-1). This agent was found to be highly effective in breast cancers that had defects in homologous recombination DNA repair pathways. After analyzing the data from the study, you and your coinvestigators concluded that the drug was minimally effective in shrinking tumor mass. Which of the following anti–breast cancer mechanisms of PARP-1 inhibition might explain the minimal effects of the drug on refractory small-cell lung cancer in your trials?

A. PARP-1 inhibitors are effective due to direct blockade of homologous recombination repair

B. PARP-1 inhibitors are effective due to blocking nucleotide excision repair

C. PARP-1 inhibitors are effective due to increased DNA methylation

D. PARP-1 inhibitors are effective due to increased double-strand DNA breaks

E. PARP-1 inhibitors are effective due to loss of cell cycle checkpoint controls

17. A 5-year-old boy, recently referred to a pediatric neuromuscular clinic at an academic medical center, presents with a chief complaint of difficulty standing. The child's family has no history of neuromuscular disease. He walked independently at 1 year of age, and his mother reported no motor defects prior to age 3, when he began to complain of pain in the lower legs accompanied by transient muscle weakness that persisted for about 1 week and resolved spontaneously. At that time, his serum creatinine kinase (CK) was found to be 3,200 IU/L (normal < 175 IU/L). A repetition of transient muscle weakness and leg pain precipitated his current referral to your clinic. On physical examination you observe no Gower's sign or pseudohypertrophy of the legs. However, an electromyogram disclosed myogenic changes. As part of your investigation, a quadriceps muscle biopsy was performed for histological and immunochemical analysis. It was determined that the boy's dystrophin protein lacked 60 amino acids at its C-terminus but was otherwise identical to the wild-type protein (total length of dystrophin is 3,684 amino acids). Which of the following categories of mutations might be responsible for the boy's truncated dystrophin protein?

A. Frameshift

B. Missense

C. Nonsense

D. Silent

E. Synonymous

14.2 Answers and Explanations

Easy	Medium	Hard

1. Correct: D. Nonhomologous end-joining repair.

The patient has chronic myelogenous leukemia featuring the characteristic translocation between chromosomes 9 and 22 (the "Philadelphia chromosome"). Ionizing radiation, which can be released from the nuclear power plant accident, causes DNA strand breaks. Repair by nonhomologous end joining (sometimes referred to as "error-prone" repair) can result in chromosomal translocations when two nonrelated DNA strands are joined together. The translocation driving his leukemia is almost certainly the result of this process.

A is incorrect. Base excision repair (BER) fixes single-base mismatches and lesions that do not distort the DNA double helix. BER cannot produce chromosomal translocations.

B is incorrect. While the double-strand breaks can be repaired by homologous recombination repair, the mechanism is high fidelity and very unlikely to produce chromosomal translocations.

C is incorrect. Mismatch excision repair addresses mismatched base pairs and cannot produce chromosomal translocations.

E is incorrect. Nucleotide excision repair fixes helix-distorting lesions such as larger DNA chemical adducts and cannot produce chromosomal translocations.

2. Correct: B. Ionizing radiation causes primarily double-strand breaks.

Hereditary nonpolyposis colorectal cancer/Lynch syndrome is an autosomal recessive disease caused by gene mutations that lead to the loss of proteins required for nucleotide mismatch repair. Ionizing radiation from medical imaging causes a range of DNA damage (primarily double-stranded DNA breaks) which are repaired by mechanisms other than mismatch repair.

A is incorrect. Although it is true that DNA adducts are fixed primarily by nucleotide excision repair, these lesions are not caused by X-rays.

C is incorrect. Lynch syndrome is a defect in mismatch repair, not a defect in DNA replication.

D is incorrect. While the statement may be true, it does not address the patient's specific concern and therefore is not a justification for the advice given to her.

E is incorrect. Though it is true that ultraviolet radiation causes primarily thymidine dimers, medical X-rays do not produce ultraviolet light.

3. Correct: D. Nucleotide excision repair.

The DNA helix is heavily distorted by the DNA adduct resulting from the reaction with the cross-linking chemotherapeutic agent with one strand of the DNA in the double helix. Lesions that distort the DNA helix are repaired by nucleotide excision repair.

A is incorrect. Homologous recombination repair fixes double-strand breaks and interstrand cross-links. The DNA lesion shown in the figure in Question 3, resulting from the reaction with the cross-linking chemotherapeutic agent, is neither of these.

B is incorrect. DNA polymerase epsilon (and delta) has 3′ to 5′ exonuclease activity to remove misincorporated nucleotides (proofreading). This activity will not repair the DNA lesion resulting from the reaction with the cross-linking chemotherapeutic agent.

C is incorrect. The DNA lesion resulting from the reaction with the cross-linking chemotherapeutic agent is an intrastrand cross-link (involves only one strand of the double helix), not a nucleotide mismatch, so mismatch repair mechanisms will not fix this lesion.

E is incorrect. Nonhomologous end-joining fixes lesions similar to those repaired by homologous recombination repair.

4. Correct: E. Nonhomologous end joining.

Ionizing radiation produces primarily double-strand breaks in DNA, which can be repaired by two different mechanisms: homologous recombination repair (HRR) or nonhomologous end-joining (NHEJ) repair (see the figure below). The two copies of a given gene must be in proximity for homologous recombination repair to fix double-strand breaks. This close proximity only occurs during S and G2 phases of the cell cycle. Since the vast majority of neurons are postmitotic (i.e., no longer dividing), opportunity for repair by homologous recombination is limited. As such, most repair of double-strand breaks in this scenario will be via the mechanism of NHEJ which has the drawback that it can join "random" ends, possibly creating mutations.

A is incorrect. BER fixes single-base mismatches and lesions that do not distort the DNA double helix. BER cannot repair double-stranded breaks.

B is incorrect. The two copies of a given gene must be in proximity for homologous recombination repair to fix double-strand breaks. This close proximity only occurs during S and G2 phases of the cell cycle. Since the vast majority of neurons are postmitotic (i.e., no longer dividing), opportunity for repair by homologous recombination is limited. As such, double-stranded breaks in the affected neurons are repaired solely by nonhomologous end joining.

C is incorrect. Mismatch excision repair addresses mismatched base pairs and cannot repair double-stranded breaks.

D is incorrect. Nucleotide excision repair fixes helix-distorting lesions such as larger DNA chemical adducts and cannot repair double-stranded breaks.

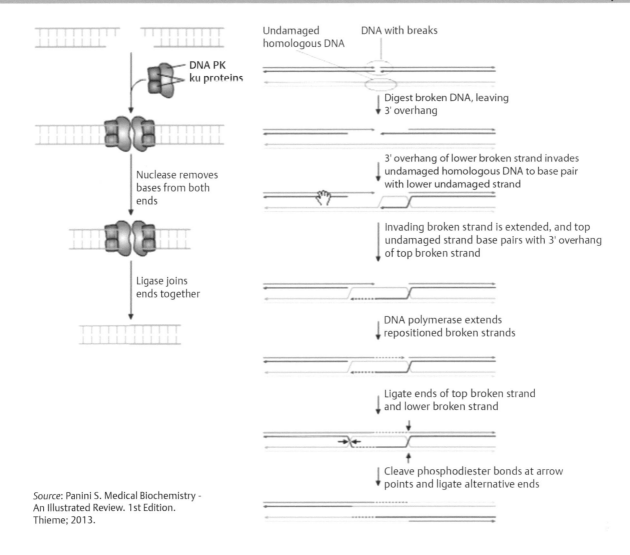

DNA PK
ku proteins

Nuclease removes
bases from both
ends

Ligase joins
ends together

Undamaged
homologous DNA

DNA with breaks

Digest broken DNA, leaving
3' overhang

3' overhang of lower broken strand invades
undamaged homologous DNA to base pair
with lower undamaged strand

Invading broken strand is extended, and top
undamaged strand base pairs with 3' overhang
of top broken strand

DNA polymerase extends
repositioned broken strands

Ligate ends of top broken strand
and lower broken strand

Cleave phosphodiester bonds at arrow
points and ligate alternative ends

Source: Panini S. Medical Biochemistry -
An Illustrated Review. 1st Edition.
Thieme; 2013.

5. Correct: B. 3' to 5' exonuclease activity of DNA polymerase epsilon.

If DNA polymerase inserts an incorrect nucleotide, pauses then "backs up" degrading the newly synthesized strand with a 3′ to 5′ exonuclease activity (proofreading). The polymerase then synthesizes new DNA to replace the DNA it just degraded, almost certainly inserting the correct nucleotide the second time around.

A is incorrect. BER can fix single-base mismatches, however, it is not the first mechanism, which is the proofreading activity of the polymerase.

C is incorrect. Homologous recombination repair fixes double-strand breaks and interstrand cross-links.

D is incorrect. Nucleotide excision repair fixes helix-distorting lesions such as larger DNA chemical adducts.

E is incorrect. Mismatch excision repair addresses mismatched base pairs and cannot repair double-stranded breaks.

6. Correct: C. Production of a truncated, nonfunctional protein.

A frameshift mutation results when a gene suffers the deletion or insertion of nucleotides that is not a multiple of three within the reading frame of the protein. The reading frame is altered by a frameshift such that random amino acids are inserted into the protein following the site of the mutation and often, shortly after the frameshift, a premature termination codon is encountered (see the figure on the next page). In either case, the protein is likely to be truncated and/or misfolded. Nonsense-mediated decay (NMD) is a mechanism that evolved specifically to prevent the production of truncated proteins from mRNAs with premature termination codons due to mutation or splice error. NMD occurs during the first round of translation, when protein complexes are still present on the exon–intron junctions of the newly synthesized and spliced mRNA. If a premature termination codon is further than about 50 nucleotides upstream of any exon–junction complexes,

CTC	CCG	TGT	CAA	CCT	GGT	GAG	CCG	CCC	CGA
LEU	PRO	CYS	GLN	PRO	GLY	GLU	PRO	PRO	ARG

CTC	CCG	TGT	CAA	CGG	TGA	GCC	GCC	CCG	A
LEU	PRO	CYS	GLN	ARG	*				

then the transcript is targeted for degradation by NMD. The net result is the loss of the active form of the protein from the cell.

A is incorrect. Based on the explanation above, a single-nucleotide deletion will not produce elevated protein levels.

B is incorrect. The alteration in the reading frame will result in multiple amino acid substitutions and most likely a termination codon shortly after the deletion. The mutation described cannot result in a single amino acid substitution.

D is incorrect. While the deletion may result in reduced levels of the mRNA by the mechanisms of NMD, it is nearly impossible that mRNA levels would be increased. NMD is a mechanism that evolved specifically to prevent the production of truncated proteins from mRNAs with premature termination codons due to mutation or splice error. NMD occurs during the first round of translation, when protein complexes are still present on the exon–intron junctions of the newly synthesized and spliced mRNA. If a premature termination codon is further than about 50 nucleotides upstream of any exon–junction complexes, then the transcript is targeted for degradation by NMD.

E is incorrect. Since termination of gene transcription by RNA polymerases is signaled by a multiple nucleotide sequence on the gene, a two-nucleotide deletion is highly unlikely to prevent termination and result in an elongated transcript.

7.   Correct: C. Fanconi's anemia.

Fanconi's anemia is an autosomal recessive double-stranded DNA break repair deficiency. Loss of functional gene product from any one of 15 different genes can lead to defective double-stranded DNA break repair. Bone marrow failure is the defining feature of Fanconi's anemia, as is elevated risk for leukemias.

A is incorrect. A-T is an autosomal recessive disorder resulting from mutation of the *ATM* gene. ATM protein is a kinase that coordinates the cellular response to double-stranded DNA breaks, including cell cycle arrest. A-T is characterized primarily by neurologic deficits.

B is incorrect. Cockayne's syndrome is an autosomal recessive disorder, caused by loss of functional *ERCC6* or *ERCC8* genes which are involved in transcription-coupled repair of DNA. Cockayne's syndrome is characterized by developmental and

neurologic delay, photosensitivity, progeria, hearing loss, and eye abnormalities.

D is incorrect. Lynch syndrome (also known as hereditary nonpolyposis colon cancer [HNPCC]) is an autosomal recessive disease caused by gene mutations that lead to the loss of proteins required for nucleotide mismatch repair. The primary outcome is significantly elevated risks for colon and other cancers.

E is incorrect. XP is an autosomal recessive disorder that results in loss of nucleotide excision repair. Homozygous mutation in any one of eight different genes can cause XP. The most characteristic feature of XP is significant increases in mutations in sun-exposed skin which leads to significant pigmentation changes and extremely elevated rates of basal cell carcinomas and other skin cancers.

8.   Correct: D. Pyrimidine dimers.

Given the location on her face, it is likely that exposure to ultraviolet (UV) light from the sun was the driver of mutations in her DNA that eventually led to her melanoma. Among the most common DNA mutations caused by UV light are pyrimidine dimers that are repaired by the nucleotide excision repair pathway.

A is incorrect. DNA adducts are typically the result of modification of the DNA molecule by chemically reactive agents.

B is incorrect. While double-stranded breaks can be indirectly produced by sunlight (e.g., unrepaired pyrimidine dimers as well as reactive oxygen species produced by sunlight can cause breaks), the direct action of UV light on DNA typically does not cause these lesions to a significant extent.

C is incorrect. Interstrand cross-links typically are the result of reactive, bifunctional chemicals with the DNA molecule. Some such agents are used as cancer chemotherapeutic agents (e.g., cisplatin).

E is incorrect. While single-stranded breaks can be indirectly produced by sunlight (e.g., unrepaired pyrimidine dimers as well as reactive oxygen species produced by sunlight can cause breaks), the direct action of UV light on DNA typically does not cause these lesions to a significant extent.

9.   Correct: D. Generation of DNA adducts.

Cigarette smoke contains thousands of carcinogenic chemicals, many of which, such as benzopyrene, react chemically with DNA, forming DNA adducts.

These adducts, if not repaired, can result in nucleotide sequence mutations. If these mutations alter proto-oncogenes (gain of function) or tumor suppressor genes (loss of function), it can lead to lung cancers such as the suspected bronchogenic carcinoma visible in the patient's radiograph.

A is incorrect. While CO from cigarette smoke binds to hemoglobin and is damaging to the patient's health, it is unlikely a direct contributor to his suspected cancer.

B is incorrect. While nicotine in cigarette smoke does increase sympathetic neurotransmission due to activation of postganglionic nicotinic receptors, it is unlikely a direct contributor to his suspected cancer.

C is incorrect. While cigarette smoking does increase levels of plasma fibrinogen and elevate the risk of thrombosis, it is unlikely a direct contributor to his suspected cancer.

E is incorrect. While cigarette smoking does reduce taste sensation and suppress appetite, which could contribute to poor nutrition, these effects are unlikely to be direct contributors to his suspected cancer.

10. Correct: B. Homologous recombination DNA repair.

BRCA1 and *BRCA2*, the genes associated with elevated breast and ovarian cancer risk, are involved in homologous recombination DNA repair pathways. These two proteins are recruited to DNA ends resulting from the break and facilitate the loading of protein factors that mediate recombination repair. Approximately 0.1% of men and women have inherited a mutation in one of their *BRCA1* or *BRCA2* genes; over time, mutation of the second, normal allele can lead to increased rate of DNA mutation and risk of the cell undergoing conversion to cancer.

A is incorrect. BER fixes single-base mismatches and nondistorting alterations. There are no known congenital defects in this pathway.

C is incorrect. Mismatch repair fixes mismatches in daughter strands, typically the result of misincorporation during DNA synthesis. Defects in this pathway are associated with hereditary nonpolyposis colorectal cancers/Lynch syndrome, which has elevated risk of colorectal and endometrial cancer, but not specifically ovarian or breast cancer.

D is incorrect. Nonhomologous end-joining repairs double-stranded breaks by joining ends haphazardly. These can sometimes result in disease-causing chromosomal translocations. There are no known congenital defects in this pathway.

E is incorrect. Nucleotide excision repair fixes chemical adducts that distort DNA. Defects in this pathway cause XP, which has significantly elevated risk of cancers of the skin, particularly in regions exposed to sunlight.

11. Correct: E. Nucleotide excision repair.

Nucleotide excision repair fixes chemical adducts that distort DNA, including pyrimidine dimers that form in response to UV light exposure. Defects in this pathway cause the disease *xeroderma pigmentosum*, which has significantly elevated risk of cancers of the skin, particularly in regions exposed to sunlight. The inability to repair these defects leads to the increased death of the patient's cells following UV light exposure, in comparison to his mother's normal cells.

A is incorrect. BER fixes single-base mismatches and nondistorting alterations. There are no known congenital defects in this pathway.

B is incorrect. Defects in homologous recombination DNA repair are associated with elevated risk of specific cancers and Fanconi's anemia.

C is incorrect. Mismatch repair fixes mismatches in daughter strands, typically the result of misincorporation during DNA synthesis. Defects in this pathway are associated with hereditary nonpolyposis colorectal cancers/Lynch syndrome, which has elevated risk of colorectal and endometrial cancer, but not specifically ovarian or breast cancer.

D is incorrect. Nonhomologous end-joining repairs double-stranded breaks by joining ends haphazardly. These can sometimes result in disease-causing chromosomal translocations. There are no known congenital defects in this pathway.

12. Correct: B. Missense.

Missense mutations within the open reading frame of a gene result in the substitution of one amino acid for another. In this case, the guanine to thymidine transversion mutation at position two of the codon coding for glycine (GLY) changed it to a codon coding for valine (VAL). This specific mutation is, in fact, commonly found in bladder cancers.

A is incorrect. A frameshift mutation results when a gene suffers the deletion or insertion of nucleotides, within the protein reading frame, that is not a multiple of three nucleotides. The reading frame is altered by a frameshift such that random amino acids are inserted into the protein following the site of the mutation and often, shortly after the frameshift, a premature termination codon is encountered.

C is incorrect. A nonsense mutation is a change in nucleotide sequence that converts a codon that codes for an amino acid into one of the three translational termination codons. Such a mutation would result in a truncated protein.

D is incorrect. A silent mutation is a change in nucleotide sequence that does not alter the amino acid specified. Because of the degenerating nature of the genetic code, a given amino acid may be specified by multiple codons. Most typically, the variation is in the third nucleotide of the codon. For example, leucine is encoded by CTA, CTG, CTT, and CCC. In the figure in Question 12 the sixth codon is CTG which encodes leucine. If this was mutated to CTT, it would still encode leucine and would be a silent mutation.

E is incorrect. A synonymous mutation is the same as a silent mutation.

13.   Correct: A. Base excision repair.

Base excision repair fixes single-base mismatches and small, nondistorting alterations such as results from methylation of single nucleotides. The mechanism of base excision repair is outlined in the figure on the right.

B is incorrect. Homologous recombination repair fixes double-strand breaks and interstrand cross-links. It does not repair small adducts such as the methylation of nucleotides by DMS.

C is incorrect. Mismatch repair fixes mismatches in daughter strands, typically the result of misincorporation during DNA synthesis.

D is incorrect. Nonhomologous end-joining repairs double-stranded breaks by joining ends haphazardly.

E is incorrect. Nucleotide excision repair fixes large chemical adducts that distort DNA, including pyrimidine dimers that form in response to UV light exposure. Small modifications such as methylation are typically recognized and repaired by base excision repair.

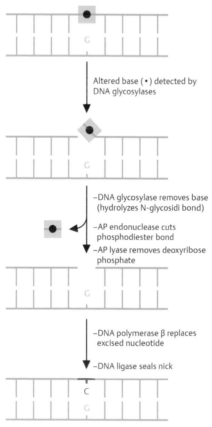

Altered base (•) detected by DNA glycosylases

–DNA glycosylase removes base (hydrolyzes N-glycosidi bond)

–AP endonuclease cuts phosphodiester bond

–AP lyase removes deoxyribose phosphate

–DNA polymerase β replaces excised nucleotide

–DNA ligase seals nick

Source: Panini S. Medical Biochemistry - An Illustrated Review. 1st Edition. Thieme; 2013.

14.   Correct: D. Lynch syndrome/hereditary nonpolyposis colon cancer.

The 3'→5'exonuclease activity of DNA polymerase is an important mechanism by which misincorporation of nucleotides during DNA synthesis is repaired. Since the drug would inhibit this activity (though less than in yeast), it would result in some of the misincorporated nucleotides not being immediately repaired. This would produce "mismatches" between the parental and daughter strands of DNA. Lynch syndrome/hereditary nonpolyposis colorectal cancer is an autosomal recessive disease caused by gene mutations that lead to the loss of proteins required for nucleotide mismatch repair. These individuals would be particularly unsuited to receive the investigational drug in a clinical trial.

A is incorrect. A-T is an autosomal recessive disorder resulting from mutation of the *ATM* gene. ATM protein is a kinase that coordinates the cellular response to double-stranded DNA breaks, including cell cycle arrest. The potentially increased number of misincorporated nucleotides due to treatment with the drug that inhibits the 3'→5' exonuclease activity of DNA polymerase would mostly be repaired by mismatch repair mechanisms, would unlikely increase the number of double-stranded breaks. Therefore, people with A-T would not be at particular risk from taking the drug.

B is incorrect. BRCA1 and BRCA2 proteins are involved in homologous recombination repair of double-stranded DNA breaks. The potentially increased number of misincorporated nucleotides due to treatment with the drug that inhibits the 3'→5' exonuclease activity of DNA polymerase would mostly be repaired by mismatch repair mechanisms and would unlikely increase the number of double-stranded breaks. Therefore, people with defective homologous recombination repair would not be at particular risk from taking the drug.

C is incorrect. Fanconi's anemia is an autosomal recessive double-stranded DNA break repair deficiency. Loss of functional gene product from any one of 15 different genes can lead to defective double-stranded DNA break repair. The potentially increased number of misincorporated nucleotides due to treatment with the drug that inhibits the 3'→5'exonuclease activity of DNA polymerase would mostly be repaired by mismatch repair mechanisms and would unlikely increase the number of double-stranded breaks. Therefore, people with Fanconi's anemia would not be at particular risk from taking the drug.

E is incorrect. XP is an autosomal recessive disorder that results in loss of nucleotide excision repair. Nucleotide excision repair fixes helix-distorting lesions such as larger DNA chemical adducts, none of which would be increased by inhibiting the 3'→5' exonuclease activity of DNA polymerase.

15. Correct: B. Homologous recombination repair.

CT involves larger doses of ionizing radiation than conventional X-ray imaging. In tissues exposed to X-rays, hydroxyl radicals (generated from X-ray interacting with water) can damage DNA bases and cause strand breaks. X-rays also damage DNA directly with double-stranded breaks being the most serious in terms of correctly repairing the breaks. Incorrectly repaired double-stranded breaks can lead to a range of mutations, including oncogenic chromosomal translocations. The repair mechanism will most likely correctly repair double-stranded breaks, and avoid mutations, is homologous recombination repair (HRR). In HRR, undamaged DNA of the homologous chromosome is used as a template in a multistep process, to carry out repair of the double-stranded break. In this mechanism, any missing DNA is replaced and the joining of correct ends is ensured. On the whole, boosting HRR would improve the odds of effective repair of the DNA damage that is most likely to increase cancer risk.

A is incorrect. BER can fix some of the types of DNA damage generated by ionizing radiation, such as small modifications of DNA bases. However, BER cannot fix double-stranded breaks which are more dangerous in terms of cancer risk.

C is incorrect. Mismatch repair (MMR) can fix some of the types of DNA damage generated by ionizing radiation, such as small modifications of DNA bases that disrupt correct base pairing. However, MMR cannot fix double-stranded breaks which are more dangerous in terms of cancer risk.

D is incorrect. NHEJ is sometimes referred to as "error-prone" repair. This is due to the fact that NHEJ has no mechanism to ensure that correct ends are joined together. In addition, DNA deletions can result from the removal of single-stranded DNA overhangs during the NHEJ process. Homologous recombination repair of double-stranded breaks is far less likely to lead to cancer-associated mutations and chromosomal translocations.

E is incorrect. Nucleotide excision repair (NER) can fix some of the types of DNA damage generated by ionizing radiation, such as large, deforming modifications of DNA bases. However, NER cannot fix double-stranded breaks which are more dangerous in terms of cancer risk.

16. Correct: D. PARP-1 inhibitors are effective due to increased double-strand DNA breaks.

The enzyme PARP-1 is involved in detecting single-stranded breaks, those generated directly by DNA damaging agents (chemical and physical) and those resulting from the process of BER. PARP-1 binds to these breaks and adds polymers of ADP-ribose to itself and nearby nuclear proteins, primarily nucleosome proteins associated with the DNA. This ADP-ribosylation serves as a "beacon" of sorts to recruit the necessary repair machinery to fix the break in the DNA. However, when PARP-1 is inhibited, the single-stranded breaks are not repaired which often leads to double-stranded breaks at these sites. Because of this, PARP-1 inhibitors are particularly useful in the treatment of cancers that have mutations that disable the homologous DNA repair pathway. In such cells, double-strand DNA breaks are repaired by the "error-prone" NHEJ pathway. The accumulation of extensive double-strand breaks repaired by this NHEJ pathway ultimately results in death of the cell.

A is incorrect. While ADP-ribosylation at double-strand breaks by PARP-1 also occurs, inhibition of PARP-1 does not directly inhibit homologous recombination repair mechanisms.

B is incorrect. Inhibition of PARP-1 does not inhibit nucleotide excision repair.

C is incorrect. The PARP-1 enzyme does not affect DNA methylation and therefore PARP-1 inhibitors will not alter this modification.

E is incorrect. PARP-1 inhibition could have a distal effect on cell cycle checkpoints, by leading to increased DNA damage. However, this effect is indirect and not the best answer to the question.

17. Correct: C. Nonsense.

A nonsense mutation is a change in nucleotide sequence that converts a codon that codes for an amino acid into one of the three translational termination codons. Such a mutation would result in a truncated protein. NMD is a mechanism that evolved specifically to prevent the production of truncated proteins from mRNAs with premature termination codons due to mutation or splice error. NMD occurs during the first round of translation, when protein complexes are still present on the exon–intron junctions of the newly synthesized and spliced mRNA. If a premature termination codon is further than about 50 nucleotides upstream of any exon–junction complexes, then the transcript is targeted for degradation by NMD. However, this particular nonsense mutation is located so close to the normal termination codon that NMD is not an issue. This specific small truncation of dystrophin must result in relatively modest defect in the protein's function, producing a milder clinical phenotype.

A is incorrect. A frameshift mutation occurs when a gene suffers the deletion or insertion of nucleotides, within the protein reading frame, that is not a multiple of three nucleotides. The reading frame is altered by a frameshift such that random amino acids are inserted into the protein following the site of the mutation and often, shortly after the frameshift, a premature termination codon is encountered. Given that the patient's dystrophin protein was otherwise identical, a frameshift could be ruled out.

247

B is incorrect. Missense mutations within the open reading frame of a gene result in the substitution of one amino acid for another. This is not the case for the patient's dystrophin.

D is incorrect. A silent mutation is a change in nucleotide sequence that does not alter the amino acid specified. This is not the case for the patient's dystrophin.

E is incorrect. A synonymous mutation is the same as a silent mutation.

Chapter 15

Gene Transcription and RNA Processing

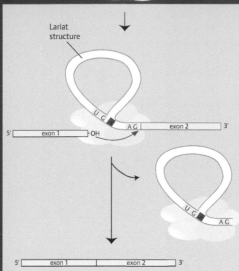

LEARNING OBJECTIVES

▶ Explain how cis-elements and trans-acting factors regulate gene transcription.

▶ Outline the biochemical steps to activate transcription of a currently silent gene.

▶ Describe how a transcription factor can be controlled by cellular signaling events and explain how defects (resulting from mutations) in signaling pathways can alter transcription factor function.

▶ Describe the roles of DNA methylation and histone modifications in regulating gene transcription.

▶ List the different functional domains of a transcriptional regulatory factor and describe how they contribute to gene regulation.

▶ Describe the biochemical nature and functional role of modifications to the 5' and 3' ends of messenger RNA (mRNA) in humans.

▶ List the types of RNA processing in human cells and describe the role of these processing events in gene expression, including production of protein isoforms.

▶ Propose mechanisms by which a single-nucleotide mutation can result in the loss of protein synthesis from an mRNA.

▶ List the basic steps and molecular components of mRNA splicing.

15.1 Questions

Easy   Medium   Hard

1. A newborn baby dies 3 days postpartum and upon autopsy cardiac malformations are observed. After reviewing the literature, you find that the baby's clinical course and postmortem findings are consistent with those described for children born with mutations in the *NKX2-5* gene. *NKX2-5* codes for a transcriptional regulatory protein involved in cardiac-specific gene regulation. You acquire the proper permissions and acquire some of the baby's tissues for analysis. As part of a research project, genetic tests indicate the baby's *NKX2-5* genes had no mutations in the protein coding sequences though the NKX2-5 mRNA was almost undetectable. Which of the following could explain the baby's pathology with respect to NKX2-5?

A. The NKX2-5 proteins were unable to bind histone deacetylase enzymes

B. The *NKX2-5* gene had a mutation in an associated transcriptional enhancer

C. The NKX2-5 proteins lacked a DNA-binding domain

D. The *NKX2-5* gene promoter was hypomethylated

2. Probands in a large family showing isolated atrial septal defects were found to have a heterozygous missense mutation in transcription factor GATA4. The mutant GATA4 protein bound DNA as effectively as the wild-type protein. However, it was observed that the mutant GATA4 protein was unable to bind to and recruit a specific protein to promoters of its target genes. Which of the following most likely represents the activity of the specific protein that GATA4 was unable to bind to and recruit to target gene promoters?

A. DNA methyltransferase

B. DNA polymerase

C. Histone acetyltransferase

D. Histone deacetylase

E. RNA polymerase

3. In all human cells, the *KLF6* gene produces multiple forms of the KLF6 protein. High levels of one specific version of the KLF6 protein, but not others, is associated with more clinically aggressive forms of epithelial ovarian cancer. Which of the following mechanisms is most likely responsible for the production of the multiple versions of the KLF6 protein?

A. Alternative splicing of KLF6 pre-mRNA

B. Increased activity of the *KLF* gene promoter

C. Regulation of KLF6 by microRNA

D. Rearrangement of the *KLF6* gene

E. Reduced activity of a transcriptional enhancer associated with the *KLF6* gene

4. The rare hereditary syndrome immune dysfunction, polyendocrinopathy, enteropathy, X-linked (IPEX) is caused by mutations in the *FOXP3* gene, which codes for a transcription factor. The *FOXP3* gene has multiple exons, all of which contain protein coding information. The figure below shows exons (*blue boxes*) and introns (*blue line*) of the human *FOXP3* gene. One particular family with a high incidence of IPEX has a curious biochemical phenotype. Affected family members have extremely low levels of normal FOXP3 protein, rather than the complete absence of the protein as normally observed in IPEX. Genetic analysis indicated one of their *FOXP3* genes was completely deleted. The remaining *FOXP3* gene had a normal protein coding sequence and was responsible for the very low levels of FOXP3 protein detected. However, analysis revealed that the mRNA transcribed from this gene has an extension of the 3' end of approximately 3,000 nucleotides, in comparison to the wild-type mRNA. The mutant mRNA was very unstable and poorly translated. A mutation in which of the following functional sequences might account for these observations?

A. Kozak sequence

B. Origin of replication

C. Polyadenylation signal sequence

D. Transcriptional silencer

E. Transcriptional enhancer

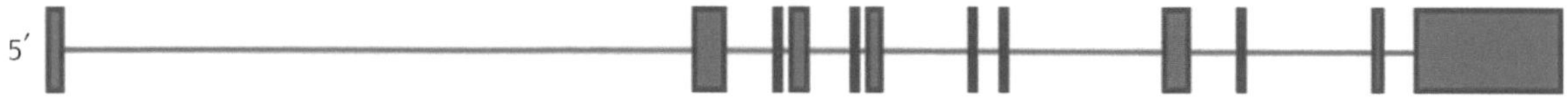

5. The nonstructural 1A (NS1A) protein, encoded by the genome of all strains of the influenza A virus, is required for productive infection by the virus. It was discovered that NS1A interacts with and inhibits the human protein CPSF30, a factor that binds the polyadenylation signal in pre-mRNAs and is required for polyadenylation of newly synthesized mRNA. Which of the following likely occurs in pulmonary epithelial cells infected by the influenza A virus?

A. An increase in proteins containing amino acid substitutions

B. A reduction in cellular protein synthesis

C. An increase in nonsense-mediated decay (NMD)

D. A reduction in new ribosome synthesis due to reduced ribosomal RNA (rRNA) synthesis

E. Excessive viral mRNA polyadenylation

6. A 41-year-old female patient presents with a chief complaint of "itchy, red ear lobes." She tells you that the problem started after she wore a new pair of earrings for an entire day, 3 days ago and has not improved, and in fact seems to have gotten worse which precipitated her visit. Physical examination reveals erythema and scaling with relatively well-demarcated, visible borders on both earlobes (see the figure below). You prescribe 0.1% triamcinolone (a glucocorticoid) cream to apply to affected areas. Which of the following biochemical events are occurring within subcutaneous immune cells in response to this drug?

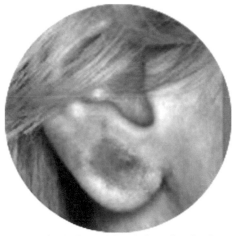

Source: Röcken M, Grevers G, Burgdorf W. Color Atlas of Allergic Diseases. 1st Edition. 2003.

A. Increased binding of RNA polymerase II to promoters of genes coding for inflammatory cytokines

B. Increased retention of glucocorticoid receptor protein in the cytoplasm

C. Reduced acetylation of nucleosomes associated with promoters of genes coding for inflammatory cytokines

D. Translocation of nuclear factor kappa B (NF-κB) to the nucleus and increased occupancy of promoters associated with genes coding for inflammatory cytokines

7. A 77-year-old woman presents in your clinic with a chief complaint of itchy, raised plaques on her chest of 3-month duration. These lesions were previously diagnosed as eczema. Since the plaque have not responded to treatment, you perform a skin biopsy which leads to a diagnosis of mycosis fungoides. Her treatment regimen includes vorinostat (Zolinza), an inhibitor of histone deacetylase enzymes. Which of the following synthetic processes is the most direct target of vorinostat on gene expression?

A. Gene transcription

B. mRNA splicing

C. mRNA export

D. mRNA polyadenylation

E. Protein translation

8. A 57-year-old female patient was brought to the emergency department by her husband with a chief complaint of weakness, nausea, vomiting, and diarrhea of 24 hours duration. Her temperature was normal. During your interview, she revealed that 36 hours earlier, she ate a salad into which she had cut up wild mushrooms. Her husband had not eaten the salad and went home to retrieve the uneaten portion. A tentative identification of the mushroom slices as *Amanita phalloides* was made. Chief among the toxins in this mushroom is the compound alpha-amanitin. She was admitted to the hospital and supporting measures begun. Over a 96-hour period, her serum aspartate aminotransferase (AST), alanine aminotransferase (ALT), and lactate dehydrogenase (LDH) continued to increase far above normal range and 4 days after admission she expired from cardiac arrest. Synthesis of which of the following biological polymers was primarily inhibited shortly after she ate the mushrooms, while the concentration of alpha-amanitin in her blood was relatively low?

A. DNA

B. mRNA

C. rRNA

D. tRNA

E. Mitochondrial RNA

9. A recent report linked a common, minor allele of the mucin 5B (*MUC5B*) gene, a single-nucleotide polymorphism (SNP) located 3-kb upstream of the *MUC5B* transcription start site, to elevated risk for familial interstitial pneumonia and idiopathic pulmonary fibrosis. With respect to *MUC5B* gene expression, which of the following could be altered in patients with the minor allele that might contribute to their disease?

A. Amino acid sequence of the MUC5B protein

B. Quantity of MUC5B mRNA

C. Polyadenylation site of the MUC5B mRNA

D. Ribosome binding of the MUC5B mRNA

E. Splicing of the MUC5B mRNA

10. A male baby, 49 days postpartum, was brought to your outpatient clinic by his parents with a chief complaint of inactivity and poor suckling of 2 weeks duration. The child had a birth weight 3.21 kg at 40 weeks of gestational age and was the first child of nonconsanguineous parents. Family history was unremarkable. The child looked alert but displayed hypotonic posture. He was sent home with monitoring and at 4 months, the child was brought to the emergency department (ED) with distressed respiration, resulting in him being admitted. His respiration continued to deteriorate resulting in him being placed on mechanical ventilation. Thorough workup revealed a genetic mutation in the gene survival of motor neuron (*SMN1*) which encodes a protein involved in the genesis of small nuclear ribonucleoproteins (snRNPs). Analysis of the RNA content of this child's motor neurons would reveal which of the following global changes in comparison to motor neurons from an unaffected child?

A. Elevated incidence of mRNAs lacking 7-methyl-guanosine cap

B. Fewer mRNAs engaged with ribosomes.

C. Increased levels of tRNAs

D. Qualitative and quantitative changes in mRNA splicing

E. Reduced levels of specific mRNAs

11. A genetic study to identify loci that increases susceptibility to type II diabetes, isolated an SNP in the fourth intron of the 17-exon gene *TCF7L2*. This gene produces a protein involved in regulating T-lymphocyte function. Examination of the molecular effect of the SNP in the fourth intron demonstrated that in addition to the full-length TCF7L2 transcript, a shorter transcript, truncated on the 3' end in comparison to the full-length transcript, was present in cells with the SNP. The truncated transcript ends not far from the location of the SNP. Which of the following was created by the SNP in the fourth intron that would explain why the SNP results in the production of a truncated transcript of TCF7L2?

A. A new exon–intron boundary (splice donor or acceptor site)

B. A new polyadenylation signal

C. A new translational initiation codon

D. A new transcriptional promoter

E. A new transcriptional regulatory protein binding site

12. A very common observation in multiple cancer types is the overexpression of the *MYC* gene. Analysis of the mechanism by which myc protein, which is a transcription factor, contributes to carcinogenesis revealed that with elevated levels of myc protein, there is an observable increase in the rate of transcriptional initiation, and mRNA levels, of essentially all expressed genes within the cell. Based on these observations, which of the following gene regulatory elements is most likely to be acted upon by the myc protein?

A. Enhancers

B. Polyadenylation sites

C. Promoters

D. Silencers

E. Splice sites

13. There is much enthusiasm about the prospects of induced pluripotent stem cells (iPSCs) as a way to repair or restore damaged, critical organs. One way to make patient-specific iPSCs is to acquire and culture fibroblasts from a patient and introduce four specific transcription factors into the cells. Following specific culturing techniques, the formally differentiated cells regain their pluripotent phenotype and can be induced to differentiate into essentially any cell type. Which of the following is one of the events that must be occurring to facilitate this remarkable conversion by the action of the four transcription factors?

A. A global increase in histone acetylation

B. Activating transcription of genes involved in inducing cell cycle arrest

C. Binding of the four iPSC transcription factors splice sites on pre-mRNAs

D. Reduction in DNA methylation at genes necessary for the pluripotent phenotype

E. Repressing transcription of genes necessary for DNA synthesis

14. Five days after a surgical procedure to remove a bone spur on his left medial malleolus, a 37-year-old male patient noted increased swelling and erythema around the site of surgical incision. He was able to make an appointment with his primary care provider the same day, where his oral temperature was 37.8°C. The patient was directed to hospital where he was admitted and started on broad-spectrum antibiotics. Cells at the site of the infection responded by rapidly activating transcription of genes encoding inflammatory cytokines (e.g., interleukin-1β). Which of the following biochemical mechanisms are part of this response to the infection?

A. Increased methylation of promoter DNA of genes encoding inflammatory cytokines

B. Rapid proteolysis of histone proteins within nucleosomes on genes encoding inflammatory cytokines

C. Recruitment of histone deacetylase enzymes to genes encoding inflammatory cytokines

D. Synthesis of additional RNA polymerase II holoenzymes

E. Translocation of specific transcription factors to the nucleus

15. A phase I clinical trial was conducted with the drug flavoperidol, proposed for the treatment of acute myeloid leukemia (AML). It kills AML cells by inhibiting gene transcription. In the preclinical work leading to this trial, investigators found that in flavoperidol-treated cultured human AML cells, RNA polymerase II was bound to promoters of genes, but the polymerase complex was stalled, unable to initiate transcription. Which of the following mechanisms for flavoperidol would explain this observation regarding RNA polymerase II in flavoperidol-treated AML cells?

A. Flavoperidol inhibits a specific kinase

B. Flavoperidol inhibits acetylation of histones within nucleosomes at promoters

C. Flavoperidol inhibits binding of a specific transcription factor to an enhancer

D. Flavoperidol inhibits DNA methylation

E. Flavoperidol inhibits histone deacetylase enzymes

16. The reciprocal translocation t(12;21)(p13;q22) is the most common chromosomal rearrangement in childhood B-cell precursor acute lymphoblastic leukemia (ALL) with an incidence of approximately 25%. This translocation event results in the production of a fusion protein made up of portions of the protein coding sequences of the *RUNX1* and *ETV6* genes. Runx1 is an enhancer binding protein that binds DNA and activates transcription from associated promoters. It was observed that in patient B-cell precursor ALL cells grown in the laboratory, the RUNX1-ETV6 fusion protein was bound to enhancers that would be occupied by RUNX1 in normal B cells. However, the gene expression pattern between the ALL cells and normal cells was significantly different: genes normally activated by RUNX1 were not expressed in the ALL cells. With respect to the nature of the RUNX1-ETV6 fusion protein, which of the following would explain the observations regarding DNA binding and gene regulation by RUNX1-ETV6 in ALL?

A. The DNA binding domain of RUNX1 is not present in the RUNX1-ETV6 fusion

B. The histone deacetylase activity of RUNX1 is not present in the RUNX1-ETV6 fusion

C. The nuclear translocation signal of RUNX1 is not present in the RUNX1-ETV6 fusion

D. The RNA polymerase II binding domain of RUNX1 is not present in the RUNX1-ETV6 fusion

E. The transcriptional activation domain of RUNX1 is not present in the RUNX1-ETV6 fusion

17. A genome-wide association study was conducted to find genetic loci associated with increased susceptibility to endometriosis. Analysis of data sets for approximately 4,000 women who developed endometriosis and approximately 8,000 controls who did not revealed a significant association for an SNP at a specific locus on chromosome 1. Women with one copy of the risk SNP had a moderately elevated likelihood of having had endometriosis; those with two copies of the risk SNP had a significantly elevated likelihood of having had endometriosis. Analysis of gene expression in normal uterine tissue samples revealed that expression of the gene cell division control protein 42 (*CDC42*) correlated with the SNP as shown in the figure below. The *CDC42* gene is located approximately 50,000 base pairs from the SNP. The CDC42 mRNA length and nucleotide content was identical in all samples, regardless of SNP. Based on these data, the risk-associated SNP on chromosome 1 likely alters the function of which of the following genetic elements?

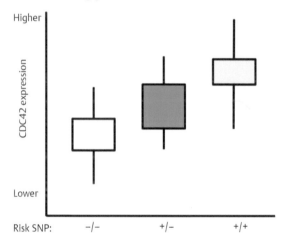

A. Kozak sequence

B. Origin of replication

C. Polyadenylation signal sequence

D. Promoter

E. Silencer

18. A patient presents in your office with a chief complain of red rash on her hands and around her nose and mouth, of 1-week duration. She reports that the rash began shortly after she began work at a print shop, where she is training as a press operator and is exposed to inks and solvents. Microscopic examination of a skin biopsy shows extensive lymphocyte infiltration (as shown in the figure below). You encourage the use of personal protective equipment while at work and prescribe an anti-inflammatory steroid ointment containing betamethasone to treat her rash. Two different versions of the protein receptor for betamethasone are produced from a single gene. Which of the following basic mechanisms is most likely directly responsible for the presence of two different steroid receptor proteins in cells?

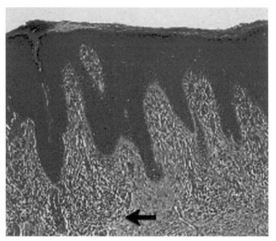

Source: Riede U, Werner M. Color Atlas of Pathology: Pathologic Principles · Associated Diseases · Sequela. 1st Edition. 2004.

A. Protein translation

B. RNA silencing

C. mRNA splicing

D. mRNA capping

E. DNA replication

19. A 23-year-old woman presents at the student health clinic at a large university complaining of intermittent abdominal cramps, diarrhea, and nausea after meals. The student has recently emigrated from Szechuan China to attend a graduate program in accounting. While taking her history, it is revealed that it is usually when eating at university functions where food is provided or at restaurants that the problems arise. Since it was her first time being outside of China, she attributed the symptoms to her system "adjusting" to Western food. Upon further questioning about the types of food she was eating prior to the episodes of gastrointestinal distress, you discover that the common factor is the presence of dairy products. She likely lacks that lactase-phlorizin hydrolase (LPH) enzyme in her gut epithelium brush border that breaks down the disaccharide lactose. Expression of this enzyme is normally downregulated once children reach the (historical) human weaning age of 3 to 5 years. Some human populations have evolved the ability to ingest milk as adults, without any gastrointestinal distress. An SNP, approximately 20,000 base pairs from the LPH gene itself, is associated with the persistence of LPH expression. The location of the SNP associated with LPH persistence into adulthood is most likely within which of the following genetic elements associated?

A. Kozak sequence
B. Polyadenylation site
C. Promoter
D. Silencer
E. Splice site

15.2 Answers and Explanations

| Easy | Medium | Hard |

1. Correct: B. The *NKX2-5* gene had a mutation in an associated transcriptional enhancer.

Enhancers and silencers are specific DNA sequences that bind regulatory factors that influence transcription from associated gene promoters. Enhancers and silencers can be within, upstream, downstream, near, and far from the gene they regulate. Transcriptional enhancers and transcriptional silencers upregulate and repress, respectively, transcription of specific genes as a part of developmental, signaling, or hormone-regulated programs in human cells (see figure below). Mutation of a distal transcriptional enhancer could result in severe reduction or loss of expression of the *NKX2-5* gene. Loss of the NKX2-5 protein in the baby resulted in loss of transcription of target genes that themselves are regulated by *NKX2-5* and are required for normal cardiac development and function.

A is incorrect. Since there were no mutations in the NKX2-5 protein coding region, the pathology could not be due to a change in NKX2-5 protein structure or function, so loss of NKX2-5 binding to a histone deacetylase enzyme could not be the cause.

C is incorrect. Since there were no mutations in the NKX2-5 protein coding region, the pathology could not be due to a change in NKX2-5 protein structure or function and so DNA binding would not be affected.

D is incorrect. Hypomethylation of a gene's promoter typically results in higher expression (if anything) of the associated gene. While excess expression of some proteins can cause cellular dysfunction, loss of expression of the protein (answer A) would definitely produce a phenotype.

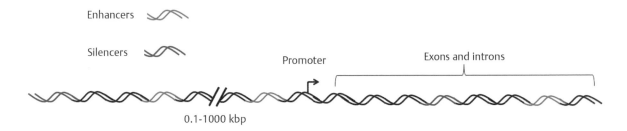

Enhancers

Silencers

Promoter

Exons and introns

0.1-1000 kbp

2. Correct: C. Histone acetyltransferase.

Transcriptional activators regulate gene transcription by several mechanisms including recruitment of histone acetyltransferase (HAT) enzymes. These enzymes acetylate lysine residues present in the *N*-terminal "tails" of histone proteins that are subunits of nucleosomes (as shown in the figure below, (i)). This acetylation results in loosening or opening of the chromatin structure, which provides access to underlying DNA by RNA polymerase II and associated factors.

A is incorrect. Methylation of guanosine residues of promoter DNA leads to silencing of gene transcription. If the mutant GATA4 protein was unable to recruit a DNA methyltransferase, the likely outcome would be an increase in gene transcription of those genes.

B is incorrect. DNA polymerase is not involved in gene transcription. It is involved in replication of genomic DNA.

D is incorrect. Just as transcriptional activators can recruit HAT enzymes which acetylate nucleosomes leading to opening of chromatin, transcriptional repressors can recruit histone deacetylases (HDAC), which carry out the reverse reaction (as shown in the figure below, (i)).

E is incorrect. Eukaryotic transcription factors, as a general rule, do not directly contact RNA polymerase enzymes.

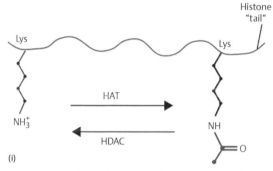

(i)

Source: Panini S. Medical Biochemistry - An Illustrated Review. 1st Edition. Thieme; 2013.

3. Correct: A. Alternative splicing of KLF6 pre-mRNA.

The primary RNA transcript of most intron-containing genes can undergo alternative splicing, where specific exons are included (or excluded) resulting in the production of multiple mRNA transcripts (as shown in the figure below, (ii)). Since protein-coding information is contained in exons, their differential inclusion/exclusion can result in the production of multiple versions of a given protein, often with very different activities.

B is incorrect. Gene promoters determine, in part, the amount of RNA produced from a gene but increasing their activity does not influence the splicing of transcripts produced by the gene. Increased activity of the KLF6 promoter would result in *more* mRNA. If a gene has multiple promoters that are associated with different first exons (which is not the case for KLF6), alternative promoter usage *can* result in transcripts with different protein coding information.

C is incorrect. Micro-RNAs (miRNAs) regulate the stability and translation of mRNAs, in a sequence-specific manner. Therefore, miRNAs affect the amount of protein produced but not the splicing of an mRNA or the nature of the protein made.

D is incorrect. Rearrangement of this gene could potentially occur, resulting in altered transcripts, but the question indicates normal cells produce multiple forms of KLF6. This rules out exceptional genetic events, like gene rearrangement, as the cause for multiple versions of the KLF6 protein being produced.

E is incorrect. Transcriptional enhancers regulate the amount of RNA produced from an mRNA, but do not influence the splicing of transcripts produced by the gene.

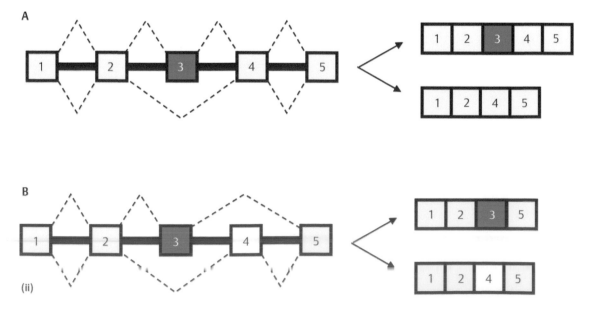

(ii)

4. Correct: C. Polyadenylation signal sequence.

The extra length of the mRNA suggests that a processing event may be malfunctioning. Splicing defects are not provided as an option and can be ruled out. The polyadenylation signal, a short AU-rich sequence, is recognized by the termination/polyadenylation machinery associated with RNA polymerase II, and results in cleavage of the nascent RNA followed by addition of 150 to 200 adenosine residues in a nontemplate-dependent manner. Loss of the polyadenylation signal sequence could result in RNA polymerase continuing to transcribe past what would be the normal termination site and continuing on to the next sequence that resembles a polyadenylation signal sequence, extending the mRNA on its 3' end. The additional sequences included in the transcript would likely result in altered function compared to the wild-type mRNA (and it indeed does in this documented case).

A is incorrect. The Kozak sequence surrounds the initiation codon (AUG) of human mRNAs and is the location where the ribosome initiates translation of the mRNA into protein. Mutation of this sequence would alter the efficiency of translation, but not the length of the mRNA.

B is incorrect. Origins of replication are the loci in the genome where the DNA replication machinery assembles. As such, it has nothing to do with mRNA length.

D and E are incorrect. Mutations of transcriptional enhancers or silencers could potentially alter the level of mRNA produced from a gene, but would not affect the length of the mRNA produced.

5. Correct: B. A reduction in cellular protein synthesis.

Inhibition of a factor (CPSF30) required for mRNA polyadenylation would prevent the addition of the poly-A tail. The poly-A tail contributes significantly to mRNA stability, export from the nucleus, and translation of mRNA by ribosomes into protein. All of these events would be severely inhibited ultimately leading to reduced cellular protein synthesis. The virus likely evolved this mechanism to inhibit the production of protein by transcriptionally induced interferon genes, as a way to evade destruction by the immune system.

A is incorrect. Loss of polyadenylation by inhibition of CPSF30 would not alter the nucleotide content of mRNA produced from a given gene. Therefore, amino acid substitutions would not result from the action of NS1A.

C is incorrect. NMD occurs when a premature initiation codon is present in a mutated gene. NMD occurs during the first round of translation, when protein complexes are still present on the exon-intron junctions of the newly synthesized and spliced mRNA. If a premature termination codon is further than about 50 nucleotides upstream of any exon-junction complexes, then the transcript is targeted for degradation by NMD. Loss of polyadenylation by inhibition of CPSF30 would not alter the nucleotide content of mRNA produced from a given gene. Therefore, introduction of premature termination codons and activation of NMD would not result from the action of NS1A.

D is incorrect. Ribosomes contain rRNAs which are transcribed by RNA polymerase I and III and are not polyadenylated. Therefore, inhibition of CPSF30 would not affect rRNA synthesis.

E is incorrect. Inhibition of CPSF30 by viral NS1A protein would result in a general reduction in polyadenylation of mRNA. It would, in any instance, lead to increased polyadenylation.

6. Correct: C. Reduced acetylation of nucleosomes associated with promoters of genes coding for inflammatory cytokines.

Glucocorticoid drugs like triamcinolone bind to the glucocorticoid receptor (GR) which is normally resident in the cytoplasm in an inactive complex with other proteins. Binding of the ligand results in the translocation of GR to the nucleus. Once there, GR regulates gene transcription in both positive and negative ways. The anti-inflammatory properties of glucocorticoids are due to (among other things) repression of transcription of genes that promote inflammation such as inflammatory cytokines. GR does this by inhibiting the activity of the proinflammatory transcription factor NF-κB. The transcriptional repression is ultimately dependent on a reduction in acetylation of histones within nucleosomes associated with the promoters of the genes repressed by GR.

A is incorrect. Reduced transcription of inflammatory cytokine genes in response to glucocorticoid treatment would be associated with less (or unchanged) RNA polymerase II bound to promoters of these genes.

B is incorrect. Binding of ligand by the glucocorticoid receptor results in homodimerization of GR proteins and translocation to the nucleus. There would be less retention of the receptor in the cytoplasm following exposure to triamcinolone.

D is incorrect. NF-κB is activated by inflammatory signals (e.g., toll-like receptor signaling) and translocates from the cytoplasm (where it is bound to the inhibitor of kappa B protein) to the nucleus. In the nucleus, NF-κB activates transcription of proinflammatory genes. Glucocorticoids do not influence this aspect of NF-κB function.

7. Correct: A. Gene transcription.

Acetylation of histone proteins within the nucleosome (the "spool" around which DNA wraps in chromatin) results in loosening or opening of the chromatin structure, which provides access to underlying DNA by RNA polymerase II and associated factors. The level of histone acetylation is determined by the relative activity of HAT enzymes which add acetylation and HDAC enzymes which remove the modification. Inhibition of histone deacetylase enzymes will result in generally increased histone acetylation; acetylation of histones within nucleosomes correlates with increased gene transcription.

B is incorrect. Histone acetylation levels have not been shown to directly influence mRNA splicing mechanisms.

C is incorrect. Histone acetylation levels have not been shown to directly influence mRNA export mechanisms.

D is incorrect. Histone acetylation levels have not been shown to directly influence mRNA polyadenylation mechanisms.

E is incorrect. Histone acetylation levels have not been shown to directly influence protein translation mechanisms.

8. Correct: B. mRNA.

Alpha-amanitin is an extremely toxic compound (LD50 < 1 mg/kg). It inhibits RNA polymerases in human cells with varying efficiency. RNA polymerase II, which transcribes mRNA, some small nuclear RNA (snRNA) and most miRNA, is most sensitive to alpha-amanitin. As such, while low concentrations of the toxin were circulating in the patient's blood, mRNA synthesis would be inhibited preferentially. Alpha-amanitin was used in classic experiments to differentiate between the different RNA polymerases in eukaryotic cells.

A is incorrect. DNA polymerases are not directly inhibited by alpha-amanitin.

C is incorrect. rRNAs are synthesized by RNA polymerase III (5S rRNA) and RNA polymerase I (all other rRNA). RNA polymerase III is inhibited at concentrations of alpha-amanitin 10-fold higher than those needed to inhibit RNA polymerase II. RNA polymerase I is not inhibited to alpha-amanitin.

D is incorrect. RNA polymerase III, which transcribes tRNAs, 5S rRNA and some snRNA, is inhibited at concentrations of alpha-amanitin 10-fold higher than those needed to inhibit RNA polymerase II.

E is incorrect. A mitochondrial RNA polymerase, structurally resembling bacterial RNA polymerase holoenzyme, transcribes mitochondrial DNA into RNA. It is not inhibited by alpha-amanitin.

9. Correct: B. Quantity of MUC5B mRNA.

Given the location of the SNP, it is possible that it is within a cis-acting regulatory element (transcriptional enhancer or silencer) that controls the transcription of the *MUC5B* gene. These regulatory elements are specific DNA sequences that are recognized by protein factors, changing the sequence can influence the efficiency of binding by the factors to the elements. This would lead to altered gene transcription. Therefore, the minor allele is most likely altering the quantity of MUC5B mRNA synthesized, which appears to be a contributing factor to the risk of familial interstitial pneumonia and idiopathic pulmonary fibrosis.

A is incorrect. Since the SNP is well upstream of the protein coding portion of the *MUC5B* gene (which is downstream of the transcriptional start site), the SNP cannot change the amino acid sequence of the MUC5B protein.

C is incorrect. The site of polyadenylation of newly synthesized mRNA is determined by sequences at the 3' end of the gene. The SNP is far upstream of this location and therefore cannot affect polyadenylation.

D is incorrect. The site of ribosome binding of mRNA is proximal to the 7-methyl-guanonise cap on the 5' end of the mRNA, downstream of the transcriptional start site. The SNP is far upstream of this location and therefore cannot affect ribosome binding.

E is incorrect. Splicing of mRNA is determined by sequences within the body of the gene, downstream of the transcriptional start site. The SNP is far upstream of this location and therefore cannot affect ribosome binding.

10. Correct: D. Qualitative and quantitative changes in mRNA splicing.

The physical findings, history, and genetic mutation confirm the diagnosis of spinal muscular atrophy, an autosomal recessive congenital disease that is the number one cause of infant death in the United States. *SMN1*, which encodes a protein necessary for the assembly of snRNPs. snRNPs are involved in pre-mRNA splicing, including recognition of splice donor and acceptor sites, creating the appropriate geometry for the splicing reaction and catalyzing the reaction itself (as shown in the figure below). Reduced snRNP availability, due to the mutation of the SMN1 protein, results in global changes in mRNA splicing that ultimately results in the physical deficits of individuals with spinal muscular atrophy.

A is incorrect. *SMN1* is not involved in the addition of the 7-methyl-guanosine cap on mRNAs.

B is incorrect. The changes in mRNA splicing resulting from the deficit of snRNPs do not influence the engagement of mRNAs with ribosomes.

C is incorrect. *SMN1* is not involved in the tRNA synthesis or processing.

E is incorrect. While altered splicing might lead to some mRNAs being degraded by NMD, this answer does not describe the most proximal biochemical event that results from reduced snRNPs levels.

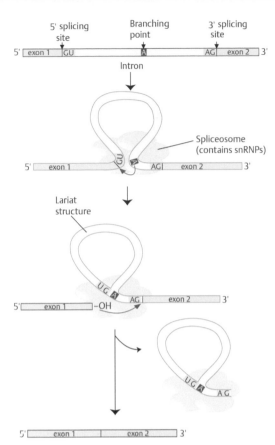

Source: Panini S. Medical Biochemistry - An Illustrated Review. 1st Edition. Thieme; 2013.

11. Correct: B. A new polyadenylation signal.

Since the TCF7L2 mRNA is truncated on the 3' end, the most straightforward explanation is that the SNP creates a new polyadenylation signal. Polyadenylation signals are relatively short, conserved nucleotide sequences that, when encountered by RNA polymerase II, result in termination of transcription followed by addition of a polyadenosine tail consisting of 150 to 200 adenosine residues, added in a template-independent manner. Since the new polyadenylation signal is within the fourth intron of the *TCF7L2* gene which contains 17 exons, utilization of this signal would result in the premature transcriptional termination and an mRNA that is significantly truncated on the 3' end in comparison to the *TCF7L2* gene that does not contain the SNP.

A is incorrect. A change in splicing, resulting from an alteration sequences at intron–exon boundaries, would be very unlikely to result in a 3' truncation of the mRNA. More likely, such a change would produce an mRNA with one more or one fewer exon included. The single, best explanation is that the SNP produces a new polyadenylation signal.

C is incorrect. The question is in regard to a change in mRNA length and therefore involves transcription, not translation. A new translation start codon would have no effect whatsoever on mRNA length.

D is incorrect. A new transcriptional promoter within the fourth intron would result in an mRNA that is altered (truncated) on the 5'-end of the mRNA, since RNA polymerase II would initiate transcription at this new promoter, downstream of the normal promoter.

E is incorrect. A new transcriptional regulatory protein binding site would alter the amount of mRNA synthesized, not the location where mRNA transcription would terminate.

12. Correct: C. Promoters.

Since myc overexpression is associated with elevation of transcription of all active genes, it must work via a conserved, genetic regulatory element present in all genes. All genes contain conserved promoter elements, conserved nucleotide sequences that are binding and assembly sites for RNA polymerase and associated factors, necessary for synthesis of RNA (as shown in the figure below).

A is incorrect. Essentially all genes are under the control of one or more transcriptional enhancers. Enhancers and silencers are specific DNA sequences that bind regulatory factors that influence transcription from associated gene promoters. Enhancers and silencers can be within, upstream, downstream, near, and far from the gene they regulate. Transcriptional enhancers and transcriptional silencers upregulate and repress, respectively, transcription of specific genes as a part of developmental, signaling, or hormone-regulated programs in human cells. There are approximately 1,500 transcription factors encoded by the human genome that bind to enhancers and silencers, which have varying nucleotide sequence identity. Mechanistically, it would be

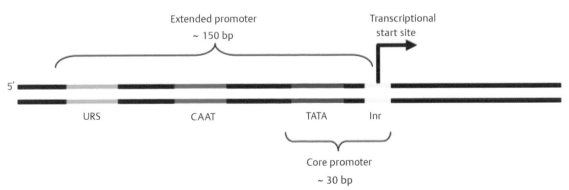

difficult for myc to utilize this wide repertoire of enhancers or silencers that have varying nucleotide sequences, to produce the observed outcome of myc overexpression.

B is incorrect. The polyadenylation signal, a short AU-rich sequence, is recognized by the termination/polyadenylation machinery associated with RNA polymerase II, and results in cleavage of the nascent RNA followed by addition of 150 to 200 adenosine residues in a nontemplate-dependent manner. Polyadenylation is not mechanistically linked to transcriptional initiation rates.

D is incorrect. Transcriptional enhancers and transcriptional silencers upregulate and repress, respectively, transcription of specific genes as a part of developmental, signaling, or hormone-regulated programs in human cells. There are approximately 1,500 transcription factors encoded by the human genome that bind to enhancers and silencers, which have varying nucleotide sequence identity. Mechanistically, it would be difficult for myc to utilize this wide repertoire of enhancers or silencers, that have varying nucleotide sequences, to produce the observed outcome of myc overexpression.

E is incorrect. The spliceosome (splicing machinery) assembles at splice sites (the junctions of exons and introns of pre-mRNA) and carries out the removal of introns and stitching together of exons. Splicing is not linked to the rate initiation of gene transcription, so myc cannot be working through this mechanism to produce the observed outcome of myc overexpression.

13. Correct: D. Reduction in DNA methylation at genes necessary for the pluripotent phenotype.

DNA methylation in humans occurs at cytosine residues that are part of CpG dinucleotides. DNA methylation of promoter DNA is associated with long-term transcriptional silencing of the associated gene. Genes that code for proteins specifically involved in maintaining pluripotency are methylated and silenced during cellular differentiation to a terminal phenotype such as fibroblasts. Thus, the DNA methylation at these gene promoters must be reversed by the action of the introduced transcription factors.

A is incorrect. The levels of histone acetylation increase at the specific target genes upregulated by the four transcription factors. Transcription factors bound to regulatory elements alter histone acetylation only at target genes associated with those elements. A global elevation of histone acetylation is not consistent with how these, or any other, transcription factors mediate transcriptional activation.

B is incorrect. iPSCs need to be able to divide, both to generate more stem cells and during the differentiation process. Thus, genes involved in inducing cell cycle arrest would not be targets for transcriptional activation by the four transcription factors that induce iPSC.

C is incorrect. Transcription factors most typically bind DNA (or bind other proteins that bind DNA) and generally do not bind mRNA.

E is incorrect. DNA synthesis is required for cell division, so transcriptional repression of gene necessary for that process is counter to the needs of iPSCs.

14. Correct: E. Translocation of specific transcription factors to the nucleus.

Bacterial surface antigens (pathogen-associated molecular patterns [PAMPs]) bind to receptors on immune and other cells and activate signal transduction cascades that result in changes in gene transcription within the nucleus. One such cascade involves NF-κB which is retained in the cytoplasm until a signal is generated. It then translocates to the nucleus and binds to DNA regulatory elements, activating transcription of genes encoding inflammatory cytokines.

A is incorrect. DNA methylation in humans occurs at cytosine residues that are part of CpG dinucleotides. DNA methylation of promoter DNA is associated with long-term transcriptional silencing of the associated gene.

B is incorrect. Proteolysis of histone proteins is not a mechanism involved in transcriptional regulation.

C is incorrect. Transcriptional repressors can recruit HDACs, which remove acetyl groups from lysine residues on histones associated with loose, transcriptionally active chromatin. This leads to chromatin compaction and transcriptional silencing.

D is incorrect. Synthesis of additional RNA polymerase II holoenzymes is not a mechanism involved in transcriptional regulation.

15. Correct: A. Flavoperidol inhibits a specific kinase.

Once the RNA polymerase II holoenzyme and associated factors are bound to a gene promoter, the enzyme must be phosphorylated on the C-terminal tail of the largest subunit for the holoenzyme to become processive. Once phosphorylated, the RNA polymerase II holoenzyme will clear the promoter and begin synthesizing RNA, entering the elongation phase of the transcriptional cycle. Cyclin-dependent kinase 9 (CDK9) in complex with a cyclin makes up the complex known as positive transcription elongation factor b (Ptefb), which is responsible for phosphorylating RNA polymerase II.

B is incorrect. The promoters in the flavoperidol-treated AML cells were bound by RNA polymerase II. Therefore, the chromatin must already acetylated and "loose," that is, the DNA is accessible to RNA polymerase II. If flavoperidol inhibited acetylation of histones within nucleosomes at promoters, then the RNA polymerase II would not be able to bind the promoter DNA.

C is incorrect. Since the promoters in the flavoperidol-treated AML cells were bound by RNA polymerase II, then all the events prior to that must have already occurred. This includes binding of specific transcription factors to enhancers which then activate associated promoters by, in part, orchestrating the acetylation of chromatin and thereby making the promoter DNA accessible to RNA polymerase II.

D is incorrect. Inhibition of histone deacetylase enzymes would lead to greater histone acetylation and open, transcriptionally competent chromatin. This is inconsistent with the observation that RNA polymerase II is bound to promoters.

16. Correct: E. The transcriptional activation domain of RUNX1 is not present in the RUNX1-ETV6 fusion.

RUNX1, like most transcription factors that bind enhancers, has a modular structure with two key domains: DNA binding and transcriptional activation. The transcriptional activation domain binds to a recruit histone-modifying enzymes, as well as other coregulators (such as the Mediator complex) that assist in assembly of the RNA polymerase II containing complex at the core promoter. The RUNX1-ETV6 fusion protein contains only part of the RUNX1 protein, including the DNA-binding domain, but lacks the transcriptional activation domain of RUNX1. As such, RUNX1-ETV6 competes for DNA binding with RUNX1 (expressed from the nontranslocated gene) at enhancers but is unable to activate transcription like RUNX1. This dominant-negative competition alters gene transcription and contributes to the development of the leukemia.

A is incorrect. The RUNX1-ETV6 must have the DNA-binding domain of RUNX1, since the fusion protein was observed bound to the same enhancers normally occupied by RUNX1.

B is incorrect. Since RUNX1-ETV6 appears to have blocked transcription of "...genes normally activated by RUNX1..." and RUNX1 occupies enhancers, it can be concluded that RUNX1 is a transcriptional activator. As such, it would not have a domain with histone deacetylase activity, since histone deacetylation results in compaction of chromatin and silencing of transcription.

C is incorrect. The RUNX1-ETV6 must have an intact nuclear translocation signal, since the fusion protein was observed bound to enhancer DNA in the nucleus.

D is incorrect. Mammalian proteins that bind enhancers or silencers and regulate gene transcription do not directly contact RNA polymerase II as part of their mechanism of action.

17. Correct: E. Silencer.

Having one copy of the endometriosis risk-associated SNP is associated with moderately higher transcription from the *CDC42* gene and two copies is associated with significantly higher expression. If the SNP is within a silencer element, substitution of one of the nucleotides could potentially reduce or disrupt DNA binding by a transcription factor that normally would repress CDC42 transcription.

A is incorrect. The Kozak sequence surrounds the initiation codon (AUG) of human mRNAs and is the location where the ribosome initiates translation of the mRNA into protein. Change in the nucleotide sequence of the Kozak would alter the efficiency of translation of the mRNA, but would have no effect on transcription.

B is incorrect. Origins of replication are the loci in the genome where the DNA replication machinery assembles. As such, it has nothing to do with gene transcription.

C is incorrect. The polyadenylation signal, a short AU-rich sequence, is recognized by the termination/polyadenylation machinery associated with RNA polymerase II, and results in cleavage of the nascent RNA followed by addition of 150 to 200 adenosine residues in a nontemplate-dependent manner. Alteration of the polyadenylation signal sequence by the SNP could potentially (though the likelihood is very small) result in RNA polymerase continuing to transcribe past what would be the normal termination site and continuing on to the next sequence that resembles a polyadenylation signal sequence, extending the mRNA on its 3' end. However, no difference in mRNA length or nucleotide sequence for the CDC42 mRNA was observed, among the samples with different endometriosis risk-associated SNPs.

D is incorrect. The endometriosis risk-associated SNP is located approximately 50,000 base pairs from the *CDC42* gene. Promoters are located (and define) at the transcriptional start site of a gene. Therefore, the SNP could not alter the nucleotide sequence and affect the function of the *CDC42* gene promoter.

18. Correct: C. mRNA splicing.

The patient's history and clinical findings indicate allergic contact dermatitis, likely arising from exposure to chemicals in the print shop. The two forms of the glucocorticoid receptor protein come from alternative splicing of the gene's RNA, utilizing one of two alternative exons.

A is incorrect. In human cells, alternative translation initiation can occur, where the ribosome skips over the first (or subsequent) start codons proximal to the 5' end of an mRNA and utilizes alternative start codons. However, this mechanism is very rare in comparison to alternative splicing.

B is incorrect. RNA silencing by microRNA reduces stability and/or translation of mRNAs present in the cell. However, it does not contribute to the presence of different mRNA isoforms produced by a gene.

D is incorrect. Addition of a 7-methly-guanosine cap to mRNA is necessary for export, stability, and translation of the mRNA. However, it does not contribute to the presence of different mRNA isoforms produced by a gene.

E is incorrect. DNA replication is not directly involved in mRNA synthesis.

19. Correct: D. Silencer.

If the SNP is within a silencer element, substitution of one of the nucleotides could potentially reduce or disrupt DNA binding by a transcription factor that normally would repress LDH transcription.

A is incorrect. The Kozak sequence surrounds the initiation codon (AUG) of human mRNAs and is the location where the ribosome initiates translation of the mRNA into protein. The SNP associated with LPH persistence is located 20,000 base pairs from the gene, so it cannot reside in the Kozak sequence.

B is incorrect. The polyadenylation signal, a short AU-rich sequence, is recognized by the termination/polyadenylation machinery associated with RNA polymerase II, and results in cleavage of the nascent RNA followed by addition of 150 to 200 adenosine residues in a nontemplate-dependent manner. A change in the polyadenylation signal would be highly unlikely to result in persistence of LPH expression; in any case, the SNP associated with LPH persistence is located 20,000 base pairs from the gene, so it cannot reside in the polyadenylation signal sequence.

C is incorrect. While an SNP in a gene promoter could potentially result in a "stronger" promoter and increase gene expression, the SNP associated with LPH persistence is located 20,000 base pairs from the gene, so it cannot reside within the promoter.

E is incorrect. Mutation of a splice site would affect the mRNA structure and quite possibly result in a defective or absent protein. In addition, the SNP associated with LPH persistence is located 20,000 base pairs from the gene, so it cannot reside within a splice site.

Chapter 16

Protein Translation

LEARNING OBJECTIVES

► Define the terms initiation (or start) codon and termination (or stop) codon.

► Apply the genetic code lookup table to deduce the amino acid sequence coded for by a nucleic acid sequence.

► List the RNA species involved in gene expression and summarize the role of each.

► Explain the role of the messenger RNA (mRNA) cap and poly-A tail in translation initiation in eukaryotes.

► Summarize the steps in the initiation of protein translation and the factors involved.

► Explain the mechanism by which ribosomes initiate translation at the correct start (AUG) codon.

► Describe the role of elongation and termination factors in protein translation, citing bacterial toxins that inhibit elongation.

► Explain the mechanisms that regulate translation during the endoplasmic reticulum stress response (unfolded protein response).

► Describe the role of microRNAs (miRNAs) and miRNA machinery in regulation of translation and potential role in diagnosis and treatment of disease.

► Explain how frameshift, missense, and nonsense gene mutations alter the reading frame of the mRNA made from the gene and how these mutations will alter the protein synthesized from the mRNA.

16.1 Questions

Easy | Medium | Hard

1. A research team working on the genetic basis of Parkinson's disease identified several gene mutations associated with significantly increased risk for developing the disease. One such gene encodes an enzyme, leucine-rich repeat kinase 2 (*LRRK2*). A number of disease-associated mutations in the *LRRK2* gene result in reduced activity of the protein compared to wild type. The most common disease-risk associated *LRRK2* gene mutation changes a specific codon in the reading frame from UCC (wild type) to GCC (disease allele). Which of the following molecular outcomes, as the result of the amino acid substitution in the LRRK2 protein, might explain why this particular mutation contributes to the development of Parkinson's disease?

Nucleotide base					
First	Second				Third
	Uracil (U)	Cytosine (C)	Adenine (A)	Guanine (G)	
Uracil (u)	F Phenylalanine (phe)	S Serine (Ser)	Y Tyrosine (Tyr)	C Cysteine (Cys)	U
	F Phenylalanine (phe)	S Serine (Ser)	Y Tyrosine (Tyr)	C Cysteine (Cys)	C
	L Leucine (Leu)	S Serine (Ser)	Stop Codon	Stop Codon	A
	L Leucine (Leu)	S Serine (Ser)	Stop Codon	W Tryptophan (Trp)	G
Cytosine (C)	L Leucine (Leu)	P Proline (Pro)	H Histidine (His)	R Araginine (Arg)	U
	L Leucine (Leu)	P Proline (Pro)	H Histidine (His)	R Araginine (Arg)	C
	L Leucine (Leu)	P Proline (Pro)	Q Glutamine (Gln)	R Araginine (Arg)	A
	L Leucine (Leu)	P Proline (Pro)	Q Glutamine (Gln)	R Araginine (Arg)	G
Adenine (A)	I Isoleucine (Ile)	T Threonine (Thr)	N Asparagine (Asn)	S Serine (Ser)	U
	I Isoleucine (Ile)	T Threonine (Thr)	N Asparagine (Asn)	S Serine (Ser)	C
	I Isoleucine (Ile)	T Threonine (Thr)	K Lysine (Lys)	R Arginine (Arg)	A
	Start (Methionine)	T Threonine (Thr)	K Lysine (Lys)	R Arginine (Arg)	G
Guanine (G)	V Valine (Val)	A Alanine (Ala)	D Aspartic acid (Asp)	G Glycine (Gly)	U
	V Valine (Val)	A Alanine (Ala)	D Aspartic acid (Asp)	G Glycine (Gly)	C
	V Valine (Val)	A Alanine (Ala)	E Glutamic acid (Glu)	G Glycine (Gly)	A
	V Valine (Val)	A Alanine (Ala)	E Glutamic acid (Glu)	G Glycine (Gly)	G

Source: Passarge E. Color Atlas of Genetics. 4th Edition. 2012.

A. Creation of an acetylation site
B. Insertion of a charged amino acid
C. Loss of phosphorylation site
D. Premature termination of translation
E. Creation of a ubiquitination site

2. A resident on the pediatric service asks you to consult on a 6-month-old female infant. She was brought to the clinic with a chief complaint of "bumps" on hands and feet and in her mouth. Her mother reports that the child has had a mild fever and been "very sleepy." At meal time, she appears cranky and disinterested in eating. Examination of the oral mucosa reveals erythematous macules approximately 2 mm in diameter, some of which appear to be ulcerated. Similar small erythematous papules are visible on her hands and feet. You reassure the mother the condition will resolve but to bring the child back if she doesn't get better in a week. The responsible pathogen, foot and mouth disease virus (FMDV), expresses an enzyme that specifically degrades the proteins in the mRNA cap-binding complex (eIF4F) in infected human cells. Which of the following processes will be diminished in cells infected with FMDV, leading in part to the lesions observed on the child's skin and mucosa?

A. Addition of the 7-methly-guanosine cap to mRNA

B. Polyadenylation of mRNA

C. Splicing of mRNA

D. Transcription of DNA into mRNA

E. Translation of mRNA into protein

3. A single-nucleotide deletion occurs in the open reading frame of a human gene that codes for an 1,100 amino acid protein. The deletion is in the part of the gene that codes for the *N*-terminal one-third of the protein. Which of the following is the most likely outcome of this mutation?

A. Production of a protein with a single amino acid substitution

B. Production of a protein with the potential for gain-of-function mutation

C. Production of moderately increased levels of the protein

D. Production of a truncated mRNA transcript

E. Production of a truncated, nonfunctional protein

4. X-linked Charcot-Marie-Tooth disease (CMTX1), one of the most common forms of inherited neuropathy, results from mutations in the gene encoding the gap junction protein connexin32 (Cx32). A newly diagnosed CMTX1 patient was found to have a point mutation that lead to complete loss of *Cx32* protein expression, though the mRNA for the *Cx32* gene was still detectable and at near-normal levels. Which of the following locations in the gene encoding *Cx32* might result in this patient's disease?

A. AUG start codon

B. Promoter

C. Enhancer

D. Polyadenylation signal sequence

5. A 47-year-old woman came to the emergency department (ED) with a chief complaint of fever and pain in her left chest when she coughs. Twelve hours before coming to the ED, she woke up with a severe, shaking chills and sweating. Taking her history, you find out that the patient has two to three alcoholic drinks on most days and has smoked one package of cigarettes daily for 17 years. Her frontal chest radiograph demonstrates a cavitary mass in the lateral aspect of the left lung base (see the figure below). Her white blood cell count was 16,000/µL (reference range: 4,500–10,000/µL). Gram stain of sputum showed many leukocytes and gram-negative rods which were confirmed to be *Pseudomonas aeruginosa*. The cellular damage producing some of her symptoms are the result of inhibition by a bacterial toxin of which of the following aspects of protein translation?

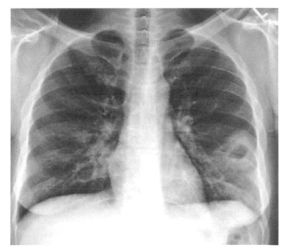

Source: Gunderman R. Essential Radiology. Clinical Presentation, Pathophysiology, Imaging. 3rd Edition. Thieme; 2014.

A. Charging of tRNAs with amino acids

B. Elongation during protein translation

C. Initiation of protein translation

D. Ribosome assembly

E. Termination of protein translation

6. A 4-year-old boy is referred to your ophthalmology clinic with a clearly visible tumor in his pupil's aperture, creating a "cat's eye" amaurosis and visual impairment (see the figure below). Following enucleation surgery, the biochemistry and genetics of the tumor was analyzed in a research laboratory with whom you collaborate. Analysis of DNA from the tumor revealed that one allele of the retinoblastoma (Rb) gene was deleted. The other Rb allele had a deletion of four nucleotides just prior to the AUG start codon. Western blot analysis of the Rb protein in these tumor cells revealed Rb protein that is smaller than predicted for a normal, wild-type protein. This smaller Rb protein did not react with a monoclonal antibody directed against the first 12 amino acids of Rb. Which of the following is the likely mechanistic reason why this smaller Rb protein is being produced?

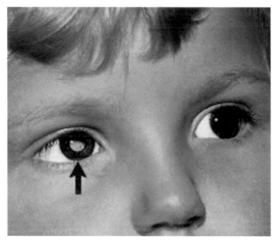

Source: Riede U, Werner M. Color Atlas of Pathology: Pathologic Principles · Associated Diseases · Sequela. 1st Edition. 2004.

A. The mutation results in incorrect polyadenylation of the mRNA during processing

B. The mutation results in the absence of 7-methyl-guanosine cap on the mRNA

C. The mutation results in the loss of binding by RNA polymerase to the Rb gene promoter

D. The mutation results in the ribosome initiating translation from an incorrect AUG

E. The mutation results in the "skipping" of the second exon during mRNA splicing

7. Recent reports have linked elevated expression of the protein eIF4E, a subunit of the mRNA cap-binding complex (eIF4F), to the aggressiveness of prostate carcinoma and diminished survival of patients. Which of the following might be the mechanism by which you are a participating investigator in a phase III clinical trials testing the efficacy and toxicity of a small-molecule inhibitor of eIF4E for the treatment of prostate cancers. Earlier phase II trials indicated that all prostate cancers, regardless of eIF4E expression status, responded to the drug, with diminished growth rates and very little toxicity. Which of the following might explain the specific efficacy of the eIF4E inhibitor drug against cancer cells?

A. Cap-independent translation mechanisms are lost in cancer cells

B. Not all mRNAs are equally dependent on cap-dependent translation mechanisms

C. Micro-RNA (miRNA) expression patterns are altered in cancer cells

D. Cancer cells typically have higher numbers of ribosomes than normal cells

8. A female infant born at term, the first child of consanguineous parents, was diagnosed with neonatal insulin-dependent diabetes at age 3 months. At 4 months of age she was hospitalized with acute liver failure, expiring 2 days later from multisystem failure. Postmortem, the child was diagnosed by a medical geneticist with Wolcott–Rallison syndrome resulting from a defect in a specific kinase. The parents were given counseling and advice for future family planning. Which of the following explains why the child's pancreatic islet cells failed shortly after birth, resulting in her diabetes?

A. Inability to alter protein translation in response to insulin signaling

B. Inability to assemble sufficient numbers of functional ribosomes

C. Inability to form disulfide bonds on newly synthesized proteins

D. Inability to phosphorylate a translational initiation factor during cellular stress

E. Inability to produce a specific amino acyl-tRNA within the mitochondria

9. Point mutation in of poly-A binding protein (PABP) prevents interaction with eIF4G—loss of translation but no difference in mRNA stability. An investigator studying the role PABP in cellular function generated a number of single amino acid substitution. One substitution at amino acid position 161 did not affect the binding of PABP to mRNA. However, it did disrupt the interaction between the cap-binding complex eIF4F and PABP. Which of the following is the most likely outcome of this mutated version of PABP on cellular physiology?

A. Reduced fidelity of protein synthesis

B. Reduced mRNA export from the nucleus to the cytoplasm

C. Reduced mRNA stability

D. Reduced initiation of protein translation

E. Reduced rate of ribosome translocation

10. A 3-year-old male child is brought to the clinic by his mother with a chief complaint of "He is standing up in an odd way." The child is within normal range for weight and height, but you notice his calf muscles are relatively large in comparison to the overall size of his legs. You ask him to stand up and he demonstrates the Gower's sign when standing from a sitting position on the floor, by placing his palms flat on the floor and "walking up" to a standing position. The patient is referred to a medical geneticist to confirm your diagnosis of Duchenne muscular dystrophy and to characterize the molecular genetics of his disease. The boy has a mutation leading to a premature stop codon within the dystrophin disease. His enrolled in a clinical trial to test the effectiveness of an aminoglycoside antibiotic derivative in treating the underlying pathophysiology of his disease. Which of the following is likely to be the target of this new drug?

A. Dystrophin protein

B. DNA polymerase

C. Ribosome

D. RNA splicing machinery

E. RNA polymerase

11. A 66-year-old woman presents with mild jaundice and upper abdominal pain with radiation to her back, unexplained weight loss, and thrombophlebitis. Following imaging studies, which lead to a diagnosis of pancreatic cancer, she is treated by surgical resection followed with combined irradiation and chemotherapy. You identify her as a candidate for a clinical trial with an investigational new drug that is a small interfering RNA (siRNA) directed against the RAS oncogene that is likely to be expressed in any remaining cancer cells she has. If the drug works as designed, which of the following processes will be most directly affected by the siRNA targeting RAS?

A. DNA synthesis

B. mRNA splicing

C. mRNA synthesis

D. Protein stability

E. Protein synthesis

12. A novel G to C mutation a few nucleotides 5' of the start codon (AUG) of the *GATA4* gene was observed in a family with a history of two different forms of atrial septal defect. Measurements of GATA4 expression of a cell engineered to contain this mutation demonstrated that the mutation resulted in a moderate reduction in GATA4 protein, as measured by Western blot. Which of the following is the most likely mechanistic explanation for the lower levels of GATA4 protein that resulted from the mutation?

A. Reduced export of the GATA4 mRNA into the cytoplasm

B. Reduced polyadenylation of the GATA4 mRNA

C. Reduced splicing of the GATA4 pre-mRNA

D. Reduced transcription of the GATA4 DNA into mRNA

E. Reduced translation of GATA4 mRNA into protein

13. A 10-year-old boy was recently admitted to your hospital service after he arrived in the emergency department by ambulance. His mother found him unconscious and unresponsive after being taken from the emergency department. The child was diagnosed at age 2 with vanishing white matter (VWM) syndrome, characterized by worsening cerebellar ataxia with mild cognitive deterioration. His condition had been stable for the previous 3 years and his recent, substantial deterioration began 3 days prior, following a modest blow to the head when he tripped on a staircase. Review of his medical records indicates that a medical geneticist had determine that the boy's VWM was due to a mutation in one of the genes of the eukaryotic initiation factor 2B (eIF2B) complex, a guanine nucleotide exchange factor. You quickly review the pathophysiology of VWM and find that the disease is often stable, for up to period of several years, but that brain trauma or infection can precipitate a rapid decline in the number and function of multiple cell types in the brain. Which of the following molecular events likely caused the cellular decline within the brain that resulted in this child's current condition and hospital admission?

A. Reduced availability of active eukaryotic initiation factor 2 alpha (eIF2alpha)

B. Reduced availability of cytosolic ribosomes

C. Reduced binding of eukaryotic initiation factor 4F (eIF4F; cap-binding complex) to mRNA

D. Reduced GTPase activity by elongation factor 2 (EF2)

E. Reduced transport of mRNA into the rough endoplasmic reticulum

14. A 35-year-old woman with systemic lupus erythematosus underwent mitral valve replacement for severe regurgitation. On day 4 after operation, a blood culture revealed vancomycin-resistant *Enterococcus faecium*. Linezolid (Zyvox) therapy was prescribed which successfully treated the infection. If mRNAs in the bacteria treated with linezolid were examined for occupancy by ribosomes, it would have been revealed that the density of ribosomes on mRNAs was significantly reduced. Which of the following activities is blocked by linezolid with respect to the mechanisms of protein translation?

A. Binds to interface between 30S and 50S ribosomal subunits and prevents translocation

B. Blocks entry of 50S ribosomal subunit into the initiation complex

C. Incorporates into growing peptide chain and acts as a "chain terminator"

D. Inhibits GTPase activity of an elongation factor

E. Prevents entry of release factor into "A" site of 70S ribosome

15. The county public health department identified a spike of gastrointestinal illnesses consisting of fever, nausea, vomiting, stomach cramps, and diarrhea. Ill people ranged in age from 16 to 77 years (median age, 28) and 61% female. Three ill people were hospitalized; no deaths were reported. Of the seven ill people who were interviewed, all reported eating or possibly eating alfalfa sprouts at restaurants the week before illness started. Traceback investigations from several different restaurants the people ate indicated that a specific supplier provided alfalfa sprouts to all locations. Testing of some remaining sprouts from the same lot indicated contamination with *Escherichia coli* 0157:H7. A toxin produced by this bacteria damaged cells and resulted in illness by targeting which of the following components of the protein translation machinery?

A. Amino-acyl tRNA synthetase enzymes

B. Elongation factor EF2

C. Initiation factor eIF4F (cap-binding complex)

D. Initiation factor eIF2alpha

E. Large ribosomal subunit (60S in humans)

16. Patients recently diagnosed with chronic myelogenous leukemia (CML) were enrolled in a study to better understand the progress of their disease from indolent phase to blast crisis. As part of the study, CML cells were isolated from blood samples during each phase of their illness, and miRNAs and mRNAs were analyzed. The graph below shows the ratio of expression of a specific miRNA in CML cells in the blast phase to CML cells in the indolent phase, plotted against the same expression ratio for the leukemogenic fusion protein BCR/ABL. Assuming there is a causal relationship between these two observations, which process is being altered by the elevated expression of the specific miRNA?

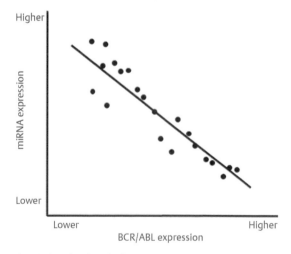

A. RNA polyadenylation

B. RNA splicing

C. RNA stability

D. RNA synthesis

E. RNA translation into protein

17. A range of strains of streptomycin-resistant strains of *Mycobacterium* isolated from clinical samples were subjected to high-throughput sequencing of their entire genomes to identify mutations that may contribute to their drug-resistant phenotype. Comparison of genome sequences between streptomycin-sensitive and -resistant strains revealed nucleotide differences in multiple genes. Mutations in genes encoding which of the following rRNAs or proteins might be responsible for the resistance phenotype in the streptomycin-resistant *Mycobacterium* strains?

A. 5S rRNA

B. 16S rRNA

C. 23S rRNA

D. Elongation factor 2

E. Initiation factor 2

18. The pathology report on a patient you suspect has iron deficiency anemia reveals mean corpuscular volume of 72 fL (reference range: 83–97 fL) and mean corpuscular hemoglobin concentration of 23 g/dL (reference range: 32–36 g/dL). Platelet count is slightly elevated and white blood cell count is within reference range. The concentration of heme in reticulocytes directly regulates the expression of globin proteins, though mRNA levels for globin proteins do not vary regardless of heme concentration. Which of the following mechanisms might account for suppression of globin protein expression in this patient's reticulocytes?

A. Reduced expression of a specific miRNA

B. Reduced histone acetylation

C. Increased DNA methylation

D. Reduced activity of eukaryotic initiation factor 2 alpha (eIF2alpha)

E. Reduced activity of eukaryotic initiation factor 4G (eIF4G; 7-methyl-guanosine cap-binding complex)

16.2 Answers and Explanations

Easy	Medium	Hard

1. Correct: C. Loss of phosphorylation site.

Using the genetic code lookup table in shown in Question 1, it can be determined that the nucleotide substitution changes a serine codon (UCC) to an alanine codon (GCC). Since serine is one of three amino acids (along with threonine and tyrosine) that can be phosphorylated, the substitution of alanine for serine could potentially lead to the loss of phosphorylation site.

A is incorrect. Acetylation occurs only on lysine residues and therefore the substitution of alanine for serine would not create a new acetylation site.

B is incorrect. The side chain of alanine is a simple methyl group and is not charged at any pH.

D is incorrect since the substituted codon, GCC, codes for alanine and is not a termination codon.

E is incorrect. Ubiquitination occurs only on lysine residues and therefore the substitution of alanine for serine would not create a new ubiquitination site.

2. Correct: E. Translation of mRNA into protein.

The mRNA cap-binding complex, eIF4F, consisting of three proteins (eIF4A, eIF4G, eIF4E) that binds the 7-methyl-guanosine cap of mRNAs and participates in the recruitment of ribosomes to mRNA for translation into protein (see the figure below). Loss of the cap binding complex would, therefore, lead to reduced protein translation and subsequent degradation of the decapped mRNA.

A is incorrect. The cap-binding complex eIF4F does not participate in the synthesis of the cap, so loss of eIF4F would not have an effect on cap addition to mRNA.

B is incorrect. The cap-binding complex eIF4F does not participate in the synthesis of the poly-A tail on mRNA, so loss of eIF4F would not have an effect on polyadenylation.

C is incorrect. The cap-binding complex eIF4F does not participate in splicing of mRNA, so loss of eIF4F would not have an effect on splicing.

D is incorrect. The 7-methyl-guanosine cap is added to the nascent mRNA shortly after initiation of transcription, an event that is independent of the cap-binding complex eIF4F.

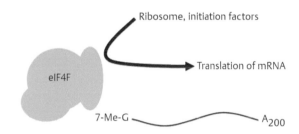

3. Correct: E. Production of a truncated, nonfunctional protein.

A frameshift mutation occurs when a gene suffers the deletion or insertion of nucleotides, within the protein reading frame, that is not a multiple of three nucleotides. The reading frame is altered such that random amino acids are inserted into the protein and often, shortly after the frameshift, a termination (STOP) codon is encountered. In either case, the protein is likely to be truncated and/or misfolded. Misfolded proteins are typically modified by polyubiquitination and then degraded by the proteasome. If the termination codon is near an exon–intron boundary, it is likely to result in the mRNA being subjected to nonsense-mediated decay.

A is incorrect. The change (but not deletion) of a base pair could produce a missense mutation which leads to an amino acid substitution. However, the deletion of a single base pair from an open reading frame will always result in a frameshift mutation.

B is incorrect. Changes in the primary sequence of a protein can alter structure and function of the protein; however, the deletion of a single base pair from an open reading frame will always result in a frameshift mutation.

C is incorrect. A frameshift mutation cannot result in higher levels of protein produced from the mutated gene.

D is incorrect. The location of transcriptional termination by RNA polymerase II is determined by the presence of a polyadenylation signal that consists of multiple nucleotides. Deletion of single nucleotide near the 5'end of the gene is unlikely, in the extreme, to result in creation of a polyadenylation signal.

4.   Correct: A. AUG start codon.

Mutation of the start codon would result in severe if not total loss of protein expression from the mRNA produced from the gene. This is because the anticodon on the initiation tRNA-Met must base-pair exactly with the start codon to initiate translation. It is possible that the ribosome scanning the mutated mRNA used the next methionine codon (AUG) in the mRNA, producing an N-terminal truncated protein that did not fold correctly and was quickly degraded and, as such, was undetectable.

B is incorrect. A single-nucleotide substitution in the core promoter could potentially reduce the levels of mRNA transcribed from the gene. The patient's findings (mRNA detected was at near-normal levels, but no protein was made) are inconsistent with a promoter mutation.

C is incorrect. A point mutation in an enhancer might lead to reduced function and lower transcription from the target gene, in this case *Cx32*. The patient's findings (mRNA detected was at near-normal levels, but no protein was made) are inconsistent with an enhancer mutation.

D is incorrect. A point mutation in a polyadenylation signal sequence might lead to reduced function and lower mRNA levels from the target gene, in this case *Cx32*. The patient's findings (mRNA detected was at near-normal levels, but no protein was made) are inconsistent with a polyadenylation signal sequence mutation.

5.   Correct: B. Elongation during protein translation.

Exotoxin A produced by *P. aeruginosa* catalyzes ADP-ribosylation of protein translation elongation factor 2 (EF2). EF2 is a G-protein that is required for the translocation of the ribosome on mRNA. For each codon-length translocation facilitated by EF2, it hydrolyses one molecule of guanosine triphosphate

(GTP). The ADP-ribosylation of EF2 blocks the ability of EF2 to hydrolyze GTP which prevents ribosomal translocation, shutting down protein translation.

A is incorrect. Exotoxin A produced by *P. aeruginosa* does not affect charging of tRNAs with amino acids by amino-acyl tRNA synthetases.

C is incorrect. Exotoxin A produced by *P. aeruginosa* does not modify or affect the activity of the factors required for initiation of translation.

D is incorrect. Exotoxin A produced by *P. aeruginosa* does not affect ribosome assembly.

E is incorrect. Exotoxin A produced by *P. aeruginosa* does not modify or affect the activity of the factors required for termination of translation.

6.   Correct: D. The mutation results in the ribosome initiating translation from an incorrect AUG.

A conserved nucleotide sequence (the "Kozak sequence") surrounds the AUG start codon of human mRNAs and is necessary for efficient initiation from a start codon. Loss of this sequence could potentially lead to the ribosome initiating from the next AUG that has a sequence more closely matching the Kozak sequence. The absence of the first 12 amino acids from the mutant protein is consistent with this explanation.

A is incorrect. The polyadenylation signal sequence is located 3' of (beyond) the protein coding region of a gene. The described mutation was prior to the protein coding sequences of the Rb gene.

B is incorrect. The addition of the 7-methylguanosine cap to the 5'ends of mammalian mRNAs is not sequence dependent and therefore a mutation will not affect capping.

C is incorrect. The mutation is not in the location where the promoter is expected, which is upstream of where transcription of the mRNA occurs. In addition, reduced binding of RNA polymerase II would result in less mRNA being produced.

E is incorrect. Since the first 12 amino acids are missing from the mutant protein, splicing out of the second exon can be ruled out as the cause. In addition, the location of the mutation is very unlikely to affect splicing further downstream.

7.   Correct: B. Not all mRNAs are equally dependent on cap-dependent translation mechanisms.

The primary reason selectivity for killing cancer cells by inhibiting eIF4E is that "weak" mRNAs (those that depend on cap-binding complex more) tend to code for proteins that contribute to the neoplastic phenotype (e.g., cyclins, vascular endothelial growth factor, the oncogene *MYC*). In contrast, many "housekeeping" genes are less dependent on eIF4F, so normal cells can withstand inhibition of eIF4E. eIF4E is the protein in the three-protein eIF4F complex that directly binds the cap. A second subunit, eIF4A has helicase activity which unwinds secondary structure (intramolecular base pairing) in 5' untranslated region of mRNAs, which are upstream of the start codon. The "weak" mRNAs, that are more dependent on eIF4F, tend to have longer, more complex 5' untranslated regions and require more helicase activity. Thus, when eIF4E is inhibited and therefore cap binding by eIF4F more limited, the "weak" mRNAs tend not to be translated as efficiently, leading to inhibition of cell growth.

A is incorrect. Cap-independent translation can occur in human cells, though it is infrequent, but it is not linked specifically to cancer cell phenotype or survival and therefore this would not provide selectivity for inhibition of eIF4E in killing cancer cells.

C is incorrect. miRNA expression patterns are often altered in cancer cells. miRNAs can inhibit translation (as well as lead to degradation of targeted mRNAs) but the mechanism by which miRNA work does not involve the cap-binding complex (eIF4F).

D is incorrect. Cancer cells do typically have more ribosomes than their normal, noncycling counterparts. However, this would not lead to a specific dependency on additional eIF4E.

8. Correct: D. Inability to phosphorylate a translational initiation factor during cellular stress.

Wolcott–Rallison syndrome is the result of loss-of-function mutations in the gene coding for the protein kinase RNA-like endoplasmic reticulum kinase (PERK) (encoded by the *EIF2AK3* gene and also known as translation initiation factor 2 alpha kinase-3). PERK is activated during the endoplasmic reticulum stress/unfolded protein response and phosphorylates the translational initiation factor eIF2alpha (as shown in the figure on the right). This results in the cell ceasing most protein translation, save for factors involved in refolding or degrading unfolded proteins which allow the cell to recover and resume normal function. Islet (insulin producing) cells of the pancreas are particularly in need of this mechanism, given the demands of insulin production, and are among the first cell types to die following birth.

A is incorrect. The inability to alter protein translation in response to insulin signaling does not cause Wolcott–Rallison syndrome.

B is incorrect. The inability to assemble sufficient numbers of functional ribosomes does not cause Wolcott–Rallison syndrome.

C is incorrect. The inability to form disulfide bonds on newly synthesized proteins does not cause Wolcott–Rallison syndrome.

E is incorrect. The inability to produce a specific amino acyl-tRNA within the mitochondria does not cause Wolcott–Rallison syndrome.

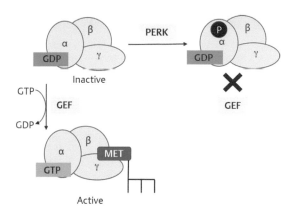

9. Correct: D. Reduced initiation of protein translation.

PABP binds to the polyadenylated 3' end of mRNAs. This interaction is important for (1) translation efficiency, (2) export of mRNA to the cytoplasm from the nucleus, and (3) mRNA stability. PABP increases translation efficiency by directly binding to eIF4F, the complex that interacts with the 7-methyl-guanosine on the 5' end of mRNA. This interaction is thought to result in circularization of the mRNA and rapid reloading of ribosomes that complete translation, back onto the 5' end of the mRNA for a subsequent round of translation. Loss of the PABP-eIF4F interaction would disrupt this mechanism, reducing protein translation globally.

A is incorrect. PABP does not have a role in ensuring fidelity of protein translation.

B is incorrect. The binding of PABP to the polyadenylated 3' end ("poly-A tail") of mRNAs is important for efficient transport of newly synthesized mRNA from the nucleus to the cytoplasm. However, this activity does not require the interaction between PABP and eIF4F, the complex that interacts with the 7-methyl-guanosine on the 5' end of mRNA.

C is incorrect. The binding of PABP to the polyadenylated 3' end ("poly-A tail") of mRNAs is important mRNA stability. Enzymatic removal of the poly-A tail is one of the first steps in the pathway for routine mRNA degradation. Binding of PABP to the poly-A tail prevents this from occurring. However, this activity does not require the interaction between PABP and eIF4F, the complex that interacts with the 7-methyl-guanosine on the 5' end of mRNA.

E is incorrect. The loss of interaction between the PABP and eIF4F, the complex that interacts with the 7-methyl-guanosine on the 5' end of mRNA, reduces initiation of translation. However, this interaction has no impact on the rate or efficiency of ribosomal translocation along the mRNA during translation.

10. Correct: C. Ribosome.

Like approximately half of all antibiotics, aminoglycosides target the bacterial ribosome to inhibit protein synthesis. Some aminoglycosides were found to also affect human ribosomes, reducing the fidelity of stop codon recognition. The new drug was developed to maximize this property, with the goal of "skipping" the premature termination codon in the child's dystrophin gene, and producing dystrophin protein. Answering this question correct would rely on recognition of the target of aminoglycoside antibiotics and/or understanding the need to resolve the problem created by the premature termination codon.

A is incorrect. Since the premature termination codon would trigger nonsense-mediated decay of the dystrophin produced by the mutated gene, there would be no dystrophin protein upon which the drug could act.

B is incorrect. Altering DNA polymerase activity would not solve the problem created by the premature stop codon.

D is incorrect. Many cases of Duchenne muscular dystrophy are caused, at the molecular level, by mutations that lead to defective splicing. However, the mutation for this child resulted in a premature termination codon and though scenarios are possible where altering splicing could result in excluding the exon containing the premature termination codon, this is not the best answer.

E is incorrect. Altering RNA polymerase activity would not solve the problem created by the premature stop codon.

11. Correct: E. Protein synthesis.

siRNAs are short (~ 20 nucleotides) RNAs that base-pair with specific sequences within target mRNAs, in this instance the mRNA for RAS. siRNAs result in degradation of the mRNAs and perhaps inhibition of translation as well. Either or both mechanisms will result in inhibition of new RAS protein synthesis.

A is incorrect. siRNAs designed to target RAS will not directly influence DNA synthesis.

B is incorrect. siRNAs designed to target RAS will not directly influence mRNA splicing.

C is incorrect. siRNAs designed to target RAS will not directly influence mRNA synthesis, though it may result in increased degradation of RAS mRNA.

D is incorrect. siRNAs designed to target RAS will not directly influence protein stability.

12. Correct: E. Reduced translation of GATA4 mRNA into protein.

The nucleotide sequence from -3 to +4, relative to the +1 AUG in an mRNA contains conserved sequences known in eukaryotes as the Kozak sequence. This sequence is required for efficient translational initiation from the associated AUG start codon. Mutation of this sequence can lead to inefficient translational initiation and reduced protein levels.

A is incorrect. Export of mRNA from the nucleus to the cytoplasm is required for translation into protein. However, the sequences surrounding the start codon are not involved in the export mechanisms.

B is incorrect. Polyadenylation of mRNA is required for stability, export, and efficient translation of an mRNA into protein. However, the sequences surrounding the start codon are not involved in the poly-adenylation mechanisms.

C is incorrect. Splicing of pre-mRNA into mature mRNA is required for generating the correct transcript to be translated into protein. However, the sequences surrounding the start codon are not involved in the splicing mechanisms.

D is incorrect. Genes must first be transcribed into RNA, and correctly processed, to ultimately be expressed as protein in a cell. However, the sequences surrounding the start codon are not involved in the transcriptional mechanisms, except in extremely rare cases where transcription regulatory DNA elements overlap the start codon.

13. Correct: A. Reduced availability of active eukaryotic initiation factor 2 alpha (eIF2alpha).

eIF2alpha is one subunit of a tripartite G-protein complex (consisting of α, β, and γ subunits) that binds methionyl-tRNA (and GTP), escorting the methionyl-tRNA to the small ribosome subunit to initiate translation. Once eIF2alpha releases the methionyl-tRNA, it hydrolyses GTP to GDP; it is inactive in the GDP-bound form. The guanosine nucleotide exchange factor eIF2B then exchanges GDP for GTP, regenerating active eIF2alpha (as shown in the figure in Answer 8). eIF2B consists of five protein subunits and mutations that lead to reduced activity in any one of the subunits can result in VWM syndrome. The episodic nature of the disease progression is due to the fact that the mutations in eIF2B reduce, but do not abolish, the GEF activity of the complex. It is only following induction of the unfolded protein response/endoplasmic reticulum stress response (e.g., from traumatic injury or infection) that the deficit in eIF2B function becomes apparent. Under stress, specific kinases phosphorylate eIF2alpha which prevents engagement of GDP-bound eIF2alpha with eIF2B; the interaction is necessary to swap GDP for GTP. As such, eIF2alpha remains in the inactive, GDP-bound form. This results in the cell ceasing most protein translation. Combining this inhibition with a mutated, ineffective eIF2B leads to much greater inhibition of protein translation than would occur with wild-type eIF2B, resulting in widespread cell death in the brain.

B is incorrect. VWM syndrome is caused by a mutation in any one of the five subunits of the guanine nucleotide exchange factor complex eIF2B, which leads to diminished activity of the complex. eIF2B is not involved in availability of cytosolic ribosomes.

C is incorrect. VWM syndrome is caused by a mutation in any one of the five subunits of the guanine nucleotide exchange factor complex eIF2B, which leads to diminished activity of the complex. eIF2B is not involved in binding of eukaryotic initiation factor 4F (eIF4F, cap-binding complex) to mRNA.

D is incorrect. VWM syndrome is caused by a mutation in any one of the five subunits of the guanine nucleotide exchange factor complex eIF2B, which leads to diminished activity of the complex. eIF2B is not involved in regulating the GTPase activity of EF2.

E is incorrect. VWM syndrome is caused by a mutation in any one of the five subunits of the guanine nucleotide exchange factor complex eIF2B, which leads to diminished activity of the complex. eIF2B is not involved in regulating transport of mRNA into the rough endoplasmic reticulum.

14. Correct: B. Blocks entry of 50S ribosomal subunit into the initiation complex.

Approximately one-half of all antibiotics inhibits protein translation. Linezolid is one of a class that works by preventing translational initiation. When the small ribosomal subunit (30S in bacteria) bound by methionyl-tRNA and initiation factors locates the start codon (AUG) on an mRNA, it pauses. At that point, the large ribosomal subunit (50S in bacteria) joins the complex, and the initiation factors are released. The complete ribosome (80S in bacteria) commences elongation. Linezolid binds to the 50S ribosomal subunit and prevents it from joining the 30S subunit bound to mRNA. As such, ribosomes that are currently translating mRNAs will complete the round of translation, but will be unable to reinitiate. This will eventually result in mRNAs in the cell being mostly devoid of bound ribosomes.

A is incorrect. If linezolid prevented translocation, the mRNAs would be found to be coated with stalled ribosomes. However, the mRNAs were found to be devoid of ribosomes indicating a block in initiation but none of the subsequent steps.

C is incorrect. Puromycin is the classic example of this type of antibiotic. It is not used clinically since it will inhibit translation by human ribosomes as well. If linezolid had this mechanism of action, the mRNAs would be expected to have ribosomes bound since they could continue to reinitiate translation.

D is incorrect. If linezolid inhibited the GTPase activity of elongation factors, the mRNAs would be found to be coated with stalled ribosomes. However, the mRNA were found to be devoid of ribosomes indicating a block in initiation but none of the subsequent steps.

E is incorrect. When a stop codon enters the "A" site of the ribosome, the peptide release factor binds to the site and disassembles the ribosome, releasing the newly synthesized protein. If linezolid inhibited release factor, the mRNAs would be found to be coated with stalled ribosomes. However, the mRNAs were found to be devoid of ribosomes indicating a block in initiation but none of the subsequent steps.

15. Correct: E. Large ribosomal subunit (60S in humans).

Shiga toxin is produced *Shigella dysenteriae* and Shiga-like toxins by shigatoxigenic strains of *E. coli* such as *E. coli* 0157:H7. Shiga toxins enter cells and then cleave a specific adenosine residue from the 28S rRNA present in the large ribosomal subunit, destroying the catalytic activity of the ribosome. The toxin ricin, derived from castor beans, works via a similar mechanism.

A is incorrect. Amino-acyl tRNA synthetases add amino acids to tRNA molecules. No known bacterial toxins function via inhibition of these enzymes.

B is incorrect. Toxins produced by some important pathogens such as *P. aeruginosa* and *Corynebacterium diphtheriae* catalyze ADP-ribosylation of protein translation EF2, inhibiting its function. *E. coli* 0157:H7 does not produce a toxin with this mechanism.

C is incorrect. Some viruses encode proteases that cleave subunits of initiation factor eIF4F (cap-binding complex), blocking cap-dependent protein translation. *E. coli* 0157:H7 does not produce a toxin with this mechanism.

D is incorrect. eIF2alpha escorts the initiator methionyl-tRNA to the small ribosomal subunit as part of the formation of the translational preinitiation complex. No known bacterial toxins function via inhibition of this protein.

16. Correct: C. RNA stability.

The figure in Question 16 shows an inverse relationship between the miRNA and the BCR/ABL mRNA levels. miRNAs anneal to complimentary sequences typically found in the 3'-untranslated regions of target mRNAs. Once bound, miRNAs (1) directly inhibit translation of the target mRNA and (2) recruit machinery to degrade target mRNA. So this particular miRNA is negative influencing the stability of the BCR/ABL mRNA.

A is incorrect. miRNAs do not directly regulate mRNA polyadenylation.

B is incorrect. miRNAs do not directly regulate RNA splicing.

D is incorrect. miRNAs do not directly regulate RNA synthesis.

E is incorrect. While miRNAs do directly inhibit translation of target mRNAs, the experimental data measured BCR/ABL mRNA levels, not protein levels. While it is possible that the decline in BCR/ABL mRNA leads to reduced protein expressed, no data supporting that possibility are presented.

17. Correct: B. 16S rRNA.

Streptomycin binds to and inhibits the small (30S) ribosomal subunit in bacteria. The rRNA component of the small ribosomal subunit is the 16S rRNA. As such, mutations in the 16S rRNA could potentially give rise to resistance to streptomycin (such mutations have been identified in streptomycin-resistant *Mycobacterium*).

A is incorrect. The 5S rRNA is a component of the large (50S) ribosomal subunit. Since streptomycin binds to and inhibits the small (30S) ribosomal subunit in bacteria, it is much less likely that mutations affecting the 50S ribosomal subunit would lead to resistance.

C is incorrect. The 23S rRNA is a component of the large (50S) ribosomal subunit. Since streptomycin binds to and inhibits the small (30S) ribosomal subunit in bacteria, it is much less likely that mutations affecting the 50S ribosomal subunit would lead to resistance.

D is incorrect. EF2 escorts amino-acyl tRNAs to the ribosome during protein synthesis. Since streptomycin binds to and inhibits the small (30S) ribosomal subunit in bacteria, mutations affecting EF2 are very unlikely to result in resistance.

E is incorrect. Bacterial initiation factor 2 (IF2) is analogous to the eukaryotic initiation factor 2 (eIF2), a tripartite G-protein that brings the initiator methionyl-tRNA to the ribosome during formation of the preinitiation complex. Since streptomycin binds to and inhibits the small (30S) ribosomal subunit in bacteria, mutations affecting IF2 are very unlikely to result in resistance.

18. Correct: D. Reduced activity of eukaryotic initiation factor 2 alpha (eIF2alpha).

Similar to the mechanism where protein kinase RNA-like endoplasmic reticulum kinase (PERK) is activated during the endoplasmic reticulum stress/unfolded protein response and phosphorylates the translational initiation factor eIF2alpha, a specific enzyme, heme-regulated eIF2alpha kinase (known as HRI) can phosphorylate eIF2alpha. This results in the cell ceasing most protein translation; in this case translation of mRNAs coding for α- and β-globin is reduced.

A is incorrect. miRNAs base-pair with specific mRNA targets and reduce their translation efficiency and/or destabilize the mRNA. Since, in this scenario, the levels of globin protein are low, if a miRNA was involved, one would expect to observe an increase in a specific miRNA.

B is incorrect. Acetylation of histones within nucleosomes associated with a gene is protranscriptional. However, the heme-dependent regulation is not at the level of transcription, since mRNA levels for globin proteins do not vary regardless of heme concentration.

C is incorrect. Increased DNA methylation is associated with long-term silencing of gene transcription. However, the heme-dependent regulation is not at the level of transcription, since mRNA levels for globin proteins do not vary regardless of heme concentration.

E is incorrect. The availability of the complex that binds the 7-methyl-guanosine cap (eIF4G) can be regulated to globally affect protein translation. However, that is not the regulatory mechanism used by heme to affect globin protein synthesis.

Chapter 17

Cell Stress and Death

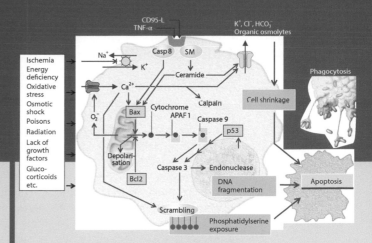

LEARNING OBJECTIVES

▶ Discuss the pathways activated during apoptosis and describe the molecular events in intrinsic and extrinsic pathways.

▶ Describe the conditions under which the unfolded protein response is activated and describe the pathways activated at the molecular level to maintain protein homeostasis.

▶ Summarize the cell's response to reperfusion injury emphasizing how reperfusion can exacerbate injury produced by ischemia.

▶ Describe the cellular homeostasis mechanisms activated following DNA damage by physical or chemical insult.

▶ Describe the cellular homeostasis mechanisms activated under hypoxic conditions.

▶ Describe the cellular homeostasis mechanisms activated under nutritional stress.

▶ List the major proto-oncogenes and tumor suppressor genes and describe their contribution to neoplastic transformation.

17.1 Questions

Easy	Medium	Hard

1. Despite the fact that about half of all patients newly diagnosed with breast cancer receive radiation therapy, not all patients derive benefit since some breast cancers are resistant to these treatments. A loss-of-function mutation that results in an inactive version of which of the following proteins is most likely to be associated with resistance to radiation therapy?

A. BRCA1 (breast cancer–associated 1)

B. MYC (v-myc avian myelocytomatosis viral oncogene homolog)

C. p53 (tumor protein 53)

D. RAS (Ras proto-oncogene, GTPase)

E. HER2 (human epidermal growth factor receptor 2)

2. A 4-year-old girl is brought to the urgent care center following 24 hours of severe diarrhea, abdominal pain, and vomiting. Her fever is 37.8°C. Her mother explains that several other children at the girl's daycare have come down with similar symptoms. You suspect it is norovirus and you recommend bed rest and hydration with pediatric electrolyte drinks. In response to the viral infection, cytotoxic T cells (Tc) are targeting infected cells through multiple mechanisms. One such mechanism involves the engagement of Fas ligand (FasL) on the surface of the Tc cells with the cognate receptor on infected cells, presenting viral antigens through major histocompatibility complex, class I. Which of the following events will occur in infected cells with the Fas ligand receptor engaged by FasL?

A. Activation of ataxia-telangiectasia mutated (ATM) kinase

B. Activation of caspase enzymes

C. Activation of cell cycle arrest

D. Release of cellular contents due to loss of membrane integrity

E. Release of cytochrome C by the mitochondria

3. A 54-year-old man was referred to you on the gastrointestinal service with a chief complaint of abdominal discomfort and tarry stool. Abdominal computed tomography (CT) revealed a soft tissue mass approximately 6 cm in diameter in his left upper abdominal quadrant. The mass has a necrotic center which you suspect is due to lack of oxygen reaching the cells in the middle of the tumor, given that the mass has poor vascularization. Which of the following changes would you predict to have occurred in any of the living cells near the necrotic interior of the tumor?

A. Decreased levels of glycolytic enzymes

B. Decreased vascular endothelial growth factor (VEGF) expression

C. Increased global protein translation

D. Increased pyruvate to acetyl-CoA conversion

E. Increased stability of the hypoxia-induced factor-1α (HIF-1α) transcription factor protein

4. An 87-year old male patient presents with a chief complaint of "my memory is shot." Following taking his history and completing physical examination, you diagnose him with moderate cognitive impairment. Recently, you read in a published report that levels of heat shock proteins (HSPs) in cells, particularly neurons on the central nervous system, declines as people age. This phenomenon may contribute to which of the following underlying pathophysiologic mechanisms related to this patient's cognitive impairment?

A. Cellular DNA integrity

B. Cellular energy production

C. Cellular membrane integrity

D. Cellular mitosis regulation

E. Cellular protein homeostasis

5. As a strategy to treat cancer, a small interfering RNA (siRNA) that targets the gene products of X-linked inhibitor of apoptosis protein (XIAP) was introduced into a cell line established from a small cell lung cancer tumor. After exposing the cells to radiation, investigators extracted genomic DNA from the cells and analyzed it by gel electrophoresis. They observed degradation of genomic DNA, visible as a "ladder" of DNA bands. The lengths of the fragments were multiples of approximately 200 base pairs in both samples, though the intensity was different in the cells treated with siRNA targeted to XIAP in comparison to cells that did not receive siRNA (as shown in the figure below). Which of the following cellular processes do the products of the *XIAP* gene likely inhibit?

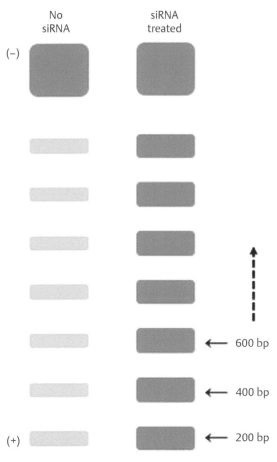

A. Apoptosis
B. DNA replication
C. Mitosis
D. Transcription
E. Translation

Consider the following case for questions 6 and 7.

A 28-month-old boy, recently emigrated from Syria as part of a refugee relocation, is brought to your clinic by his mother as a new patient. His mother relates a medical history including delayed walking (21 months), ataxic gait with frequent falls, and delayed speech characterized by dysarthria. The boy has had many respiratory and ear infections and psychomotor delay but his somatic growth was otherwise normal. On examination, florid bulbar conjunctiva telangiectasia was visible bilaterally (as shown in the figure in Question 7).

6. In addition to the current issues the child faces, he also has an increased risk of which of the following diseases, due to his genetic mutation?

A. Aneurysms
B. Coronary artery disease
C. Diabetes mellitus
D. Leukemia
E. Rheumatoid arthritis

7. Excessive exposure to which of the following medical imaging techniques might be best avoided for this patient?

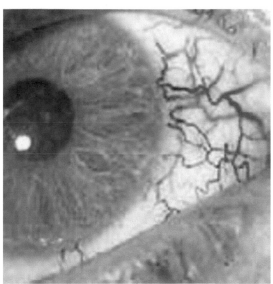

Source: Passarge E. Color Atlas of Genetics. 4th Edition. 2012.

A. Computed tomography
B. Magnetic resonance imaging (MRI)
C. Positron emission tomography (PET)
D. Ultrasound

8. A 23-year-old, male, African-American medical student is preparing for an upcoming medical mission in Nicaragua over spring break. He is prescribed mefloquine to take prior to and during the trip as a prophylactic against malaria. Prior to filling his prescription, he reads in the news that mefloquine might be associated with neurologic side effects. He mentions this to a resident in the clinic. The resident says he can write Mr. Hughes a prescription for a different drug, primaquine. The student fills the primaquine prescription at a very busy pharmacy and begins taking the pills that day. The following day he feels tired and skips his workout at the gym. He is alarmed when he sees his urine appears very dark and schedules an appointment at the student health clinic. After hearing his history and reviewing his medications, the physician in the clinic suspects the student may have a glucose-6-phosphate dehydrogenase deficiency (G6PD). A deficit in which of the following metabolites in his red blood cells accounts for this student's symptoms?

A. Adenosine triphosphate

B. Flavin adenine dinucleotide (FAD)

C. Glucose

D. Iron

E. Nicotinamide adenine dinucleotide phosphate, reduced (NADPH)

9. Following hypoxic brain injury due to ischemia, additional neuronal death can occur following restoration of blood flow (reperfusion). Cellular stress response pathways, including persistent activation of c-jun N-terminal kinase (JNK), are associated with ischemia-reperfusion cell death. Testing of an inhibitor of JNK in a rodent model of ischemia reperfusion revealed increased survival of neurons and reduced decline in postinjury functional deficits. Which one of the following events was elevated in the neurons of animals treated with the JNK inhibitor, versus those untreated, during ischemia reperfusion?

A. Apoptosome formation

B. Bcl2 activity

C. Pro-caspase cleavage

D. Cytochrome C release

E. DNA fragmentation

10. A 24-year old woman has come to your clinic with a chief complaint of "help deciding to take the test for Huntington's disease." She is the only child of a mother aged 48 and a father aged 51. Five years ago, her mother was diagnosed with Huntington's disease, an autosomal dominant congenital disease that destroys neurons in the basal ganglia of the brain causing progressive deterioration. The disease is caused by an expansion of a trinucleotide repeat in the protein coding region of the huntingtin (*HTT*) gene, expanding a tract of glutamine residues in the encoded protein, resulting in aggregation of the protein. In neurons expressing the huntingtin protein with the expanded glutamine tracts, which of the following events most directly results in the death of the neurons within the basal ganglia of Huntington's patients?

A. Decreased transport of proteins out of the endoplasmic reticulum

B. Decrease in almost all protein translation

C. Increased expression of chaperone proteins within the endoplasmic reticulum

D. Increased expression/activity of specific transcription factors

E. Increased phosphorylation of translational initiation factors

17.2 Answers and Explanations

Easy	Medium	Hard

1. Correct: C. p53 (tumor protein 53).

p53 (tumor protein 53) is a tumor suppressor protein that is activated by DNA damage, including DNA damage produced by ionizing radiation. Activated p53 produces cell cycle arrest and, if damage is significant, can activate pathways leading to apoptosis (as shown in the figure on the next page). Loss of p53 would lead to severely reduced or absent induction of apoptosis in cancer cells exposed to radiation, reducing its effectiveness in the treatment of cancer.

A is incorrect. Loss of BRCA1 (breast cancer–associated 1), either through inherited or spontaneous

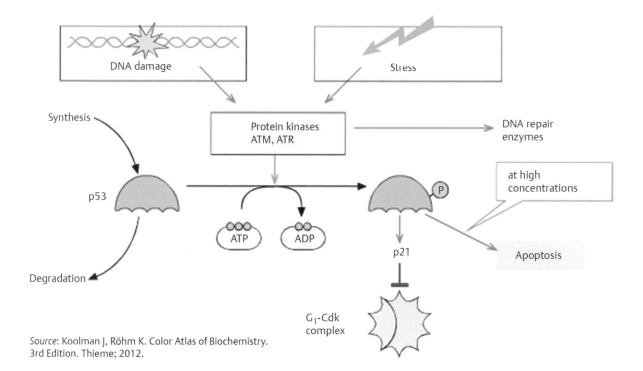

Source: Koolman J, Röhm K. Color Atlas of Biochemistry. 3rd Edition. Thieme; 2012.

mutation, disables specific DNA repair pathways. This would, in general, make cells more sensitive to radiation therapy.

B is incorrect. MYC (v-myc avian myelocytomatosis viral oncogene homolog) is a proto-oncogene that is overexpressed (via multiple mechanisms) in many cancers, thus gain of function is associated with its cancer-causing ability. Loss of MYC is not associated with carcinogenesis.

D is incorrect. RAS (Ras proto-oncogene, GTPase) is a proto-oncogene that typically has specific, single amino acid substitutions in many cancers that result in gain of function. Loss of RAS is not associated with carcinogenesis.

E is incorrect. HER2 (human epidermal growth factor receptor 2) is a proto-oncogene that typically has specific, single amino acid substitutions in several cancers (particularly breast cancers) that result in gain of function. Loss of HER2 is not associated with carcinogenesis.

2. Correct: B. Activation of caspase enzymes.

Binding of the FasL on the surface of T cells to the Fas receptor (FasR) induces the extrinsic pathway of apoptosis (as shown in the figure on the next page).

This involves cleavage of initiator pro-caspases (pro-caspase 8) to the enzymatically active caspase 8. Caspases are protease enzymes that cleave at a motif containing two aspartic residues in target proteins. Caspase 8 cleaves effector pro-caspases 3, which then carries out degradation of cellular proteins and other effector enzymes (including caspases 6 and 7) to achieve apoptosis.

A is incorrect. The ATM kinase is not activated FasL engaging the FasR. ATM is activated by double-stranded DNA breaks.

C is incorrect. Activation of the FasR does not specifically inhibit cell cycle arrest, rather causing the death of the cell via apoptosis.

D is incorrect. Apoptosis is programmed cell death, that is a specific, ordered process. A key feature of apoptosis is the fragmentation of cells into smaller, membrane-encased components that does not induce inflammation. Loss of membrane integrity and release of cellular contents is characteristic of cell death by necrosis.

E is incorrect. Release of cytochrome C by the mitochondria occurs in the intrinsic pathway of apoptosis activation (as shown in the figure on the next page).

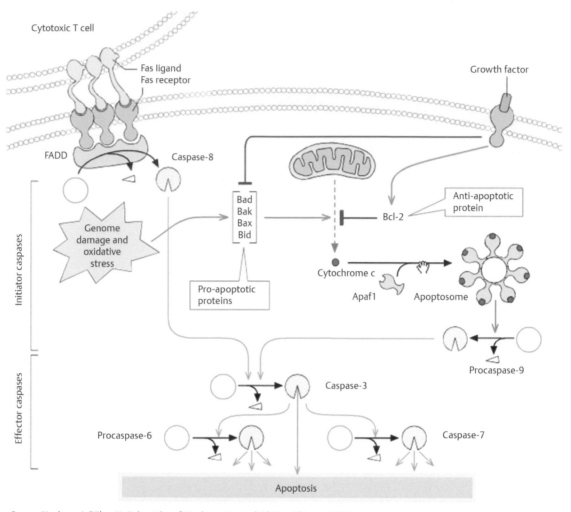

Source: Koolman J, Röhm K. Color Atlas of Biochemistry. 3rd Edition. Thieme; 2012.

3.   Correct: E. Increased stability of the hypoxia-induced factor-1a (HIF-1a) transcription factor protein.

Under normoxic conditions, specific proline and asparagine residues in the HIF-1α transcription factor are hydroxylated by enzymes requiring oxygen and α-ketoglutarate, an intermediate of the citric acid cycle (both are indicators of oxidative metabolism) (as shown the figure on the next page). The hydroxylated residues are bound by the von Hippel–Lindau (VHL) protein which leads to the degradation of HIF-1α. Hypoxia results in decreased proline and asparagine hydroxylation of HIF-1α and loss of binding by the VHL protein. This stabilizes HIF-1α, which then translocates to the nucleus and, along with HIF-1β, binds to DNA targets in the genome and regulates transcription of appropriate target genes to respond to the low-oxygen conditions.

A is incorrect. One cellular response to hypoxia is increased expression and activity of glycolytic enzymes (the transcription of which is induced by HIF-1α) to help maintain sufficient adenosine triphosphate (ATP) production in the absence of respiratory metabolism.

B is incorrect. Chronic hypoxia can result in increased production of VEGF by affected cells as a long-term adaptation to increase blood supply and, presumably, oxygen availability.

C is incorrect. Hypoxia can induce the endoplasmic reticulum stress response, which results in inhibition of global protein synthesis.

D is incorrect. Under hypoxic conditions, conversion of pyruvate to acetyl-CoA is inhibited and conversion of pyruvate to lactate increases to regenerate nicotinamide adenine dinucleotide oxidized (NAD^+).

4.   Correct: E. Cellular protein homeostasis.

HSPs are protein chaperones and chaperonins involved in ensuring and maintaining protein folding. Chaperones protect newly synthesized unfolded proteins as they emerge from the ribosome and help them fold into its proper tertiary structure. They can also interact with unfolded proteins to refold them into their correct structure. Chaperonins are barrel-shaped channels with two compartments that admit unfolded proteins and catalyze their folding in an ATP-dependent manner. With fewer HSPs available, protein homeostasis is disrupted with subsequent negative effects on cellular function. In the case of the patient, this may be contributing neuronal dysfunction or death, leading to his cognitive impairment.

A is incorrect. Lower levels of HSPs may indirectly influence cellular DNA integrity, but it is the general negative effect on cellular protein homeostasis that is the basic cellular dysfunction.

B is incorrect. Lower levels of HSPs may indirectly influence cellular energy production, but it is the general negative effect on cellular protein homeostasis that is the basic cellular dysfunction.

C is incorrect. Lower levels of HSPs may indirectly influence cellular membrane integrity, but it is the general negative effect on cellular protein homeostasis that is the basic cellular dysfunction.

D is incorrect. Lower levels of HSPs may indirectly influence cellular mitosis regulation, but it is the general negative effect on cellular protein homeostasis that is the basic cellular dysfunction.

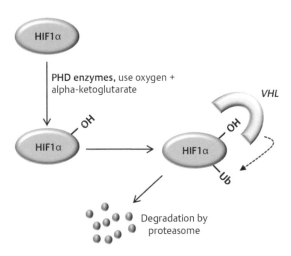

5. Correct: A. Apoptosis.

XIAP binds to and inhibits caspases, the proteolytic enzymes involved in signaling and execution of apoptosis. XIAP is an E3 ubiquitin ligase that ubiquitinates caspases, targeting them for protein degradation by the proteasome. siRNAs are short RNAs that base-pair and lead to the degradation of their messenger RNA (mRNA) targets. Therefore, an siRNA that specifically targets XIAP would result in less XIAP protein in the cell. This, in turn, would produce higher levels of apoptosis following exposure of cells to radiation. The mechanisms of apoptosis includes activation of nucleases that degrade DNA. The approximately 200 base pair ladder is characteristic of DNA degradation during apoptosis, reflecting the fact that the DNA between adjacent nucleosomes is preferentially degraded, leaving the approximately 200 base pairs of DNA that wrap around the nucleosomal particles mostly intact. Since inhibition of XIAP by siRNA resulted in more cells going through apoptosis, the size/intensity of the bands in the DNA ladder is greater.

B is incorrect. XIAP does not directly affect DNA replication.

C is incorrect. XIAP does not directly affect mitosis.

D is incorrect. XIAP does not directly affect transcription.

E is incorrect. XIAP does not directly affect translation.

6. Correct: D. Leukemia.

The child has ataxia-telangiectasia (A-T), which is caused by a mutation in the ataxia-telangiectasia mutated (*ATM*) gene which codes for a protein kinase. The ATM kinase is activated by DNA double-strand breaks and initiates an integrated response including cell cycle arrest (through p53 activation) and DNA repair mechanisms. The deficit in DNA repair response is responsible for the deficits of A-T and an elevated risk of cancers (~ 25% lifetime risk) and in particular leukemias and lymphomas.

A is incorrect. Individuals with A-T do not have a specific, elevated risk of aneurysms.

B is incorrect. Individuals with A-T do not have a specific, elevated risk of coronary artery disease.

C is incorrect. Individuals with A-T do not have a specific, elevated risk of diabetes mellitus.

E is incorrect. Individuals with A-T do not have a specific, elevated risk of rheumatoid arthritis. They do have immune defects which is consistent with the child's repeated respiratory and ear infections.

7. A. Computed tomography.

CT utilizes X-rays which is a type of ionizing radiation. Such radiation will produce double-stranded DNA breaks. People with A-T lack the ATM kinase which is activated by DNA double-strand breaks and initiates an integrated response including cell cycle arrest (through p53 activation) and DNA repair mechanisms. CT and X-rays are used with A-T patients when necessary, but it is possible that excessive use might elevate a patient's risk of cancer more so than an individual without A-T.

B is incorrect. MRI does not expose an individual to radiation and does not damage DNA.

C is incorrect. The most common form of PET employs a positron emitting tracer, fluorodeoxyglucose (^{18}F-FDG). However, this type of radiation does not appear to cause significant DNA damage.

D is incorrect. Ultrasound does not expose an individual to radiation and does not damage DNA.

8. Correct: E. Nicotinamide adenine dinucleotide phosphate, reduced (NADPH).

The medical student has a G6PD deficiency. Approximately 10 to 15% of African-American men (the gene is found on the X chromosome) have a variant G6PD isoenzyme with reduced activity. Oxidative stress (in this case the drug primaquine) generates free radicals which are scavenged by glutathione in erythrocytes. With the medical student, his erythrocyte glutathione was depleted, leading to hemoglobin denaturation and precipitation from the nonscavenged free radicals, producing anemia. When glutathione is oxidized by a free radical, it can be reduced subsequently by NADPH, which is converted to NADP$^+$ in the process. NADPH is generated by either mitochondrial-based pathways or by the pentose phosphate shunt (also called the phosphogluconate pathway), which generates ribose and NADPH. The pentose phosphate shunt requires the action of glucose-6-phosphate. Since erythrocytes lack mitochondria, they are fully dependent on the pentose phosphate shunt to regenerate NADPH. Since the medical student has a defective version of G6PD, he cannot regenerate NADPH efficiently, leading to oxidative destruction of his red blood cells.

A is incorrect. Low ATP is not responsible for the medical student's anemia.

B is incorrect. Low FAD is not responsible for the medical student's anemia.

C is incorrect. Low glucose is not responsible for the medical student's anemia.

D is incorrect. Low iron is not responsible for the medical student's anemia.

9.   Correct: B. Bcl2 activity.

JNK is activated by cellular stresses including inflammatory mediators (cytokines and chemokines) and physical or chemical stressors (e.g., reactive oxygen species). Like essentially all cell stress response pathways, JNK increases activity of both prosurvival and proapoptotic responses. Very high and/or persistent activation of JNK results in the proapoptotic pathways succeeds in initiating programmed cell death. Activation of the intrinsic pathway of apoptosis by JNK (or other effectors) involves the activation of proapoptotic proteins (Bad, Bak, Bax, Bid) and *inhibition* of the antiapoptotic protein Bcl2 (as shown in the figure in Answer 2). The proapoptotic proteins cause release of cytochrome C from mitochondria (Bcl2 normally inhibits this release), which leads to formation of the apoptosome, a higher-order structure constructed of subunits of the Apaf1 protein. The apoptosome activates the initiator pro-caspase 9, which then cleaves and activates downstream effector caspases. JNK activity of the magnitude that initiates apoptosis would normally inhibit Bcl2 activity; treatment of animals with an inhibitor of JNK during ischemia reperfusion would result in elevated Bcl2 activity compared to the nontreated animals.

A is incorrect. Formation of the higher-order apoptosome from Apaf1 protein subunits is a key event in the intrinsic apoptosis pathway (as shown in the figure in Answer 2). Inhibition of JNK would result in reduced apoptosome formation during ischemia reperfusion in comparison to the nontreated animals.

C is incorrect. Pro-caspases are inactive until cleaved into their active, proapoptotic form (as shown in the figure with Answer 2). Inhibition of JNK would result in reduced pro-caspase cleavage during ischemia reperfusion in comparison to the nontreated animals. Inhibition of JNK would result in reduced apoptosome formation during ischemia reperfusion in comparison to the nontreated animals.

D is incorrect. Cytochrome C release from mitochondria initiates events in the intrinsic apoptosis pathway (as shown in the figure with Answer 2). Inhibition of JNK would result in reduced cytochrome C release during ischemia reperfusion in comparison to the nontreated animals.

E is incorrect. DNA fragmentation into fragments that are multiples of approximately 200 base pairs is a hallmark of apoptosis (as shown in the figure in Question 5). Inhibition of JNK would result in reduced DNA fragmentation during ischemia reperfusion in comparison to the nontreated animals.

10.   Correct: D. Increased expression/activity of specific transcription factors.

The aggregations of mutant huntingtin protein result from the incorrect folding of huntingtin due to the expanded glutamine tracts. Unfolded huntingtin will activate the unfolded protein response (UPR; also referred to as the endoplasmic reticulum stress response [ERSR]). The UPR/ERSR has multiple signaling branches involving increased activation of specific transcription factors and inhibition of most protein translation (but not of the factors necessary for the UPR/ERSR and for apoptosis) due to phosphorylation of a translational initiation factor. Persistent activation of the UPR/ERSR, as occurs with the continuous presence of the unfolded mutant huntingtin, ultimately results in the activation of apoptosis. Apoptosis is driven by the accumulation over time of a specific transcription factor, C/EBP homologous protein (CHOP), which activates the apoptotic program.

A is incorrect. Decreased transport of proteins out of the endoplasmic reticulum does occur during the UPR/ERSR but is not a direct driver of apoptotic pathways.

B is incorrect. Phosphorylation of eukaryotic initiation factor 2 alpha (eIF2alpha) by PERK kinase leads to a global decline in protein translation with the exception of factors necessary for the UPR/ERSR and apoptosis. However, decreased protein translation during UPR/ERSR is not a direct driver of apoptotic pathways.

C is incorrect. Increased expression of chaperone proteins within the endoplasmic reticulum does occur during the UPR/ERSR but is not a direct driver of apoptotic pathways.

E is incorrect. Increased phosphorylation of translational initiation factors does occur during the UPR/ERSR but is not a direct driver of apoptotic pathways.

Chapter 18

Biochemical and Molecular Techniques

LEARNING OBJECTIVES

▶ Outline the steps of the polymerase chain reaction (PCR) and reverse transcriptase quantitative PCR and defend the choice of these methods when used in a diagnostic clinical test.

▶ Outline the steps of assays based on antibody–antigen recognition (Western blot and enzyme-linked immunosorbent assay [ELISA]) and defend the choice of these assays in a diagnostic clinical test.

▶ Explain the potential utility of information obtained via gene expression profiling by microarray or RNA sequencing in clinical diagnosis.

▶ Defend the choice of DNA sequencing when used in a diagnostic clinical test.

▶ Describe the type of information available from how high-throughput sequencing (next-generation sequencing) and explain how it might be used in prognosis, diagnosis, therapy, and risk assessment.

▶ Discuss the use of transgenic mice to model human disease, citing their strengths and weaknesses.

▶ Explain how recombinant DNA techniques allow production of proteins used in medical therapies.

18.1 Questions

Easy	Medium	Hard

1. A 27-year-old man presents at a local free clinic with a chief complaint of "white patches" on his tongue. Taking his history, you determine that he is an intravenous drug user with a history of homelessness. You suspect his candidiasis may be the result of immune dysfunction secondary to infection with human immunodeficiency virus (HIV). A rapid, in-office test indicates he is HIV positive. To confirm this test, you order a Western blot that will utilize the patient's serum as part of the procedure. Which of the following describes the manner in which the patient's serum is used in the Western blot procedure?

A. RNA is extracted from the serum and converted to complementary DNA (cDNA)

B. Serial dilutions of the serum are coated onto plastic wells in a 96-well plate

C. The serum is allowed to hybridize to HIV proteins bound to a filter paper

D. The serum is separated on a denaturing gel sodium dodecyl sulfate polyacrylamide gel electrophoresis (SDS-PAGE)

E. The serum is separated on a nondenaturing gel (agarose gel electrophoresis)

2. A male infant was born to a HIV-infected mother who received no prenatal care or prophylactic antiretroviral therapy to prevent transmission of the virus to the child in utero. The infant tested positive for HIV and a decision made to immediately begin aggressive, antiretroviral therapy. Following the child longitudinally, at 30 months, it appeared that his viral load had dropped below the level of detection. A detection method based on which of the following technical methods would provide the strongest evidence to support this remarkable claim?

A. Enzyme-linked immunosorbent assay

B. Viral enzyme activity assay

C. Polymerase chain reaction

D. Western blot

E. Northern blot

3. A new diagnostic test has been proposed to assess colon cancer risk by measuring changes in gene expression in intestinal epithelial cells present in fecal samples. The number of cells in a given fecal sample is very small, numbering in the hundreds. In the test, the expression level of a specific gene is measured and compared to a standardized, normal control sample. Which of the following technical approaches is best suited to measure the expression levels of the five genes in this diagnostic assay?

A. Enzyme-linked immunosorbent assay

B. Gene expression profiling by high-throughput RNA sequencing

C. Quantitative real-time reverse transcriptase polymerase chain reaction (qRT-PCR)

D. Western blot

E. Whole genome sequencing

4. You have obtained surgical samples from patients with hepatocellular carcinoma (HCC) undergoing liver resection with perihepatic lymphadenectomy. You hope to study these samples to understand why lymph node metastases from primary HCC is relatively low, in comparison to other cancers such as lung cancer, renal cancer, gastric cancer, and intrahepatic cholangiocarcinoma. To address this problem, you wish to identify genes that are differentially expressed when comparing the primary HCC to the HCC cells that have metastasized to perihepatic lymph nodes. Which of the following techniques would be most appropriate to achieve the goals of your planned study?

A. Gene expression profiling (microarray)

B. Enzyme-linked immunosorbent assay

C. Western blot

D. Quantitative real-time reverse transcriptase polymerase chain reaction

E. Whole genome sequencing

Consider the following case for questions 5 and 6:

A 72-year-old female patient is referred to a regional comprehensive cancer center for treatment of her recently diagnosed metastatic colorectal cancer. In addition to irinotecan with fluorouracil (5FU) and folinic acid (FOLFIRI) for her first-line treatment, the oncologist considers including cetuximab (Erbitux). The prescribing information for cetuximab includes the notation that it should be used for "...*K-Ras* wild-type, EGFR-expressing, tumors...." *K-Ras* mutations found in cancers typically result in single amino acid substitutions. They can occur at dierent amino acid positions, though a given tumor generally only has one such amino acid substitution in each *K-Ras* gene.

5. A Food and Drud Administration (FDA)-approved, diagnostic test employing which of the following techniques would be the best approach to determine the status of the *K-Ras* gene in biopsy material from this patient's tumors?

A. Enzyme-linked immunosorbent assay

B. Gene expression profiling by microarray

C. Gene expression profiling by high-throughput RNA sequencing

D. Sanger DNA sequencing

E. Whole genome sequencing

6. An FDA-approved, diagnostic test employing which of the following techniques would be the best approach to determine whether the patient's tumors express protein from the *EGFR* gene?

A. Enzyme-linked immunosorbent assay

B. Gene expression profiling by microarray

C. Gene expression profiling by high-throughput RNA sequencing

D. Sanger DNA sequencing

E. Whole genome sequencing

7. A 61-year-old woman presents in your outpatient clinic with a chief complaint of persistent fatigue and occasional blurry vision. Upon examination and history, you determine she has weakness in her right leg that has caused her to stumble occasionally. Following additional diagnostic tests, you prepare a treatment plan which includes a weekly intramuscular injection of interferon (IFN) β-1a (IFN-β-1a). Which of the following was necessary for production and manufacture of a recombinant version of this drug?

A. Biochemical isolation of IFN-β-1a from bovine tissue

B. Cloning of the cDNA for IFN-β-1a

C. Identification of a hybridoma producing a monoclonal antibody against IFN-β-1a

D. Isolation of a small molecule that mimics the binding of IFN-β-1a to its receptor

E. Polymerase chain reaction amplification of the gene encoding IFN-β-1a

8. Tissue samples from a patient with cutaneous melanoma, including the primary lesion as well as adjacent, normal tissue were analyzed for the presence of a mutation in the gene *B-Raf* proto-oncogene, serine/threonine kinase encoding the BRAF protein. The most common driver mutation in BRAF found in melanoma cells is a gain-of-function mutation where aspartic is substituted for valine at amino acid position 600 (BRAF-V600E). In the normal tissue of this patient, only the normal BRAF was detected; in the melanoma, both the normal and BRAF-V600E alleles were detected. The raw data from the clinical laboratory test are shown in the figure below. Given the nature of these data, which of the following techniques was employed in the clinical laboratory to analyze the melanoma and adjacent normal tissue?

A. Gene expression profiling by microarray

B. Northern blot

C. Quantitative real-time reverse transcriptase polymerase chain reaction

D. Western blot with polyclonal antibody recognizing entire BRAF protein

E. Whole genome sequencing

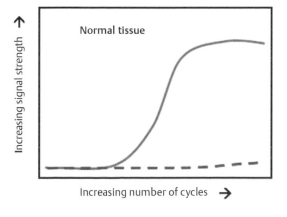

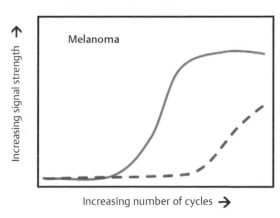

9. A 55-year-old man with dysphagia and a mediastinal mass was referred to a regional comprehensive cancer center for assessment and treatment. Computed tomography with oral and intravenous contrast medium revealed a soft tissue mass (~ 5 cm diameter) adjacent to the distal esophagus and significant, wide spread lymphadenopathy, and numerous small (~ ≤ 1 cm) nodules in the left lung. He consented to be enrolled in a clinical trial to expand his treatment options. The approach of the trial is to identify the full range of gene mutations that are present in biopsied tumor tissue as part of a cancer genomics study. The benefit to the patient is that identified mutations in specific genes may allow application of currently available mutation-targeted therapies. Which of the following technical approaches would provide the most comprehensive, nonbiased approach to cataloging all mutations in the DNA isolated from this patient's tumors?

A. Gene expression profiling by high-throughput RNA sequencing

B. Gene expression profiling by microarray

C. Quantitative real-time reverse transcriptase polymerase chain reaction

D. Sanger DNA sequencing

E. Whole genome sequencing

10. A recent study claimed to demonstrate a link between global changes in alternative splicing of mRNA and an elevated risk of schizophrenia. Planning a large-scale study to confirm these results, a research group will collect postmortem tissue samples from the frontal lobe and the CA1 region of the hypothalamus, from patients who died with schizophrenia and age-matched controls who died in the absence of mental illness. The investigators wish to assess the expression levels of tens of thousands of mRNA splice variants in these two samples. Which of the following technical approaches is most useful to achieve this goal?

A. Gene expression profiling by high-throughput RNA sequencing

B. Quantitative real-time reverse transcriptase polymerase chain reaction

C. Sanger DNA sequencing

D. Western blot

E. Whole genome sequencing

Consider the following case for questions 11 and 12:

Friedreich's ataxia is an autosomal recessive disease is most commonly caused by the expansion of a trinucleotide repeat (GAA) in the first intron of the frataxin gene. This results in a loss-of-function mutation due to the expansion causing silencing expression of the frataxin. The next two questions address two different patients suspected of having Friedreich's ataxia.

11. The differential diagnosis of a 26-year-old man with progressive limb and gait ataxia included Friedreich's ataxia. A PCR assay was performed, using DNA from the patient and both his parents and his healthy 39-year-old sister as template. The PCR primers flanked the location of the intronic GAA repeats. The PCR products were subjected to agarose gel electrophoresis and the DNA in the gel visualized by fluorescent stain. Assuming the patient has Friedreich's ataxia, which of the following marked lanes in the gel represent the PCR on the DNA sample from the patient?

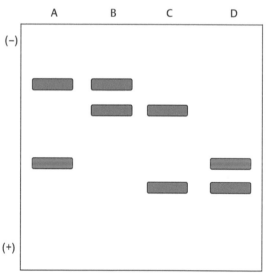

A. A

B. B

C. C

D. D

12. Another patient, this time a 29-year-old female patient, is suspected of also having Friedreich's ataxia. The same PCR-based test was performed on her DNA and the DNA of both her parents (she is an only child). The agarose gel electrophoresis of these reactions is shown in the figure below. Based on neuroimaging, physical examination, and history, you are very confident the patient has Friedreich's ataxia. Based on the outcome of the PCR-based test, additional testing based on which of the following techniques, would you request to define the genetic cause of this patient's Friedreich's ataxia?

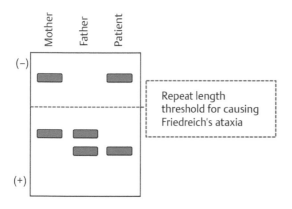

A. Gene expression profiling by high-throughput RNA sequencing

B. Quantitative real-time reverse transcriptase polymerase chain reaction

C. Sanger DNA sequencing

D. Western blot

E. Whole genome sequencing

18.2 Answers and Explanations

Easy	Medium	Hard

1. Correct: C. The serum is allowed to hybridize to HIV proteins bound to a filter paper.

The serum is allowed to hybridize **to HIV proteins bound to a filter paper.** The patient's serum contains antibodies directed against proteins expressed by HIV. In the Western blot technique, proteins are size-separated by denaturing SDS-PAGE and transferred to nylon membrane. In this specific case, proteins from HIV are separated on the gel and transferred to the membrane. The patient's serum is allowed to hybridize to the proteins bound to the filter paper, that is, the patient's serum provides the primary antibody in the Western detection assay. Antibodies against HIV proteins will only be in the serum if the patient's immune system has been exposed to the virus. Following extensive washing, a secondary antibody is added which specifically binds to human immunoglobulin. The secondary antibody is "tagged"; it has a detection reagent covalently bound to it, either a fluorescent moiety or an enzyme that can cleave a light-producing or colorimetric substrate. The signal is visualized either directly (colorimetric) or through electronic detection (light or fluorescence). If the patient's serum lacks antibodies against HIV, no signal will be detected.

A is incorrect. Western blot assays for proteins, not RNA.

B is incorrect. The step described is used in some types of ELISA but not Western blot.

D is incorrect. The patient's serum is used in solution to probe (hybridize) viral proteins immobilized on nylon filter paper. The serum proteins are not run on a gel.

E is incorrect. The patient's serum is used in solution to probe (hybridize) viral proteins immobilized on nylon filter paper. The serum proteins are not run on a gel. Nondenaturing agarose gels are primarily used for separating nucleic acids, and typically are not used for proteins.

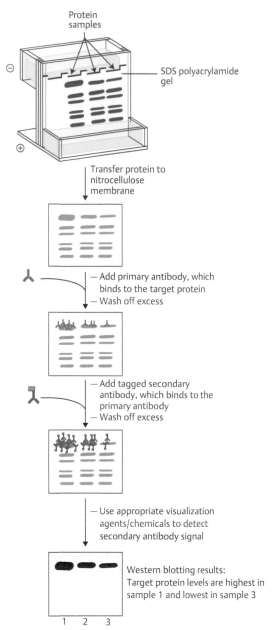

Protein samples

SDS polyacrylamide gel

⊖

⊕

Transfer protein to nitrocellulose membrane

— Add primary antibody, which binds to the target protein
— Wash off excess

— Add tagged secondary antibody, which binds to the primary antibody
— Wash off excess

— Use appropriate visualization agents/chemicals to detect secondary antibody signal

Western blotting results: Target protein levels are highest in sample 1 and lowest in sample 3

1   2   3

Source: Panini S. Medical Biochemistry - An Illustrated Review. 1st Edition. Thieme; 2013.

2. Correct: C. Polymerase chain reaction.

PCR is an exquisitely sensitive method for detecting nucleic acids in biological samples. The technique amplifies DNA through a repeated series of specifically primed DNA synthesis reactions that result in exponential increases in the amount of the amplified product. Even a single copy of the viral RNA converted to cDNA or a proviral DNA integrated into the genome of the infected infant would be detected by this technique. Importantly, PCR would detect a quiescent "reservoir" of proviral DNA, suppressed by the antiretroviral drugs, that could produce virus at a later time.

A is incorrect. ELISA is based on immunodetection of a protein in a biological sample and as such ELISA cannot detect quiescent, proviral DNA. Additionally, PCR is far more sensitive, capable of detecting a single copy of the proviral DNA.

B is incorrect. An assay based on detection of viral enzyme activity protein in a biological sample cannot detect quiescent, proviral DNA. Additionally, PCR is far more sensitive, capable of detecting a single copy of the proviral DNA.

D is incorrect. Western blot is based on immunodetection of a protein in a biological sample, or the presence of antibodies in human serum directed against HIV, and as such Western blot cannot detect quiescent, proviral DNA. Additionally, PCR is far more sensitive, capable of detecting a single copy of the proviral DNA.

E is incorrect. Northern blot detects the presence of specific RNAs using radiolabeled or enzyme-linked detection of nucleic acid probes that hybridize to target RNAs. It requires the presence of significant levels of viral mRNAs and cannot detect quiescent, proviral DNA. Additionally, PCR is far more sensitive, capable of detecting a single copy of the proviral DNA.

3. Correct: C. Quantitative real-time reverse transcriptase polymerase chain reaction (qRT-PCR).

qRT-PCR is useful for measuring expression of one or a few genes. Importantly, it is a highly sensitive technique based on PCR, able to amplify and detect extremely small amounts of RNA in a sample, making it particularly well-suited for this specific application. To conduct this procedure, RNA in the recovered intestinal epithelial cell would be first converted to cDNA via reverse transcription. The cDNA is used as the template for PCR, specifically targeting the gene of interest for this assay. Included in the PCR reaction is a fluorescent DNA probe directed each of the target gene sequences. As more of the target gene DNA is synthesized, more fluorescent signal is generated. Following each extension phase, the fluorescent signal is detected, that is, in "real time." The number of PCR cycles required for the fluorescent signal to reach a predetermined threshold (cycle threshold or Ct) is proportional to the amount of starting template, that is, the RNA for the target gene that was present in the original tissue sample.

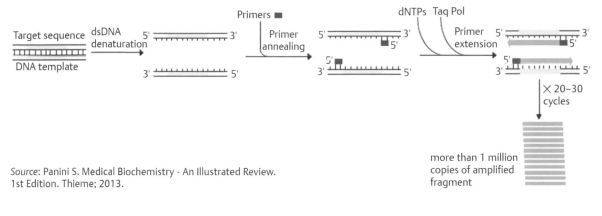

Source: Panini S. Medical Biochemistry - An Illustrated Review.
1st Edition. Thieme; 2013.

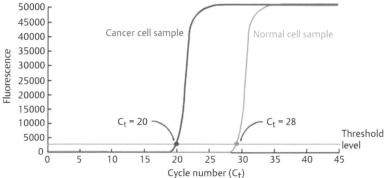

Source: Panini S. Medical Biochemistry - An Illustrated Review. 1st Edition. Thieme; 2013.

A is incorrect. ELISA is based on immunodetection of a protein in a biological sample. It is insufficiently sensitive to detect, reliably, specific proteins from such a small sample size (a few hundred cells).

B is incorrect. Gene expression profiling by high-throughput RNA sequencing quantifies the number of transcripts for all approximately 24,000 human genes present in the samples analyzed, in addition to providing qualitative information regarding the mRNA present (e.g., the relative levels of mRNA splice variants). It is technically complex to perform and analyze the data and is very expensive. Since the proposed diagnostic test for colon cancer risk requires information on only one gene, the expense and effort for gene expression profiling by high-throughput RNA sequencing are not necessary.

D is incorrect. Western blot is based on immunodetection of a protein in a biological sample. It is insufficiently sensitive to detect specific proteins from such a small sample size (a few hundred cells).

E is incorrect. Whole genome sequencing does not yield information about gene expression. Rather, it provides the sequence of the genomic DNA present in cells. In addition to being technically complex to perform and analyze the data, and very expensive, the information it yields is not what is required for the proposed diagnostic test.

Gene expression profiling by microarray is the best technique of those listed to achieve global comparisons of gene expression patterns between two samples. Completion of this technique will yield a list of all known human genes with their relative expression levels among samples tested (i.e., expression in the primary HCC and in the HCC cells that have metastasized to perihepatic lymph nodes). The figure below outlines the technical details of gene expression profiling by microarray.

B is incorrect. ELISA is based on immunodetection of a specific, defined protein in a biological sample. It is not suited to the goals of the proposed study, which needs to compare global gene expression patterns to discover differences between two tissues.

C is incorrect. Western blot is based on immunodetection of a specific, defined protein in a biological sample. It is not suited to the goals of the proposed study, which needs to compare global gene expression patterns to discover differences between two tissues.

D is incorrect. qRT-PCR is useful for measuring expression of one or a few genes that have been specifically chosen. However, since the goal of the proposed study is to compare global changes in gene expression (i.e., all ~ 22,000 human genes) qRT-PCR is not the best choice.

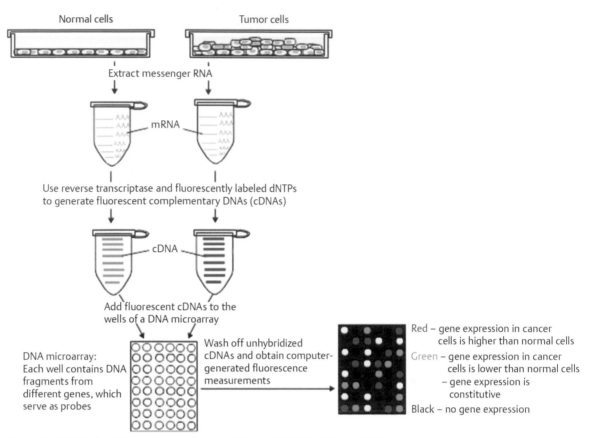

Source: Panini S. Medical Biochemistry - An Illustrated Review. 1st Edition. Thieme; 2013.

E is incorrect. Whole genome sequencing does not yield information about gene expression. Rather, it provides the sequence of the genomic DNA present in cells. The information it yields is not what is required for the proposed study.

5. Correct: D. Sanger DNA sequencing.

Since the information required to prescribe cetuximab is whether a single gene (*K-Ras*) or wild type is mutated, Sanger DNA sequencing is the best choice, since the technique will provide the nucleotide sequence of a specific locus in the genome. Sanger DNA sequencing utilizes primer extension to determine the sequence of a specific locus, in this case the *K-Ras* gene. In automated Sanger sequencing, a single sequencing reaction is assembled containing the target DNA (in this case, DNA extracted from the colorectal cancer tumor biopsy), locus-specific primer, all four deoxyribonucleoside triphosphates (dNTPs), and all four dideoxyribonucleoside triphosphates (ddNTPs) which lack a hydroxyl group on both the 3' and 5' carbons of the ribose moiety. Each of the ddNTPs is labeled with a unique fluorescent color tag. As the DNA polymerase extends the primer, it occasionally incorporates a ddNTP, which terminates extension of the DNA chain, due to the absence of a hydroxyl group on the 3' carbon. Since the ddNTP that produced the termination has a specific colored label, it can be read using an automated detection system.

A is incorrect. ELISA is based on immunodetection of a specific, defined protein in a biological sample. An antibody that specifically recognizes the *K-Ras* mutant epitope, but not the wild-type *K-Ras* protein, could potentially be used to determine if the mutation was present by ELISA. However, given that multiple *K-Ras* mutations have been observed in cancers, it would require Western blots with each and every antibody developed against the range of mutations observed in cancers. Sanger DNA sequencing is far more direct and efficient for the stated purpose.

B is incorrect. Gene expression profiling by microarray is useful for making global comparisons of gene expression between two or more samples. It is a relatively expensive technique, both in terms of execution in the clinical laboratory as well as subsequent analysis of the data. Since the information required to prescribe cetuximab is whether a single gene (*K-Ras*) or wild type is mutated, the expense of microarray is not justified, since it will give far more information than is necessary to treat this patient.

C is incorrect. Gene expression profiling by high-throughput RNA sequencing will provide the sequence as well as the level of all expressed RNAs in a sample. It is a relatively expensive technique, both in terms of execution in the clinical laboratory as well as subsequent analysis of the data. Since the information required to prescribe cetuximab is whether a single gene (*K-Ras*) or wild-type is mutated, the expense of RNA sequencing is not justified, since it will give far more information than is necessary to treat this patient.

E is incorrect. Whole genome sequencing provides the sequence of the genomic DNA present in cells. While this would reveal whether the *K-Ras* genes had mutations, whole genome sequencing is a relatively expensive technique, both in terms of execution in the clinical laboratory as well as subsequent analysis of the data. Since the information required to prescribe cetuximab is whether a single gene (*K-Ras*) or wild type is mutated, the expense of whole genome sequencing is not justified, since it will give far more information than is necessary to treat this patient.

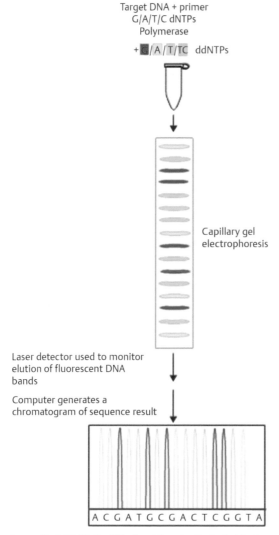

Source: Panini S. Medical Biochemistry - An Illustrated Review. 1st Edition. Thieme; 2013.

6. Correct: A. Enzyme-linked immunosorbent assay.

ELISA is based on immunodetection of a specific, defined protein in a biological sample. An ELISA employing an antibody that specifically recognizes the EGFR proteins could determine if, and how much of, the EGFR protein is present in the sample. See the figure below for an explanation of the technical aspects of ELISA.

B is incorrect. Gene expression profiling by microarray is useful for making global comparisons of gene expression between two or more samples. It measures RNA levels, is complex and expensive, and provides far more information than is necessary to achieve the goal of determining if the tumor expresses EGFR.

C is incorrect. Gene expression profiling by RNA sequencing is useful for making global comparisons of gene expression between two or more samples. It measures RNA levels, is complex and expensive, and provides far more information than is necessary to achieve the goal of determining if the tumor expresses EGFR.

D is incorrect. Sanger DNA sequencing provides the DNA sequence of a chosen locus. It does not provide any information on gene or protein expression.

E is incorrect. Whole genome sequencing provides the sequence of the genomic DNA present in cells. It does not provide any information on gene or protein expression.

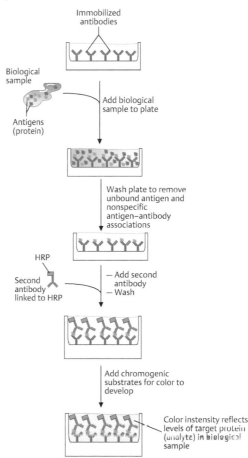

Source: Panini S. Medical Biochemistry - An Illustrated Review. 1st Edition. Thieme; 2013.

From the presentation and the treatment plan, the patient has multiple sclerosis. Production of recombinant proteins typically is from cDNA reverse transcribed from the mRNA produced by the gene of interest. Since most human genes have introns and can be quite large, cloning the gene is difficult as well as unnecessary to produce the desired protein. The cDNA is typically cloned into an expression plasmid, which contains the genetic elements necessary for expression of the cDNA into mRNA and then protein within host cells. The host cells for production of recombinant protein can be bacterial, insect, or mammalian.

A is incorrect. Biologically active proteins can be purified from animal tissues, and retain activity when used in humans. However, these are not recombinant, which employ the use of recombinant DNA techniques.

C is incorrect. The drug being used with the patient is the IFN-β-1a cytokine itself, not an antibody directed against that protein. A blocking antibody is used to inhibit the activity of tumor necrosis factor α (TNF-α) in certain inflammatory diseases might be produced in this way.

D is incorrect. Such a procedure is not required for production of a recombinant protein. However, this approach can be used to produce a drug that mimics the biological activity of the recombinant protein.

E is incorrect. Since most human genes have introns and can be quite large, cloning the gene is difficult as well as unnecessary to produce a protein of interest.

qRT-PCR measures levels of specific mRNAs in a sample. In this instance, two primer pairs were employed in the reaction: one pair that amplifies the normal allele of BRAF and a second pair that amplifies the mutant (BRAF-V600E) allele. In the RNA from the normal tissue, only mRNA for the normal BRAF allele is present, indicated by the fluorescent signal that rises as the number of PCR cycles increases. However, with the mRNA from the melanoma, signal for the mutant allele of BRAF is present in addition to a signal for the normal BRAF allele. The information that allows determination of the correct answer is (1) the signal increased with cycle number (PCR has multiple cycles), (2) the quantitative nature of the assay, (3) the specific detection of a slight variant (one nucleotide) of the target gene, BRAF. Only qRT-PCR is characterized by all three features.

A is incorrect. Gene expression profiling by microarray is useful for making global comparisons of gene expression between two or more samples. The data in the figure below are not the output from gene expression profiling by microarray, which are either presented as heat-maps or as tabular data. In addition, microarray uses hybridization of nucleic acid probes which cannot efficiently detect single-nucleotide differences between targets, making it a poor choice for detecting the BRAF-V600E mutation.

B is incorrect. Northern blot detects RNA molecules in samples using hybridization of nucleic acid probes to membrane-bound RNA samples. The Northern blot technique cannot efficiently detect single-nucleotide differences between targets, making it a poor choice for detecting the BRAF-V600E mutation.

D is incorrect. Western blot is based on immunodetection of a specific, defined protein in a biological sample. While an antibody that specifically recognizes the BRAF-V600E epitope, but not the wild-type BRAF protein, could potentially be used to determine if the mutation was present by Western blot; the data presented in the figure below are not consistent with the Western blot.

E is incorrect. Whole genome sequencing provides the sequence of the genomic DNA present in cells. While this would reveal whether the mutation coding for BRAF-V600E is present, whole genome sequencing is a relatively expensive technique, both in terms of execution in the clinical laboratory as well as subsequent analysis of the data. In addition, the data presented in the figure in question 8 are not consistent with whole genome sequencing.

Whole genome sequencing provides the sequence of the entire genome present in a sample. This includes not only the protein coding regions of genes (the exon portion of the genome or "exome") but also DNA in introns and intergenic regions. As such, any mutations, including those in regulatory elements such as transcriptional enhancers and promoters, will be identified. Mutations are identified by first sequencing the genome through one of multiple high-throughput techniques and then aligning the "reads" from the sequencing to a reference human genome. Using advanced computational methods, potential mutations are identified and then curated manually to determine if any are actionable.

A is incorrect. Gene expression profiling by high-throughput RNA sequencing will provide the sequence as well as the level of all expressed RNAs in a sample. However, only sequences derived from RNAs are read, so any mutations outside these transcripts will not be detected. The goal of the study is to identify *all* mutations which include sequences outside of RNA coding regions.

B is incorrect. Gene expression profiling by microarray provides a global measure of gene expression (mRNA) in a sample. Since it is based on hybridization between cDNA produced from mRNA isolated from a sample and defined nucleic acid probes, it will not lead to discovery or identification of mutations in DNA.

C is incorrect. qRT-PCR measures levels of specific mRNAs in a sample. As such, it will not lead to discovery or identification of mutations in DNA.

D is incorrect. Sanger DNA sequencing utilizes primer extension to determine the nucleotide sequence of a specific locus. As such, it will not lead to discovery or identification of mutations in DNA.

10. Correct: A. Gene expression profiling by high-throughput RNA sequencing.

Gene expression profiling by high-throughput RNA sequencing provides qualitative and quantitative information about the RNA purified from cells or tissues. The RNA is first converted to cDNA and subject to sequencing through one of multiple high-throughput techniques. The short sequences obtained "read" are then aligned to a reference human genome. Using advanced computational methods, the number of reads for a given exons, as well as how often specific exon–exon pairs are present. From this analysis, a quantitative assessment can be made regarding which mRNA splice variants produced by a given gene are present in the sample. Comparisons between the control brains and the brains from those with schizophrenia would address whether consistent, global changes in splicing are associated with greater disease risk.

B is incorrect. qRT-PCR can be designed to detect and quantify the presence of mRNA splice variants. However, each splice variant would require a separate primer pair and reaction, making it completely impractical for the global analysis of all genes, which is the goal of the study outlined.

C is incorrect. Sanger DNA sequencing provides the DNA sequence of a chosen locus. It does not provide any information on what mRNA is synthesized in a given cell from that gene. It is also not a high-throughput technique.

D is incorrect. Western blot is used to detect specific proteins. As such, it is unsuited to the goals of the study outlined.

E is incorrect. Whole genome sequencing does not yield information about the mRNAs produced from the genome. Rather, it provides the sequence of the genomic DNA present in cells. As such, it is unsuited to the goals of the study outlined.

11. Correct: B. B.

Agarose gel electrophoresis is typically run horizontally. The samples (in this case, the completed PCR reactions containing amplified DNA) are loaded into wells embedded near one end of the gel. The gel is submerged in buffered electrolyte solution and current applied such that the cathode is closest to the sample wells and the anode at the other end of the gel. The DNA is negatively charged at the buffer's pH and so migrates through the gel toward the anode. The DNA molecules are separated by size, with shorter molecules running "faster" than larger molecules. Once the electrophoresis is complete, the gel is soaked in a fluorescent stain that preferentially stains the DNA, so it can be visualized as "bands" on the gel.

Trinucleotide repeat syndromes have some common characteristics. First, the number of trinucleotide repeats can be variable. Second, there is typically a threshold number of repeats above which disease occurs. Friedreich's ataxia is an autosomal recessive disease most commonly caused by the expansion of a trinucleotide repeat (GAA) in the first intron of the frataxin gene, which significantly reduces the gene's expression. The parents' samples are in lanes A and C. Both parents have one copy of the frataxin gene with larger numbers of repeats, which are the bands higher on the gel, nearer the cathode. Each parent also has frataxin gene with a smaller number of repeats, which are the bands lower on the gel, nearer the anode. Since they are asymptomatic, the "smaller" frataxin gene must have a repeat number below the pathogenic threshold. Note, however, that even though these "smaller" alleles are below the threshold, there is variation between the number of repeats that each parent has. By chance, the patient's healthy sister inherited the alleles with length below the disease-causing threshold from each parent. The patient inherited alleles with trinucleotide repeat expansion beyond the disease-causing threshold from each parent and thus developed Friedreich's ataxia.

A is incorrect. The DNA for the PCR reaction in lane A came from a parent who is heterozygous for the trinucleotide repeat expansion.

C is incorrect. The DNA for the PCR reaction in lane C came from a parent who is heterozygous for the trinucleotide repeat expansion.

D is incorrect. The DNA for the PCR reaction in lane D came from the patient's healthy sister. She inherited the alleles with length below the disease-causing threshold from each parent.

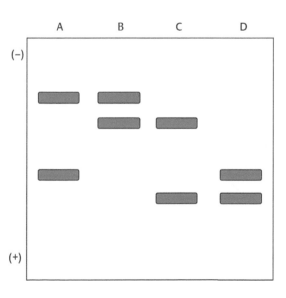

12. Correct: C. Sanger DNA sequencing.

The patient has only one allele, inherited from her mother, that has a trinucleotide repeat expansion consistent with developing Friedreich's ataxia. Friedreich's ataxia is an autosomal recessive disease is most commonly caused by the expansion of a trinucleotide repeat (GAA) in the first intron of the frataxin gene. This results in a loss-of-function mutation due to the expansion causing silencing expression of the frataxin. Based on the PCR results, this patient has only one expanded repeat but apparently still lacks the frataxin protein, since she has the disease. The allele she inherited from her father must have some other loss-of-function mutation, such as a nucleotide substitution or insertion that leads to a missense or nonsense mutation. To determine if this is the case, Sanger DNA sequencing would be the most direct and cost-effective approach to locating a small mutation in the protein coding sequence of the frataxin gene the patient inherited from her father.

A is incorrect. Gene expression profiling by high-throughput RNA sequencing will provide the sequence as well as the level of all expressed RNAs in a sample. It is a relatively expensive technique, both in terms of execution in the clinical laboratory as well as subsequent analysis of the data. Since the information required is the sequence of a single gene (frataxin), the expense of RNA sequencing is not justified, since it will give far more information than is necessary.

B is incorrect. qRT-PCR is useful for measuring expression of one or a few genes. It does not provide sequence information of the amplified regions, which is what is required to define the genetic cause of this patient's Friedreich's ataxia.

D is incorrect. Western blot is based on immunodetection of a protein in a biological sample. It will not provide information about the genetic cause of this patient's Friedreich's ataxia.

E is incorrect. Whole genome sequencing provides the sequence of the genomic DNA present in cells. While this would reveal whether the frataxin gene had a small mutation, whole genome sequencing is a relatively expensive technique, both in terms of execution in the clinical laboratory as well as subsequent analysis of the data. The expense of whole genome sequencing is not justified, since it will give far more information than is necessary to define the genetic cause of this patient's Friedreich's ataxia.

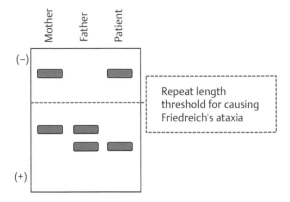

Index